The face of medicine

MANCHESTER
1824
Manchester University Press

rethinking
art's histories

SERIES EDITORS
Amelia G. Jones, Marsha Meskimmon

Rethinking Art's Histories aims to open out art history from its most basic structures by foregrounding work that challenges the conventional periodisation and geographical subfields of traditional art history, and addressing a wide range of visual cultural forms from the early modern period to the present.

These books will acknowledge the impact of recent scholarship on our understanding of the complex temporalities and cartographies that have emerged through centuries of world-wide trade, political colonisation and the diasporic movement of people and ideas across national and continental borders.

Also available in the series

Art, museums and touch Fiona Candlin

The 'do-it-yourself' artwork: Participation from fluxus to relational aesthetics Anna Dezeuze (ed.)

After the event: New perspectives in art history Charles Merewether and John Potts (eds)

Photography and documentary film in the making of modern Brazil Luciana Martins

Women, the arts and globalization: Eccentric experience Marsha Meskimmon and Dorothy Rowe (eds)

Flesh cinema: The corporeal turn in American avant-garde film Ara Osterweil

After-affects|after-images: Trauma and aesthetic transformation in the virtual Feminist museum Griselda Pollock

Vertiginous mirrors: The animation of the visual image and early modern travel Rose Marie San Juan

The newspaper clipping: a modern paper object Anke Te Heesen, translated by Lori Lantz

Screen/space: The projected image in contemporary art Tamara Trodd (ed.)

Timed out: Art and the transnational Caribbean Leon Wainwright

Performative monuments: Performance, photography, and the rematerialisation of public art Mechtild Widrich

The face of medicine

Visualising medical masculinities in late nineteenth-century Paris

Mary Hunter

Manchester University Press

Published by Manchester University Press
Altrincham Street, Manchester M1 7JA

www.manchesteruniversitypress.co.uk

British Library Cataloguing-in-Publication Data
A catalogue record for this book is available from the British Library

Library of Congress Cataloging-in-Publication Data applied for

ISBN 978 0 7190 9757 7 hardback

First published 2016

Typeset
by Frances Hackeson Freelance Publishing Services, Brinscall, Lancs
Printed in Great Britain
by TJ International, Padstow

Contents

Figures

Acknowledgements

Teachers, friends, colleagues, archivists, institutions, funding bodies, and family have made writing this book possible. Many thanks are due to the following. Tamar Garb and Tom Gretton nurtured *The Face of Medicine*'s early stages as a dissertation at University College London, with the help of funding from the University of London and the Wellcome Trust. Their intellectual rigour, infectious fascination with French culture, and sense of humour made them excellent advisers and mentors. My dissertation examiners, Caroline Arscott and Richard Thomson, gave crucial advice about how to transform the thesis into a book and the encouragement to do so. Years later in the manuscript stage, Mechthild Fend and Fae Brauer were attentive and generous readers. I owe special thanks to Mechthild for reading the final draft and for her inspired comments and conversation. Manchester University Press's Emma Brennan was perfectly patient as an editor for a first-time author, and I am grateful to her, Polly Bentham, and Frances Hackeson for their help.

Multi-year funding from the Social Sciences and Humanities Research Council of Canada, Le Fonds de recherche du Québec – Société et culture, and McGill University have supported the research and writing of this book, and the hiring of students as research assistants. For research help and practical assistance, I must thank Sylvie Boisjoli, Shana Cooperstein, Amanda Clarke, Alexandra Kelebay, and Lexi Stefanatos. I am also thankful to the following institutions, museums, and archives for giving me access to their holdings and the permission to reproduce images and objects from their collections: Institut Pasteur, Wellcome Library, Hôpital Saint-Louis, Hôpital de la Salpêtrière, Archive de l'Assistance Publique, Osler Library for the History of Medicine at McGill University, the New York Academy of Medicine, and the Bibliothèque Nationale de France.

At McGill, I have benefited from an environment that encourages interdisciplinary research, and the support of my colleagues in the Art History and Communication Studies Department: Darin Barney, Jenny Burman, Gabriella Coleman, Chriscinda Henry, Cecily Hilsdale, Matthew Hunter, Amelia Jones, Becky Lentz, Charmaine Nelson, Jeff Moser, Marc Raboy, Carrie Rentschler,

Christine Ross, Jonathan Sterne, Will Straw, and Angela Vanhaelen. I have also enjoyed and profited from conversations about medical cultures with colleagues in different departments and faculties, particularly Annmarie Adams, Nick Dew, Jennifer Fishman, Abe Fuks, Chris Lyons, Wendy Owens, Tabitha Sparks, Lisa Stevenson, Tamar Tembeck, and George Weisz. I would particularly like to thank Thomas Schlich for looking over my manuscript and helping an art historian with the particularities and peculiarities of the history of medicine.

Over the past decade, I have presented parts of this work at many conferences and invited lectures. I am thankful for the advice and encouragement I have received from scholars and friends whose work I admire: Masha Belenky, Marta Braun, Kathryn Brown, Anthea Callen, Holly Clayson, Terry Dolan, Elizabeth Emery, Michelle Facos, Briony Fer, Michael Finn, Michael Garval, Sander Gilman, Susan Hiner, Ludmilla Jordanova, Serena Keshavjee, Marni Kessler, Rachel Mesch, Linda Nochlin, Michel Pierssens, Todd Porterfield, Lise Schreier, Vanessa Schwartz, Willa Silverman, Abigail Solomon-Godeau, Alexandra Wettlaufer, and Richard Wrigley.

For their camaraderie and enthusiasm for trying out ideas, I have many people to thank: Scott Allan, Simon Baker, Stina Barchan, Juliet Bellow, Fran Berry, Sam Bibby, Anja Bock, Warren Carter, Nancy Walbridge Collins, Colette Curran, Keren Hammerschlag, Karen Ho, Kristen Hutchinson, Ed Krcma, Amy Mechowski, Allison Morehead, Hans Nichols, Emily Richardson, Harriet Riches, Tamara Trodd, Kaija Vogel, and Terri Wills. A heartfelt thank you to Jo Applin, Catherine Clinger, and Richard Taws for their friendship, advice, and fresh eyes whenever I needed them. I am also grateful to Natasha Ruiz-Gómez and Tania Woloshyn, my fellow art/medicine buffs, for reading parts of this book with great care. I am particularly thankful for the friendship of the late Lisa Smirl, whose inventive approach to interdisciplinary scholarship with social impact has changed the way I look at the world.

A special thank you to two pioneering scholars – Tamar Garb and Amelia Jones – whose examples have been a source of inspiration and support, particularly as I ventured into the early years of academia and motherhood.

A network of family and friends too numerous to name have supported this work in important ways. In particular, I wish to thank Willa Leus and Nick Martire for helping to make Montreal our home and for the wonderful fresh air at Prout's Neck; Judy Sorensen and Pierre Pitre for listening and advising; my aunts for their encouragement; and Fran and Neil Macmillan for their considerable help.

Family support has provided the backbone to my work, particularly as much of the research of this book took me away from Canada and brought me to London, Paris, and Amsterdam over the course of ten years. Chris and Sarah, my older siblings, may have mocked my 'artsy' ways but have always stood by me. My parents, John and Dette Hunter, were unwavering devotees, as always, even though this project was not the type of art history they learned at school. My mother, who died a year before I completed this book, was an inspiring role model who fostered my curiosity about art from the start. My two daughters, Phoebe and Eliza, have been as patient as one can expect from young kids familiar with the term 'tenure clock'. They are my joy and reality.

But it is to Stuart Macmillan – encouraging, calm, and with a greater knowledge of nineteenth-century diseases than he ever wanted – that I dedicate this book.

Introduction

The 1887 Salon in Paris was a site of illness, addiction, and inoculation, according to art critic Chamillac. A 'pictorial virus' had infected the world of art:

> Young men, old men, women – blonde or red, brunette or green – decorated people, panic-stricken and anaemic poets and merchants, showing all the signs of the deepest dejection as they leave the Palais de l'Industrie. Stooped and expressionless, wobbling along on their weakened legs, they struggle mightily to carry a red booklet, a distinctive sign of their current state, intended to warn healthy people to move away from them as fast as they can. These unfortunates have in effect just been infected with the germ of painting.
>
> This terrible vaccine, which certain princes of science consider fatal, has entered into their standard practices … to such an extent that they couldn't live without it, and every year they ask for more. That and morphine! Will our race withstand it? Time will tell.[1]

Chamillac's review was accompanied by an illustration showing frail and nauseated spectators stumbling out of the Salon as if they had received a lethal injection (Figure 1). He described the viewers as patients and the paintings as infectious microbes to illustrate his theory of inoculation: unlike the actual procedure, in which one's dosage gradually increased until immunisation, these 'patients' were forced to swallow up to 2,500 'germs' on their first visit, receiving smaller doses until the end of Salon. Through visual ingestion, visitors were infected and cured. By using inoculation as a metaphor for viewing modern paintings, Chamillac linked art and scientific medicine to question their roles in France's future. Could the French body endure mass inoculation? Would the art 'microbes' kill the nation or ensure its survival?

Chamillac's medical metaphors exemplify the entanglement of art, science, politics, and popular culture in the early Third Republic.[2] They also allude to the three large oil paintings of famous men from the Parisian medical and scientific elite on display that year at the Salon. The famed microbiologist Louis Pasteur (1822–95) was portrayed by his relative, the emerging artist

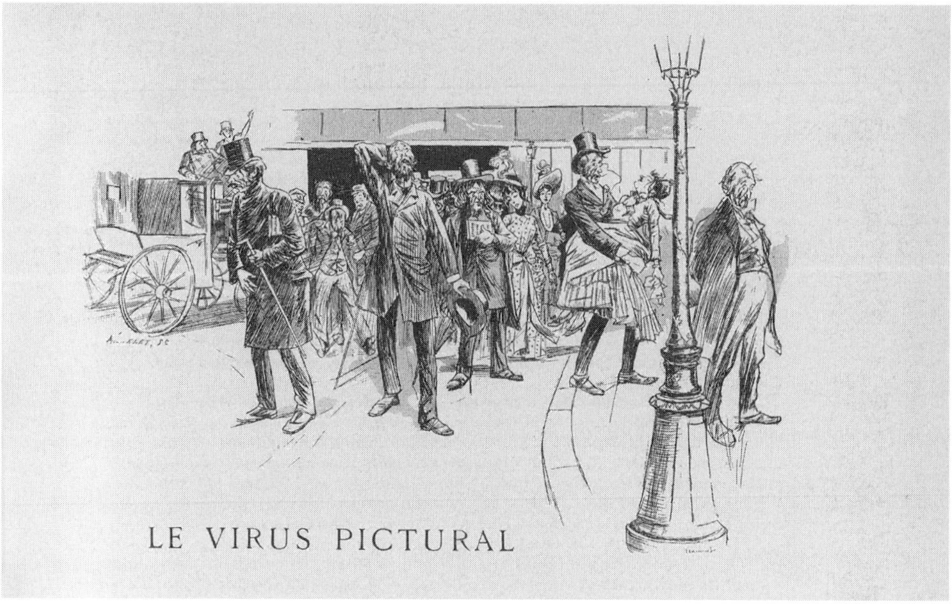

1 Illustration from 'Le Virus pictural', *La Revue illustrée*, I, 1887, p. 337.

Laurent Lucien-Gsell (1860–1944), surrounded by scientific colleagues as they prepared to vaccinate French and foreign patients with Pasteur's newly invented rabies vaccine (Figure 2). Henri Gervex (1852–1929), known as the painter of the scandalous nude *Rolla* (1878), depicted the wealthy surgeon Jules-Émile Péan (1830–98) pontificating about his new surgical tool before an attentive crowd while a bare-breasted young woman lies unconscious on an operating table (Figure 3). The third painting, by André Brouillet (1857–1914), shows renowned neurologist Jean-Martin Charcot (1825–93) lecturing to Parisian personalities from medical, artistic, and political fields about the hypnotic state of a salaciously dishevelled hysteric swooning in the arms of one of his handsome protégés (Figure 4).

These life-size paintings attracted Salon visitors and critics; reviews were written, reproductions made, and prints sold. Often discussed together in Salon criticism, these works – which merged and complicated the genres of portraiture and history painting – formed a thematic group that symbolised the importance of the sitters and the greatness of their occupations.[3] Significantly, the works owed much to the three paintings of Pasteur displayed at the Salon the previous year and to the related art criticism that debated how scientific heroes should be pictured in art that could serve as trustworthy historical documents for future viewers. The most discussed paintings were by the established academic Léon Bonnat (1833–1922) – who portrayed a serious Pasteur and his well-dressed

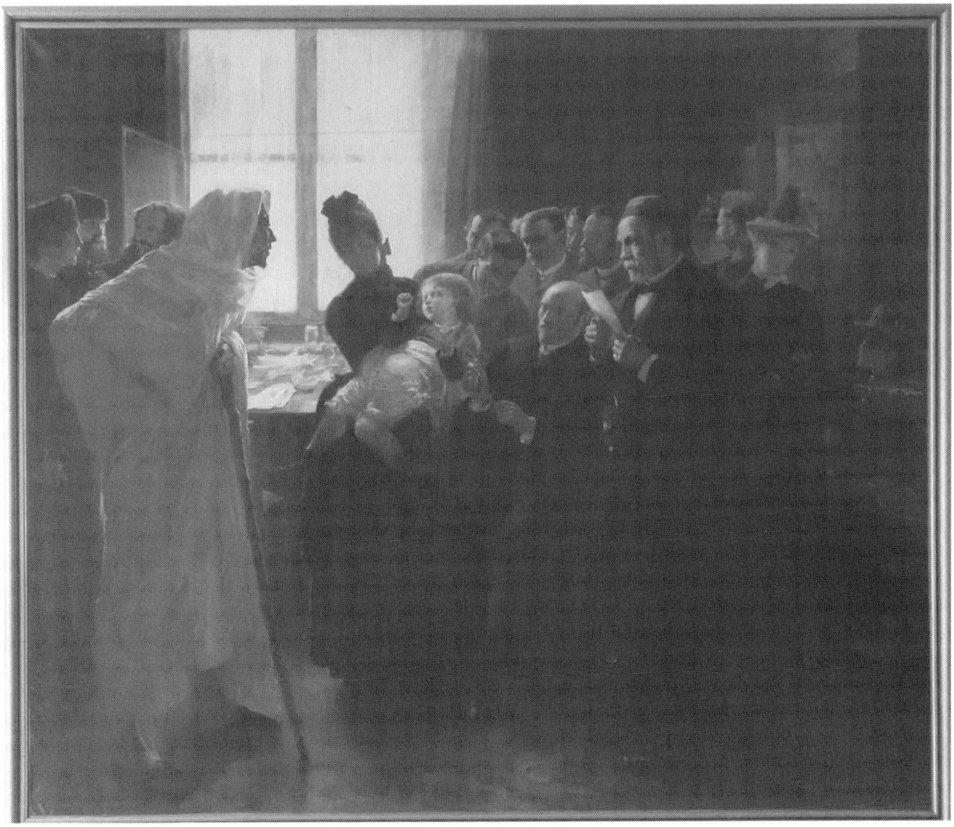

Lucien Laurent-Gsell, *La Vaccine contre la rage au laboratoire de M. Pasteur* (1887), oil on canvas, 250 x 290cm. 2

granddaughter against a dark backdrop – and the young Finnish painter, Albert Edelfelt (1854–1905), who depicted a focused Pasteur working alone on his cure for rabies in a laboratory (Figures 5 and 6). Gsell's small painting, which shows his relative hard at work amongst other men, received little attention: it was small, hung high, and hard to see (Figure 7).

This book argues that these 1886 and 1887 paintings are crucial to the visualisation of elite medical masculinities in the late nineteenth century. They exemplify the medical community's social and political uses of art and aesthetics, and are vital for investigating artists' cultural appropriation of scientific and medical principles in the last decades of the nineteenth century. Each of the three chapters is anchored in an examination of a portrait of Pasteur, Péan or Charcot, and expands to analyse lesser-known depictions of bodies that the men commissioned and collected for professional and personal gain, including anatomical wax models, photographs, stained-glass windows, and

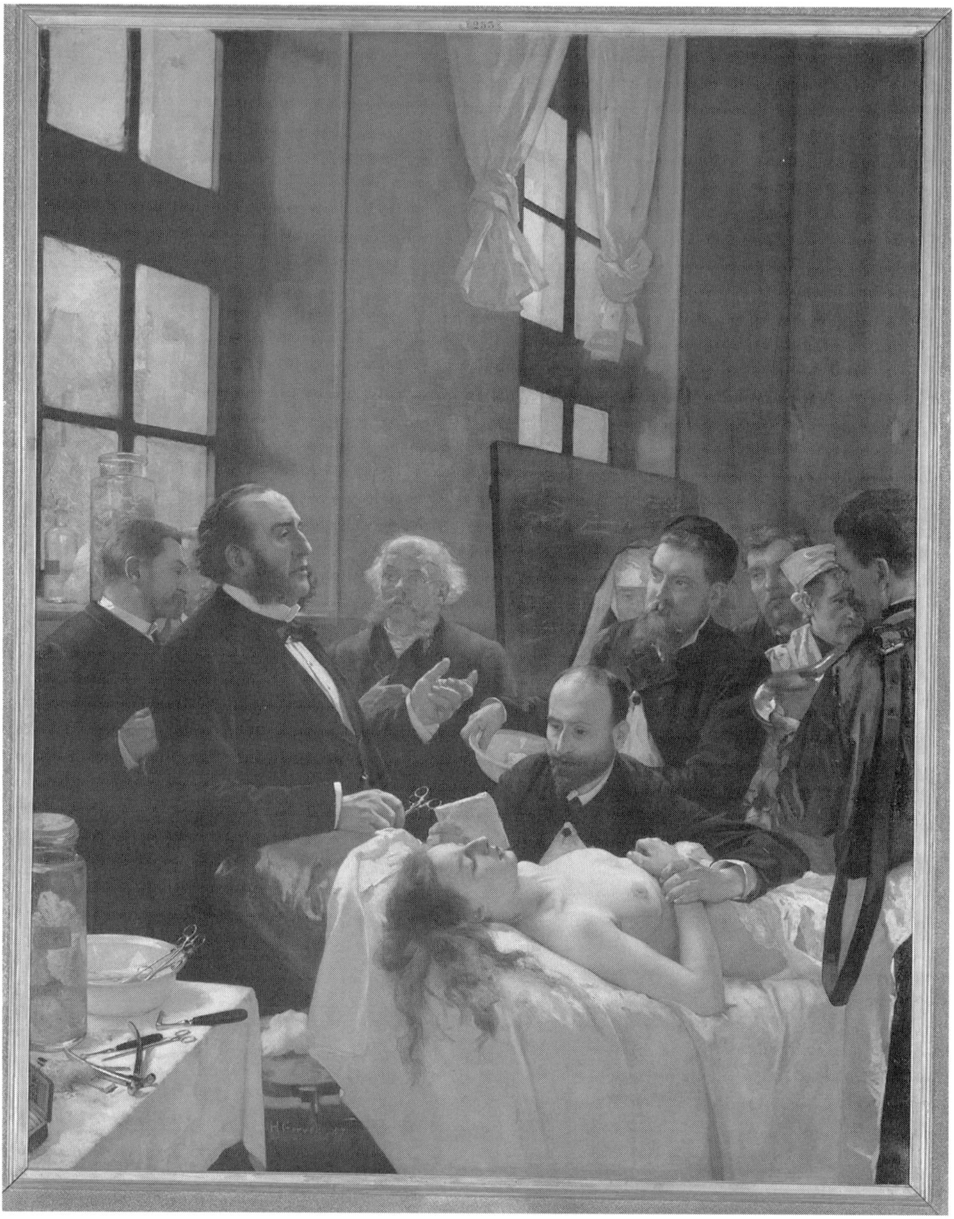

3 Henri Gervex, *Avant l'opération: le Docteur Péan enseignant à l'hôpital Saint-Louis sa découverte du pincement des vaisseaux* (1887), oil on canvas, 242 x 188cm.

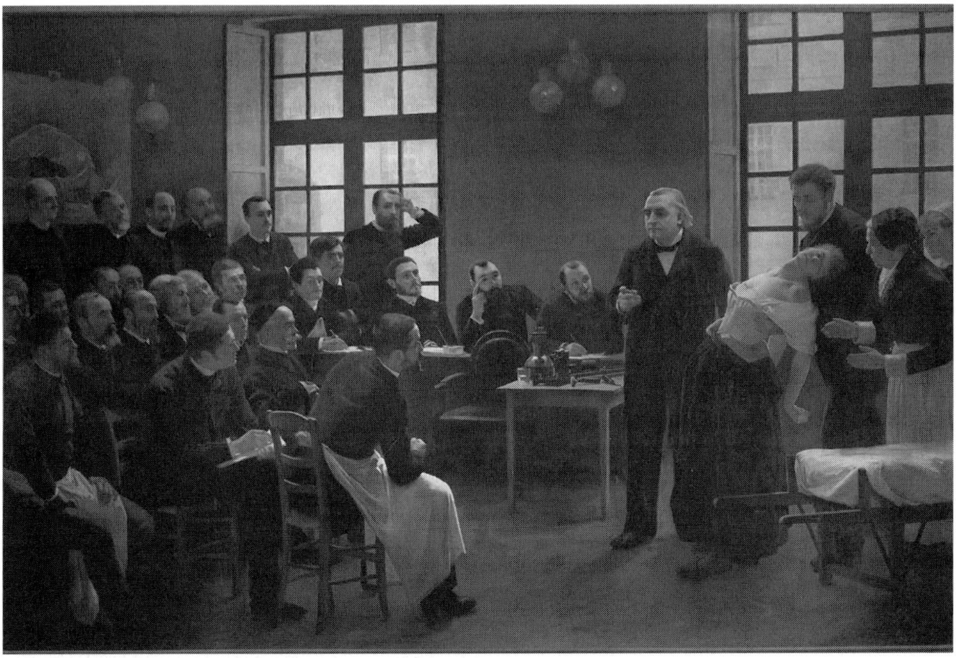

André Brouillet, *Une leçon clinique à La Salpêtrière* (1887), oil on canvas, 290 x 430cm. 4

funerary monuments. Images and objects were central to social and professional exchanges, the performance of individual and collective identities, and the production of knowledge in medical and scientific worlds. *The Face of Medicine* explores how, why, and where artists and medical men worked collectively by examining archival sources surrounding the production, display, and reception of these works. It considers how doctors, artists, and scientists – as well as journalists, art critics, and art historians – partook in the diverse rhetorics of realism, nationalism, and scientific and medical objectivity to varying degrees and different ends.

The Face of Medicine sheds new light on the relevance of the visual in medicine and science, and the relationship between artistic and medical practices and imagery. By examining previously unstudied sources across disciplinary boundaries – oil paintings, medical textbooks, popular caricatures, personal letters, Salon criticism, and waxworks – it rethinks the politics of medical representations and their social impact. In this sense, it departs from standard models of the social history of art and feminist scholarship by focusing not only on the portrayal of specific male physicians and scientists, but also on the role of images, objects, inventions, and procedures in the making of what Lorraine Daston and Otto Sibum call 'scientific personae'.[4]

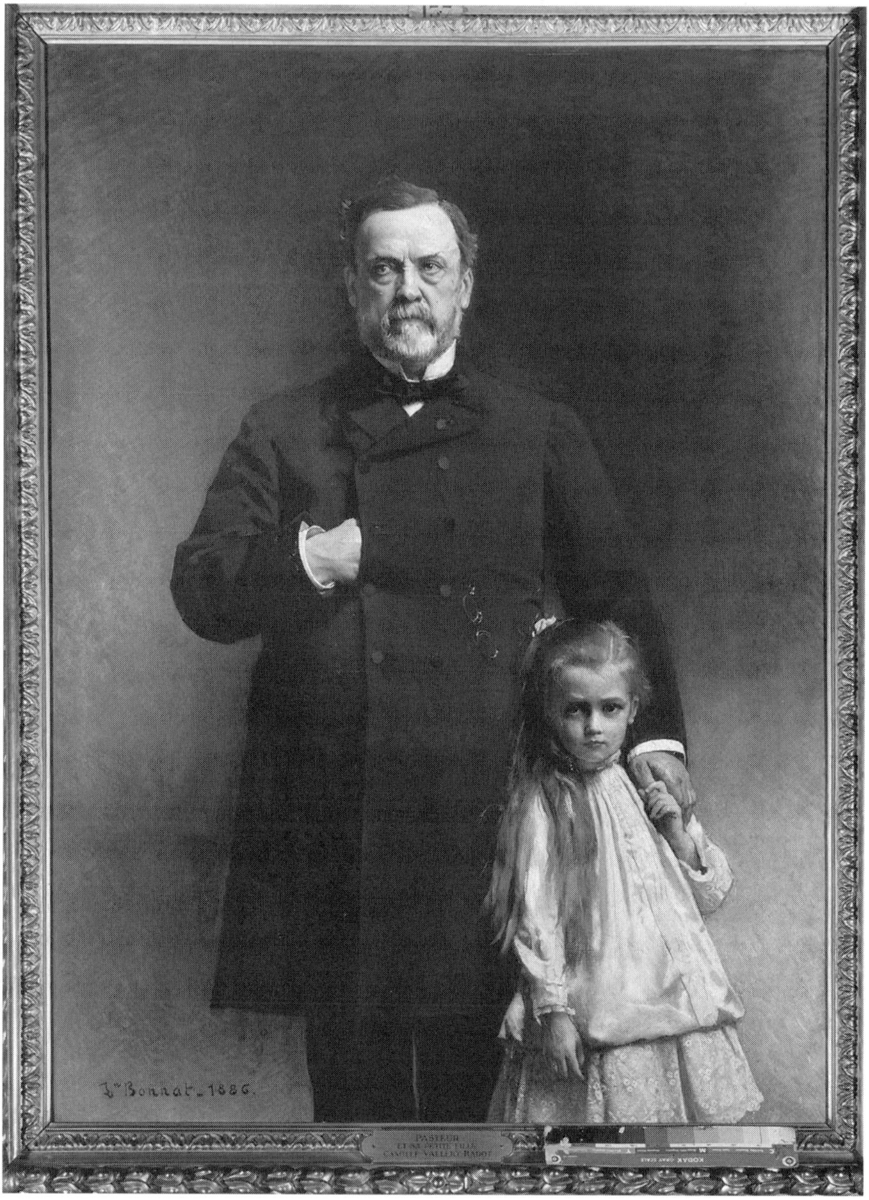

5 Léon Bonnat, *Pasteur et sa petite fille Camille* (1886), oil on canvas, approx. 160 x 130 cm.

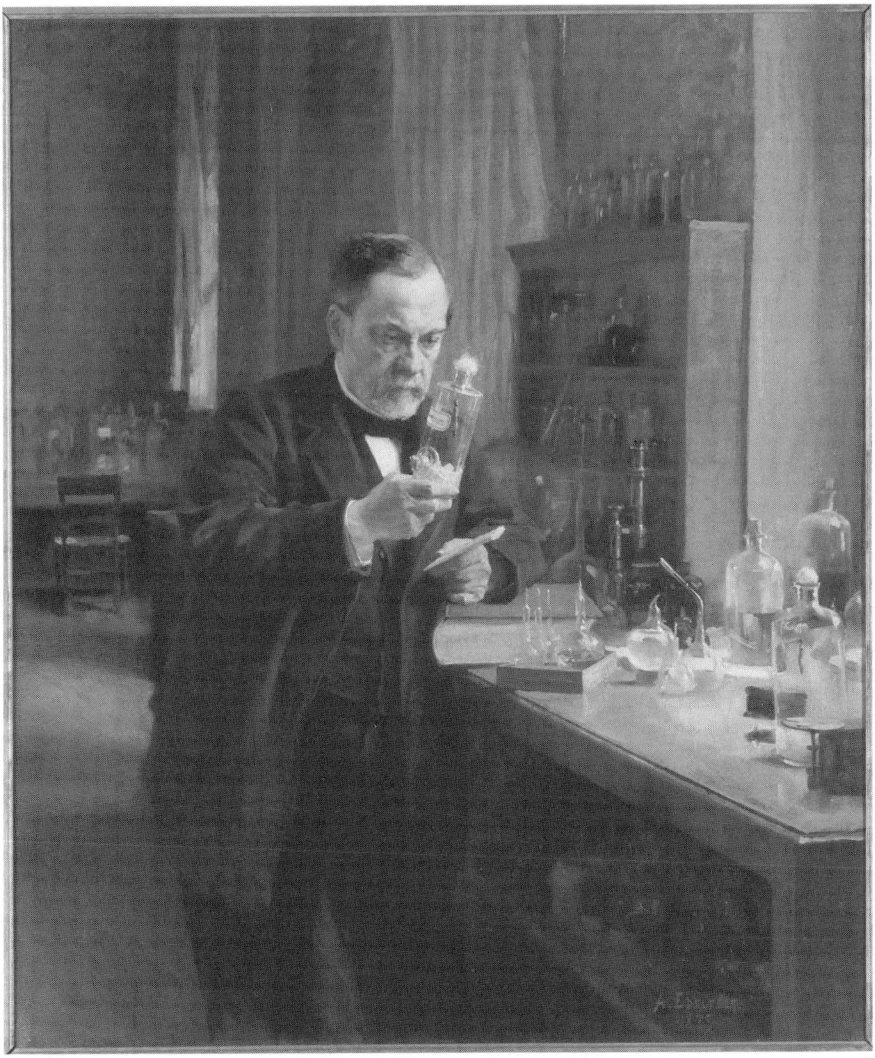

Albert Edelfelt, *Louis Pasteur* (1885), oil on canvas, 154 x 126 cm. 6

The popular and political cultures of medicine

The scientific themes of these 1886 and 1887 Salon paintings and the corresponding criticism show how medical thinking permeated the culture of late nineteenth-century Paris. Like Émile Zola's Rougon-Macquart series, Charcot's famous lectures at the Hôpital de la Salpêtrière, and the rise of entertainment venues showing disease and deformity, to name but a few contemporary cultural

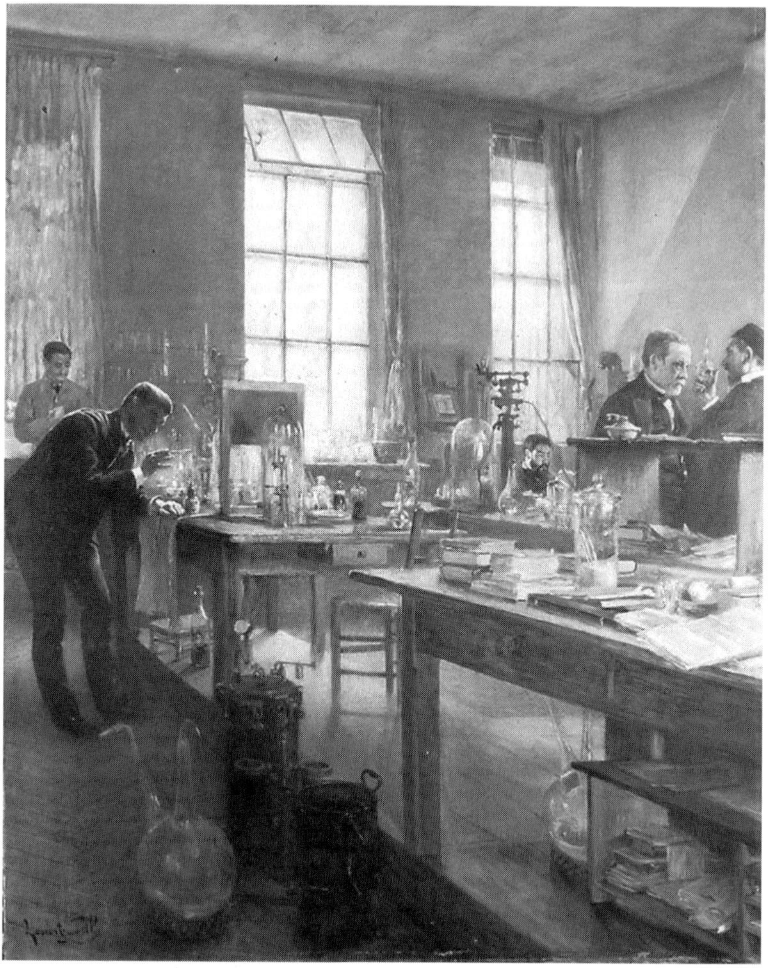

7 Lucien Laurent-Gsell, *Le Laboratoire de M. Pasteur* (1886), oil on canvas, 91 x 78cm.

manifestations, these paintings encouraged a shared fascination with medicine that familiarised the public with the leading men of the scientific and medical elite.[5] The popularity of these artworks was the product of great social, political, and economic change. The new visibility of medical men and the success of their experiments contributed to their rise in status. As more patients survived modern procedures, public confidence grew. Scientific and medical advances provided France with strength and power: medicine cured the sick, vaccinations protected soldiers from infection, and newly patented procedures and technologies increased economic and intellectual prowess. Although Chamillac described the illness provoked by paintings, French art, like French medicine, was simultaneously associated with strength because of its long-standing role as a prominent cultural force. Both were necessary for the formation – and promotion – of a healthy French nation.[6]

Scientific knowledge was essential to the capitalist world order of late nineteenth-century Europe. French technological advances in photography, electricity, bacteriology, and surgery, as well as newly invented vaccinations and medical treatments had wide-ranging financial consequences that increased not only the incomes of scientists and physicians, but also those of industrial leaders, lawyers, trade merchants, and others whose work was tied to these fields. With their increase in wealth, many men of this new elite attempted to secure their recently acquired social positions through displays of status. The production of portraits, sculptures, political positions, ceremonies, and professional collections reinforced the authority of this new group, and linked scientific advancement to national identity and personal gain.

These associations were grounded in concrete cultural and political conditions, since the newly established republican administrations of the early Third Republic heralded modern science and medicine as prerequisites for national salvation.[7] While the particular politics of republicanism evolved over the Third Republic's seventy years, its guiding tenets of liberty, equality, and fraternity, and its rejection of the monarchy, clericalism, and Bonapartism, were consistent. Fuelled by patriotic sentiment and a desire for national preservation after defeat by Prussia in 1870 and the brutal suppression of the Commune in spring 1871, the French Republic stressed the national, military, and industrial importance of scientific medicine. Between 1871 and 1914, 358 physicians became government deputies and senators. These men – who predominantly aligned themselves with the republican left – had a disproportionately large political influence.[8] This was especially the case after January 1879, when republicans achieved a majority in the Senate and Chamber of Deputies, and when Jules Grévy, the first unequivocally republican politician, became president. The republican physician-legislators supported further funding of the sciences, major institutional reforms in education and health, and the establishment of new social laws. By utilising their social authority, these medical men passed laws that brought healthcare to the public and began to rid hospitals of clerical influence. As Philip Nord argues, by the 1880s, the Latin Quarter – the neighbourhood containing many institutions of higher learning, including the Paris medical school – was a 'republican territory outright' where the 'republicanisation' of academic life was complete.[9]

Pasteur, Péan, and Charcot all benefited from republican policies (though their personal politics and religious beliefs differed), particularly as the government increasingly funded laboratories, academic chairs, hospital photographic studios, and medical museums. These medical collections – some of which were publicised in the popular press, such as Charcot's museum at the

Salpêtrière – contributed to the wide-ranging visual culture of medicine that fulfilled republican aims of collectivity, education, and world leadership.

Medical masculinities

'Today's doctor has been placed at the very top of our social ladder, a rank he merits because he is one of our great educators and one of the active leaders of our civilisation', wrote Horace Bianchon (Maurice de Fleury) in *Nos grands médecins d'aujourd'hui* (1891).[10] As opposed to the so-called quacks of the past, whose interventions often caused more harm than good, these 'new' doctors were regarded as trustworthy modern heroes (generally).[11] They provided new models of masculinity as their occupations became associated with the positive traits attributed to the male sex; the ideal medical persona comprised reason and objectivity whether the actual men had any of these defining virtues or not.

The Face of Medicine examines how the masculinities of medical men were conceptualised visually, and explores how these men provided archetypes of health and virility to which other bodies and sexualities could be compared.[12] These ideals could never be fully realised, but they were aspirational models, roles to enact and heroic masculinities to perform. While examining the historical commonalities of medical manhoods and scientific personae are key components of the book, particularly in the first chapter on Pasteur, masculinities are not considered unified or stable. As Robert Nye argues, 'Masculine scripts, however widely supported by the wider culture, are inherently unstable because they have to be performed.'[13] Masculinities are, after all, numerous and constantly renegotiated. They are 'configurations of practice' produced through social action and vary in accordance to gendered exchanges in specific social situations, as R.W. Connell and James W. Messerschmidt argue.[14] These plural masculinities (and femininities) are related to hierarchical positions occupied by the hegemonic gender norms.[15] Established medical leaders, like Pasteur, Péan, and Charcot, were representative of the masculine elite. However, as my analyses of medical men and their collections of images and objects demonstrate, relationships amongst men were complex. While some associations produced alliances and bonds, others were marked by competition and subordination.[16] The republican underpinnings of medical culture indicated a desire for democracy even though scientifically justified racism and misogyny also informed medical manhoods, masculine norms, and their visualisation.

By focusing on the medical male elite, this book departs from the majority of recent studies on nineteenth-century medical culture that concentrate on the female body, with a particular emphasis on hysteria.[17] While the intense focus on this 'female malady', particularly during the 1980s and 1990s, enabled productive methodologies for studying the construction of sexuality and disease, other components of nineteenth-century French medicine have gone largely ignored. This book offers a focused investigation of male doctors and scientists, and provides a detailed analysis of the role of visual images and practices in the formation of these identities. Salon paintings and criticism point to the anxieties surrounding masculinities, scientific occupations, and medicine's role in modern life. By exploring the moments when the assumed stability of masculinity and the seemingly undisputed objectivity of medical practice were questioned, *The Face of Medicine* moves beyond treating representations of male doctors as one-dimensional heroic characters who define female patients as 'other' (man vs. woman, rational vs. irrational, health vs. sickness, sanity vs. madness). While these binaries were surely prevalent and played out in nineteenth-century medical and artistic discourse – particularly in visual images – they were not static or rigid. French feminism's development, women's integration into medical schools, and Marie Curie's rise to prominence in the 1890s destabilised gender norms. Furthermore, some female patients displayed agency. The celebrity performer Jane Avril (who was once a Salpêtrière patient), for example, transformed the signs of female illness associated with hysteria into cutting-edge artistic practice; pathology was re-appropriated as a form of subversion. By studying the intricacies and fabrication of male scientific and medical personae, my approach examines the prevalence of 'othered' female bodies in histories of art and medicine, while also acknowledging the centrality of this 'othering' to contemporary cultural discourse. Indeed, the instances when the focus on the female body went beyond the requirements of artistic and medical duty, and challenged the rationality and reason often associated with ideal medical masculinity and realist aesthetics, demonstrate the complexities and contradictions of gender.

It has been well documented that the male mind and body – bourgeois, working-class, and aristocratic – came under intense scrutiny after the Franco-Prussian war (1870–71).[18] French fears of degeneracy, depopulation, heredity, and illness were conflated with those surrounding modern masculinity and, as is evident in Chamillac's criticism, they persisted for well over a decade after the war's end. Medical texts and images, scientific experiments, and government studies focused on the male body to produce models of ideal and degenerate manhood: the perceived weaknesses of men had to be transformed for the sake of the nation.[19] Standards of masculinity were disseminated through newspaper articles, popular phrenological studies, and collected photographs, as well as statues and books that commemorated France's *grands hommes*.

As a paradigm of ideal manhood, the masculinity of the Parisian medical elite was regarded as heterosexual, intelligent, normative, courageous, virile, and rational. In his 1902 book, *La Profession de médecine*, Peinard (Dr Noël Raynauld) claimed, 'the attributes of virility inspire, in general, respect in the weak, confidence in women, and the public will have only pity and suspicion of a limp and frail doctor not in the most flourishing and robust health!'[20] Nye, in his detailed account of male honour codes in nineteenth-century French medical culture, shows how personal integrity and professional ability were not only desirable characteristics for physicians, but intricately linked to their abilities: a doctor's personal honour and morals were benchmarks of his professional reliability.[21]

Objectivity was of particular concern in art, science, and medicine of the period.[22] These fields shared a desire to study the visible world undistorted by emotional or personal bias. Objectivity was an essential virtue of ideal masculinity, especially for men in scientific and medical spheres whose education, intellectual skills, and class position contributed to their status as detached observers. As Lorraine Daston and Peter Galison argue, objectivity was a key facet of the scientific self – although this concept and the specificities of its understanding changed as the century progressed.[23] It was increasingly understood as a defining quality of the man (not woman) of scientific medicine.[24] Debates on the acceptance of women into medical schools in France combined a new ethos of scientific detachment with popular beliefs about the relationship between biological sex and intellectual competence; it was widely argued that women had neither the mental ability, nor the emotional distance for medical vocations.[25]

The concept of objectivity has long been the focus of feminist critiques of scientific culture. Nancy Chodorow, Donna Harraway, Lorraine Daston, and Catharine MacKinnon, amongst many others, have explored how the ideal of scientific objectivity is gendered since it was formed in opposition to the supposedly feminine characteristics of sensitivity and irrationality.[26] Many argue that the perceived inability to be objective restricted women's success in scientific fields. However, medical objectivity was not always praised or accepted at face value in the late nineteenth century, despite the celebratory tone of medical literature.[27] The efficacy of medicine, the truthfulness of its claims and the neutrality of physicians were often questioned. Doctors faced a paradox: their occupation centred on curing, but their livelihoods depended on suffering. Public mistrust of medical practice erupted when a physician's personal finances and ambitions appeared to overshadow his patient's well-being.

From the public's viewpoint, medical men's professionally sanctioned ability to observe and touch naked bodies threatened their assumed neutrality, as did their fascination with what was popularly perceived as grotesque. As *The Face of Medicine* argues, a sense of desire existed behind the rational veneer of medical practices and personae. The unrelenting drive to be purely objective – itself an impossible goal – is an example of this madness. Numerous contemporary French caricatures and critiques portrayed physicians as lascivious men who preyed on innocent women, or as dishonest crooks who capitalised on sickness and death. Honoré Daumier's mid-century illustration, *To Operate or Not to Operate: Medicine Has to Bring in the Money*, shows a doctor charging a patient for both the medical procedure and the patient's misery. Similarly, a 1905 cartoon from *L'Assiette au beurre* depicts a husband exclaiming, 'I hope he's not going to charge me for this operation!', while watching his wife in a physician's embrace (Figure 8). The conflicting conceptions of medical men illuminate anxieties about medical occupations at the time. Medical objectivity, like masculinity, was always vulnerable to critique and thus needed constant reassertion. For this reason, the ideal of masculine trustworthiness was of the utmost importance: professional and personal identity and integrity, as well as economic stability, were at stake.

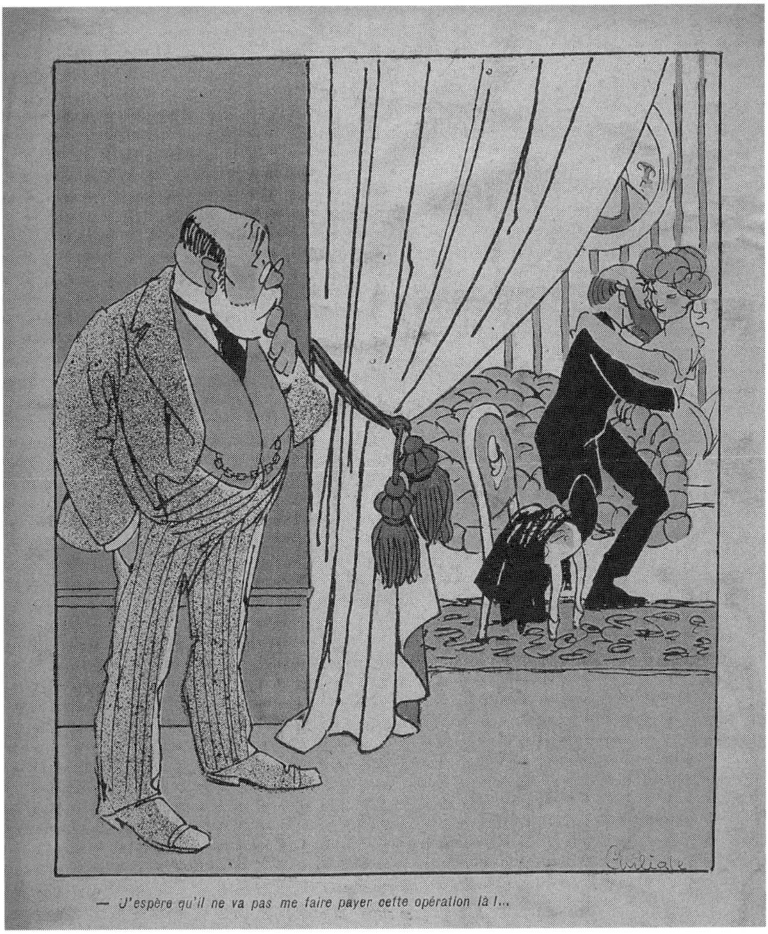

Culiale, 'J'espère qu'il ne va pas me faire payer cette opération là!', from *L'Assiette au Beurre* (c.1905), colour lithograph, 25.8 x 20.8cm. 8

Portraiture in the 1880s

Changes in the creation and reception of portraiture during the second half of the nineteenth century have been amply documented.[28] The 1876 essay by Edmond Duranty, champion of the Impressionists, which called for modern portraits to show people in contemporary surroundings, in everyday dress, and in the midst of social habits, is the most cited of many reviews that demanded a change in portraiture in light of the increase of cheap photographs and the decline of the official Salon system.[29] Thirteen years later, in 1889, the Salon critic Maurice Hamel was still following Duranty's lead in his critique of the artifice of official portraiture: 'Although it follows different stylistic tendencies, portraiture nowadays is more and more concerned with intimate truth, disdainful of flattering approximations and official lies. People want to see the whole man and his inner thoughts.'[30] As Duranty's and Hamel's texts suggest, many critics wanted portraiture to provide depictions of modern people that were sincere and accurate, rather than contrived. The desire to document the present realistically was a key characteristic of the culture; portraiture and modern history paintings provided a perfect means to do so. 'The nineteenth century, as it was ending, was beginning to draw attention to this period in our history', the artist of Péan's portrait, Henri Gervex, reminisced in his memoirs. 'We were recollecting its important dates, reviewing its important facts, portraying its important men.'[31]

It is challenging to categorise the 1886 and 1887 paintings of Pasteur, Péan, and Charcot, since some are quite clearly portraits (Bonnat and Gervex were commissioned to make portraits), while others blur the boundaries between portraiture and history painting. They are all aligned with portraiture because they are concerned with likeness, identity, and status, but, with the exception of Bonnat's work, they are also modern history paintings: they provide narratives of contemporary scenes focused on important people and events. The performative element of scientific personae is exemplified by these paintings: life-sized images filled with the hustle of modern Paris provided ideal stages for showcasing celebrity and invention. These paintings demonstrate how, to borrow Robert Rosemblum's phrase, 'the facts of portraiture turn into the artifice of theatre'.[32] In this respect, they are linked to the *portrait historié*, a term coined in eighteenth-century France to refer to portraits that showed known individuals as historical, biblical, literary, or mythological notables. However, while the 1886 and 1887 paintings do contain historical references, the men portrayed do not assume the identities of other personages, nor are they placed in a past time. These works clearly concern the identities and contemporaneity of the men portrayed. In fact, they are historically significant because they are the first French portraits to show recognisable contemporary doctors and scientists at work in specific contemporary spaces.[33] They differ from earlier precedents that depict scientists and physicians as learned men in library-like settings or as historical protagonists in genre scenes or as figures against nondescript backgrounds. While the paintings can be understood as products of the major shifts in popular understandings of scientific medicine, they also demonstrate art historical changes: these images, and the accompanying art criticism, show the breakdown of boundaries between portrait, genre, and history painting that began in earlier periods in French art (particularly in the eighteenth century) and continued in the 1880s. Significantly, Salon critics spent little time discussing the specific genre of each painting; official categories were no longer as important. Rather, critics focused on which work would provide the most truthful and sincere historical document for future viewers.

Salon criticism, particularly that surrounding the 1886 portraits of Pasteur, provides a crucial introduction to concerns about how men of science and medicine were rendered in the late nineteenth century. For this reason, I have drawn upon it extensively in this book. Criticism has its own conventions and problems, but nonetheless provides accounts that are vital to our understanding of artworks and the popular perceptions of the people and events portrayed. Crucially, the language used in Salon criticism is often similar to that of medical books and atlases, particularly the introductions to illustrated volumes, which describe the works within using a descriptive and flattering vocabulary while stressing veracity. Both relied on the rhetoric of objectivity to instil their visual representations with verisimilitude. Furthermore, understandings of what constituted healthy bodies, admirable morals, and proper sexualities were often analogous in medical and artistic texts and images, and thus became mutually reinforcing.

Scientific medicine

The terms science and medicine encompass a wide range of practices, theories, approaches, histories, and objects of study. While certain components of science were – and continue to be – quite separate and disparate from medicine, *The Face of Medicine* focuses on a historical moment and on historical figures that embody complex intersections.[34] The advances of laboratory science, exemplified by Pasteur's work, had a huge effect on medical practice and thought. The term 'scientific medicine' has its roots in germ theory and the discoveries of laboratory practice.[35] For example, Pasteur's research on microbes influenced surgical methods (though Péan disputed many of the chemist's claims), Charcot spoke publicly in support of Pasteur's rabies vaccination, and Pasteur was familiar with Charcot's studies on hysteria. Furthermore, as the present study shows, many doctors, including Péan and Charcot, were followers of scientific medicine, while Pasteur was considered a medical scientist because his work also focused on human beings and viruses. All of their work, although very different, was informed by (or, in Pasteur's case, contributed to) scientific advances in chemistry, hygiene, and microbiology, as well as modern clinical practices. Medical identities were increasingly tied to scientific ones, and vice versa. As Chapter 1 argues, the portraits of Pasteur became prominent models for depicting chemists and other laboratory scientists, and were integral to future representations of physicians, surgeons, and other medical men.

A shared focus: imaging the body

Medical discourse, as an authoritative force of the nineteenth century, formed and influenced conceptions of bodies, sexualities, and diseases. However, precise medical and scientific understandings intended for educated audiences often took on different assumptions and meanings when filtered through lay minds and outside motivations. Artistic circles were familiar with many of the emerging theories of modern medicine, and medical and scientific communities were aware of the power of artistic conventions. Both artistic and medical training focused on visual examination of the human body.[36] As Anthea Callen argues, art, and its pictorial customs and idealising traditions, enabled medicine to visualise normal and pathological bodies, while medical ideas became equally embodied in artists' depictions.[37] Artists often appropriated and imitated the medical model to create representations of bodies that were considered real and truthful; they partook in scientific culture to elevate art's status to that of science. By drawing on medical discourse, they rendered bodies as deviant or normal, and contributed to discourses on regulation that permeated the public sphere through popular novels, advertising, magazines, newspapers, and artworks. Conversely, medicine worked with cultural and commercial interests to communicate standards about bodies. The increased surveillance of bodies was institutionally implemented through state programmes in medicine, hygiene, law, education, and military training. The classification of bodies was also socially executed by the public who, armed with popularised medical knowledge and a sophisticated awareness of its visual codes, participated in defining normative bodies and behaviours.

Pasteur, Péan, and Charcot contributed to the circulation of representations of bodies, not only through the portrayals of their own bodies in portraits, but also through the many depictions they commissioned for their homes, workplaces, and publications. Like other doctors and scientists, they collaborated with artists to create lifelike models of bodies, diseases, and sexualities. In this book, I engage in debates on the visualisation of these bodies – male and female, healthy and sick, clothed and unclothed, sentient and unconscious – to consider how sex, health, race, gender, and class were inscribed onto images in medical and artistic spheres. This approach, which is built upon theoretical work in art history, gender studies, discourse theory, and the history of medicine, as well as history and visual culture, expands from and engages with the now widely explored understanding of the body as a socially constructed category, and sex, gender, and identity as performative. The human body is a biophysical entity, but nonetheless formed and shaped by society, history, and power.[38]

Rethinking the visual culture of medicine

The Face of Medicine rethinks art's histories through its consideration of the history and visual culture of medicine and its analysis of previously unexamined archival medical sources. It departs from 'traditional' art history through a study of 'non-art' images and texts. By rethinking disciplinary categories and conventions, this book provides a new account of a scrupulously researched period. Yet, it draws on art historical models through a focus on Salon criticism and oil paintings, and a concentration on conventional artistic categories such as realism, portraiture, and history painting. By investigating basic components of nineteenth-century art, I propose novel ways of looking at these oft-studied years. Furthermore, my focus on artists – Gervex, Brouillet, Gsell, and Bonnat – who were popular in their period, but who have since been overshadowed by the scholarly focus on Impressionism, allows us to reconsider the Impressionists by putting their work in dialogue with their contemporaries.[39] This approach demonstrates how our understandings of modern art have privileged too narrow a base of artists and practices.

While the topic of this book requires a cross-disciplinary approach to account for the multiple ways that medicine infiltrated and shaped visual culture, it also necessitates close readings of specific images and objects in order to analyse the relationship between medicine and art in this historical period and location. By broadening the objects of study beyond traditional art historical categories, my approach initiates new ways to explore these issues. It engages with a visual culture approach, since it examines 'high' and 'low' forms of art, treats medical objects with the same attention as Salon paintings, considers representations in varying media, and examines both texts and images. It does not see these images and objects as having equal social, cultural, or economic value. Rather, the differences between them, their modes of production, cultural status, theoretical make-up, materiality, audiences, and historical standing are understood as essential to their meaning. These differences are crucial factors in the fabrication and performance of identities, histories, and realities, as each object, medium, style, theme, and narrative is embedded in a socially and culturally produced system of meaning and value.[40] The current study does not exist outside of these parameters: I do not presume to write an objective history, though my approach is entangled in the historian's desire to do so through the use of archival material and critical modes of analysis.[41] By exploring the ways in which medical men competed with one another and used visual culture to secure personal and occupational interests, *The Face of Medicine* argues that these men, their actions, and their collections were far from apolitical. The men actively engaged in shaping the public's understanding of their identities as they provided the public face of modern medicine.

Rethinking realisms

This book is concerned with the competing claims to truth and objectivity made by mediums, narratives, genres, and styles, particularly those that were considered realist in nineteenth-century art and medicine.[42] Rethinking definitions of realism is necessary if we are to account for the variety of realisms, and understand it as a pluralistic and diverse category. Reconsidering realism encourages us to question the naturalised association of nineteenth-century French realism (particularly that associated with Gustave Courbet, Édouard Manet, and the impressionist circle) with modernism in the history of art and with truth and 'mechanical objectivity' in the history of science (like realism and objectivity, truth is a complex and changing concept). Generally, paintings, prints, and sculptures were described as realist or naturalist when they imitated the visible world accurately, despite differences in formal and technological strategies.

Portraying the world realistically was a central concern for artists, scientists, and physicians in the second half of the nineteenth century, although what that meant and how it manifested visually varied greatly. Realism as an artistic style or category was variable and difficult to define. To this day its definition is notoriously problematic, its omnipresence, contradictions, and paradoxes are, at times, downright bothersome. 'Like a garden weed', Abigail Solomon-Godeau wrote, 'realism would seem to stubbornly resist elimination; … even the newest technologies of image production are generally assimilated to realist codes, particularly if we loosely define them as systems of representation that efface their own material production, the signifier treated as identical to a (pre-existent) signified'.[43] In 1875, Pierre Larousse's *Grand dictionnaire universel du XIXe siècle* explained that *réalisme* eludes a precise definition: 'We do not pretend to define exactly what might fittingly be called realism, from the point of view of art. The supposed inventor of the system of painting that has been named realism, Courbet, ingenuously declared, in a manifesto published in 1855, that he did not understand the meaning of the word'.[44] The lengthy entry that follows discusses the multiple styles, subject matters, theories, and permutations of realist projects: realism indicated the sincere, the ugly, the immoral, and the truth in art. Larousse named Carolus-Duran, Ernest Ange Duez, Jean-Jacques Henner, and Henri Fantin-Latour (amongst other artists whose styles vary greatly) as realists. Although his name was included in the list, Édouard Manet was described as an 'eccentric realist'.[45] The adjectives and personal names used to describe the different forms, modes, and types of realism attest to its diversity.

Like realism, the term naturalism was – and continues to be – defined in many ways. The two are often regarded as different in many art historical and literary debates: naturalism is regularly associated with detailed representations and the rejection of the idealisation of experience, whereas realism is defined as the rejection of the beautiful in favour of unidealised depictions of contemporary life. The ease with which many nineteenth-century Salon critics used them interchangeably in the 1880s demonstrates that they were both ascribed to images that were believed to picture visual reality accurately. Larousse's *Grand dictionnaire* explained that *naturalisme* was often simply another word for *réalisme*.[46]

Realism's association with modernism is paramount, as is shown in the influential yet diverse work of Linda Nochlin, Michael Fried, Klaus Herding, Stephen Eisenman, and Gabriel Weisberg, amongst others.[47] Michael Fried demonstrates in *Courbet's Realism*, *Menzel's Realism,* and *Manet's Modernism* how different artists had their own realisms; realistic styles and theories were part of an artist's subjective and idiosyncratic practice even though they were related to wider representational systems and debates.[48] Richard Thomson's recent book, *The Art of the Actual*, examines an assortment of work beyond the 'modernist masters' and aptly explores the ties between naturalism and the mentality of exactitude, consensual collectivism, and objectivity that were central to republican ideology during the early Third Republic.[49] For Thomson, such work is always politically charged.

Although some critics and artists believed that images could make greater claims to reality by being filtered through an artist's subjective experience, others thought art should strive to be purely objective and detached. Many from both camps turned to the sciences for a language with which to produce 'the real'. As we well know, many mid-century theorists and artists admired and imitated the scientific model, which, they believed, was often based on direct and documented visual observation and experience. This empiricist approach to truth was supported by the conviction that scientific theories were verified or disproven by their relationship to an independently existing reality. Artists used science as a model for truth, though their understandings of truth often varied. The Goncourt brothers wrote in 1860, 'The true is the basis of all art; it is its foundation and its conscience',[50] Jules Castagnary claimed in 1863 that naturalist art was 'truth bringing itself into equilibrium with science',[51] and Pierre-Joseph Proudhon argued in 1865 that 'art cannot subsist apart from truth and justice; science and morality are its leading lights'.[52] For these authors, science held a moral superiority and access to truth that artistic practice needed to follow to achieve a similar status.[53] Although scientific study was not as obviously concerned with morality as philosophy and religion, its intellectual advances and guiding principles were increasingly understood as part of France's moral progress. Scientific reasoning and objectivity carried the possibility of moral benefit, and were considered part of a scientist's moral character.[54]

The success of contemporary scientific endeavours, such as Pasteur's work on germ theory and the rabies vaccine, and the authority granted to scientific models, was desired and appropriated by many in the art world as the century progressed.[55] Paul Lenoir wrote in his 1889 book on the history of realism and naturalism that 'Truth, reality, and nature are the common ground where different expressions of human feeling must coexist. Out of their alliance, masterpieces are composed.'[56] He also wrote, 'Science – such is the last word of our current aspirations. Science carries within it fact, reality, truth and the immensity of the infinite.'[57] For many artists and writers, such an alliance provided art with its greatest successes. Science furnished art with an authoritative model by which to claim mastery over the realm of the truthful, while art increasingly gave science a visual language and aesthetic conventions. In turn, the positive moral virtues attributed to science – honesty, sincerity, and authenticity – took visual form in the aesthetics of realist practice. Realist formal strategies (i.e., the learned artistic techniques and strategies used to produce images and objects that resembled visual reality) were subtly imbued with an understood neutrality and objectivity for some art critics, while other styles were consigned to the realm of the imaginary, fantastical, and unreal. Realist painterly techniques were applied to scientific subject matter because nineteenth-century artists, scientists, and viewers thought such themes required the most 'impartial' of styles.

Although realism was often used as a metaphor for neutrality and visual accuracy, especially in Salon criticism about medically themed paintings, realist strategies were no more objective than any other artistic practice; all styles are intricately bound to professional, institutional, cultural, political, and personal imperatives.[58] In her now canonical text, *Realism*, Nochlin discusses the myth of realism as the 'styleless style'.[59] By simply assuming that representations are true because of art's mimetic capacity to reflect reality, the powerful influences of convention and history, as well as conscious and unconscious intentions and aspirations (be they institutional, individual, or societal), are ignored. Such assumptions also disregard how artists' perceptions, and subsequent artworks, were conditioned by media's properties and abilities. Despite claims to reality made by the optical details of certain materials and procedures, and the cultural associations drawn between the assumed sincerity of modern science and realist works during the nineteenth century, the 'reality effect' was forged by strokes of paint, coloured pigments, photographic chemicals, malleable wax, and other media and techniques. Formal conventions and particular materialities produced this effect. For example, perspectival norms created by painterly lines and marks were regarded as neutral visions of the world, and black-and-white photography was praised for its all-encompassing details despite its two-dimensionality and lack of colour. The *mise-en-scènes* of realist paintings evince representational conventions, particularly since the scenes depicted were often staged in studios. As Peter Brooks claims, realism is a 'form of play that uses carefully wrought and detailed toys' in order to reproduce 'the look and feel of the real thing'.[60]

The juxtaposition of different brushwork, the use of shadows and highlights, the application of perspective, and the mixing of pigments to form lifelike colours allowed artists to produce convincing pictures of the world. Yet, as Roland Barthes argues, these elements all signify the real but are not reality; a realist sign attempts to efface itself in order to create an illusion of the real but it can never *be* reality.[61] James Elkins also questions the claims to reality made by painterly marks by arguing that we should not consider these realist techniques as a simple 'alphabet of realism' but must recognise that pictorial elements are both semiotic and non-semiotic.[62] Furthermore, in our current global age, we know that an image's degree of realism and claim to truth are not historically or geographically secure since people from different cultures and historical periods read and produce reality in different ways. 'Realism is relative', Nelson Goodman argues; it is dependent upon the representational systems of particular places, societies, and times.[63]

I have chosen to use the word realist, as opposed to naturalist, *juste-milieu*, or *pompier* to analyse the works by Bonnat, Edelfelt, Gsell, Gervex, and Brouillet because that was the term most used by the 1886 and 1887 Salon critics to describe these artists and their diverse works.[64] It was also the term most used to describe photographs, drawings, and sculptures in medical contexts. Although other art historians may prefer to keep the word realist for 'modernist heroes', like Courbet and Manet, such an approach does not account for the wide-ranging definitions of and approaches to realism in the last decades of the nineteenth century, nor does it recognise the flexibility of the term and its different conceptions in specific historical periods and fields. Thomson argues that 'naturalism' is the most apt term because it was the most commonly used over the twenty-year period of his study (he claims that 'realism' was declining in its use in artistic discussions).[65] Yet Thomson does not examine medical or scientific images produced outside of the art world – this is not his book's aim – nor does he focus exclusively on the late 1880s. He does, however, draw upon Gabriel Monod's notion of *réalisme scientifique* to explore how the academic coined the term to show the ties between art and literature, and between art and science. As Monod suggested, the desire for truth and scientific realism was found in all facets of intellectual culture.[66] Although his notion was not conceived until 1894, it evidences how a contemporary thinker conceptualised the intermingling between artistic and scientific spheres in the preceding years.

Revisiting realism via portraits of Pasteur, Péan, and Charcot, as well their collections, promises a radical rethinking of its theorisation. By taking into account artistic, scientific, and medical understandings and manifestations of realism, it is evident that realisms were flexible and multifarious. Even within the confines of nineteenth-century French painting, realism was not a static term: by the end of the nineteenth century, the realisms of Courbet and Manet (which were primarily understood as revolutionary and avant-garde during the mid-century) came to symbolise the semi-official style of the early Third Republic.[67] Certainly the realism of Courbet's 1855 *Atelier du peintre. Allégorie réelle déterminant une phase de sept années de ma vie artistique et morale* ('The painter's studio: a real allegory summing up seven years of my artistic and moral life') – an allegorical painting that shows both recognisable portrayals of known figures along with symbolic characters – differs greatly from the works discussed here. For the artists of the 1886 and 1887 paintings of medical men, legibility and easily recognisable people, settings, and identities were more important than pushing the boundaries of the art world, critiquing the Salon system, or exposing human suffering. The realisms of Bonnat, Gervex, Brouillet, Gsell, and Edelfelt were contingent upon the commercial art market, the Salon system, new views of science and medicine, and republican politics and policies.

Art and science, objectivity and subjectivity

The fields of art, medicine, and science overlapped, but were distinct. The scientific self was, generally, diametrically opposed to the artistic self, as Daston and Galison posit: objectivity was most often aligned with science and subjectivity with the arts.[68] This divide, however, was not always clear, particularly when one considers how so many artists and critics utilised the rhetoric of scientific objectivity to promote their work, and how often doctors and scientists relied on visual practices borrowed from art. Natasha Ruiz-Gómez explores these blurred boundaries in her analysis of the images and objects made by Dr Paul Richer for the Hôpital de la Salpêtrière. They were products of a deliberate 'dialogue between scientific and artistic selves', she argues; they are 'scientific artworks' that purposely collapse the binary between subjective and objective to produce a 'hybrid of the indexical and the artistic'.[69] *The Face of Medicine* takes a similar approach by examining the instances where artists, physicians, scientists, and patrons worked together to produce a variety of works that merged the fields of art, medicine, and science.

The medium most discussed in terms of its status as art or science was photography. In the nineteenth century, it utilised fine art's conventions to legitimate its status as art. However, as a seemingly indexical medium tied to its referent and thus reality, photography was invested with the authority of science (the camera's technological properties and chemical processes contributed to this as well).[70] The mechanics of cameras appealed to scientists, since they offered visual representations with ostensibly little human involvement. Photographs conceived as objective evidence were perfect for empiricist projects. This ideal of 'mechanical objectivity' (a term coined by Daston and Galison) promised images untainted by subjectivity and mediation, and fitted with scientists' and physicians' aspirations of impartiality.

Recent studies on the history of photography, influenced by the pioneering work of John Tagg and Allan Sekula, have critiqued the alleged 'mechanical objectivity' of photography to analyse how a photograph's ability to signify the real was based on specific historical and cultural belief systems. Jennifer Tucker argues that there was great scepticism about photography's truth claims during the nineteenth century: a photograph's indexicality alone did not produce its authoritative power as social and material circumstances related to photographic production and consumption shaped perceptions of it as a medium of truth and reality. Human agency, technique, skill, and judgement, as well as the gendered and class dynamics of photographic labour, informed understandings of photography's evidentiary status. As she argues, we need to 'combine the study of the ideal of mechanical objectivity in photography with analysis of the actual process through which people mobilized and used photographic evidence'. [71] Tanya Sheehan also suggests that photography's authority was not solely based on its purported objectivity and the 'disembodied gaze' of the camera. Rather, a photographer's bodily involvement in the studio laboratory was not only definite, but in some cases desirable.[72]

While 'mechanical objectivity' and the distancing effects of a camera were often sought, this was not always the case in artistic and medical realms. Collaborating with artists, touching up photographs, applying hair to wax models, and drawing from life did not always fall easily into the categories of objectivity or subjectivity, or artistic or scientific. Often, subjectivity was needed to make an object appear real and objective; an expert's mark could evince reality and stand for truth as equally as it could point to the fictional and idiosyncratic.

New technologies of vision – microscopes, stereoscopes, cameras, and telescopes – further altered the ways in which the real was understood and imaged.[73] Studies on the history of theories of vision show how anatomical examinations of the microstructure of the retina proposed that vision was a physiological process.[74] Conceptions of vision, along with novel visual experiences, formed modern observers, including physicians, scientists, and artists. 'Ways of scientific seeing are where body and mind, pedagogy and research, knower and known intersect', Daston and Galison have argued. 'Yet historized, collective ways of seeing undeniably produce knowledge, and therefore qualify as the stuff of epistemology.'[75]

Realisms: overlaps and intersections

The Face of Medicine provides neither a historiography of realism, nor an in-depth critique of its numerous philosophical musings, but rather explores the permutations and modifications of a variety of realist projects. Realism – in its various forms – was a site of overlap between artistic and medical spheres. By drawing on diverse conceptions of realism in nineteenth-century French medical and artistic discourses, I explore the characteristics, intricacies, and troubles of realist representations, procedures, and methods. I examine how realisms competed and converged in the construction of reality as an image's or object's degree of realism was dependent on cultural, historical, literary, artistic, and scientific notions of what constituted 'reality'. Terry Eagleton shows that simply describing 'something as realist is to acknowledge that it is not the real thing'.[76] However, Nicholas Green argues that there is a problem not only with the belief that 'some modes of discourse *can* approximate the "real", but that there is a real – out there – to be approximated'.[77] Nonetheless, visual and textual conventions, such as descriptive prose, detailed brushwork, and professional affiliations – particularly modern scientific medicine's cultural association with truth – produced and performed 'reality' through historically specific codes that signified reality to nineteenth-century audiences. Yet, the manufacturing of what Roland Barthes calls the 'reality effect' was often covert, as codes were naturalised, and often invisible.[78]

Theories of mimesis are useful for studying imitations of the visible world. They alert us to the codified representational systems through which the world is filtered and open up the possibilities of interdisciplinary analysis. We become aware of the complex roles that notions of resemblance, imitation, similarity, and mimicry play in the formation of realisms: how they work to produce the belief that an image, text, performance, or object is an accurate simulation of a thing, person, or event. By studying the changing conceptions of realism in artistic, medical, and scientific works, *The Face of Medicine* considers how realism came to signify social reality in nineteenth-century culture.[79] It demonstrates how ideologies of realisms – far from being neutral and descriptive – are inflected by social processes and attitudes, including professional cultures and beliefs. Mimesis is 'a history of disputes over the power to make symbolic worlds; that is, the power to represent the self and others and interpret the world', Gunter Gebauer and Christoph Wulf claim.[80] By focusing on mimesis in terms of power, they provide a model that is not concerned with the traditional boundaries between art and science. Rather, they explore those that allow for the entanglement of art, science, literature, philosophy, and aesthetics, seeing these links as the productive side of mimesis. In this book, I take advantage of the flexibility of the concept, and draw on what Christopher Prendergast refers to as the 'inherent conceptual ambiguity' of mimesis.[81] By focusing on realism's correspondence with other discourses of verisimilitude, particularly those of scientific medicine, I explore the processes of inclusion and exclusion that are integral to this correspondence and, subsequently, to the ways in which this process creates meaning. As Lawrence R. Schehr argues, interruptions in realism's ability to represent should not be regarded as realism's failure, but as integral to the realist project.[82] Mimesis should never be understood as a homogeneous term, for although it is linked to similarity, it is always open to the opposite. It is, as Arne Melberg points out, a 'meeting-place' for opposing forces: proximity and distance, presence and absence, similarity and difference.[83] This more flexible approach accounts for the changing views and forms of realism across disciplines.

Collections and displays

How medical professionals sought to make sense of the world by creating, collecting, and cataloguing lifelike depictions of bodies and illnesses is central to *The Face of Medicine*.[84] These images and objects were thought to attest to the truthfulness of their discoveries and inventions, as well as strengthen their claims to the reality of diseases and diagnoses. They were crucial to the performance of individual and collective identities, and were products of collective and individual methods of scientific observation. Men of science, art, and medicine often shared these items, and gave them as gifts to one another. These exchanges were vital to the homosocial circles of artistic, medical, and scientific culture – they provided a means of sharing knowledge, skills, and sociability, established professional ties, and facilitated self-promotion and male collectivity.[85]

The Face of Medicine investigates how the medical and scientific elite used images and objects both publicly and privately – be it through exhibiting sculptures in medical museums, exchanging personal photographic portraits, or commissioning paintings for the Salon or the home. Certainly Charcot's and Péan's medical collections, and the photographic studios in their respective hospitals, owe much to the support of republican policies. Intended for medical education, these medical displays were considered modern, objective, and truthful even though they were informed by individual taste, personal ambition, and professional rivalries.

Georges Didi-Huberman argues that the assembling and cataloguing of collections is a form of fabricating reality as the knowledge generated by collecting practices becomes aligned with truth.[86] The medical establishment's production and authentication of reality through the creation and collection of renderings of bodies – as well as the subjective fantasies involved in amassing objects for personal ownership – at times manifested a desire for the real that undermined the claims to objectivity assigned to these collected medical objects.

This book concentrates on these troubled moments. While these images and objects served to portray personal and professional identities as rational and reasonable, they also fulfilled desires that exceeded the necessities of scientific duty, particularly when a naked female patient was the focus of male attention.[87]

Gender was always implicated in collecting practices, particularly when sexual stereotypes inflected the collected images and objects. As Jonathan Crary suggests in his discussion of the overlapping figure of collector, detective, consumer, and fetishist, there is a perversion at the core of the search for fact and truth.[88] Michel Foucault has also pointed out this link between the production of knowledge and pleasure in his account of the history of sexuality. He argued that the nineteenth-century construction of a *scientia sexualis* – a Western practice for finding the truth about sex based in forms of knowledge-power, such as a physician's interrogation of a patient – has always functioned as a type of *ars erotica* (what he argued was the manifestation of Eastern approaches that elicit sexual knowledge through pleasure) despite its seeming contradistinction.[89] Behind the ostensibly neutral naming, ordering, and cataloguing of bodies and behaviours in nineteenth-century medicine, exists an intensified pleasure intrinsic to that very practice.[90]

Three case studies

Each chapter of *The Face of Medicine* centres on a painting that portrays a celebrated man associated with the Parisian medical elite that was exhibited at the 1886 or 1887 Salon, and then expands to consider the representations of bodies that these men collected, commissioned, and/or created. Like medical case studies, they focus on the individual and then expand to situate these men, their popular personae, and their collections in wider debates.

Chapter 1 investigates portraits of Pasteur, including the 1886 Salon paintings by Bonnat, Edelfelt, and Gsell, as well as portrayals of scientists in the popular press and the images and objects on display in Pasteur's home, laboratory, and the Pasteur Institute. Through an examination of Pasteur's various personae, it analyses modern male professionalism and masculinity in scientific spheres, and considers how the 1886 and 1887 Salon portraits of the chemist served as templates for future representations of medical men. It illuminates what was at stake in these images, particularly as they pertained to promoting Pasteur's identity as a humanitarian leader and global scientific saviour.

Chapter 2 centres on Gervex's portrait of Péan, *Avant l'opération: le Docteur Péan enseignant à l'hôpital Saint-Louis sa découverte du pincement des vaisseaux* (Before the operation: Dr Péan at the Hôpital Saint-Louis presenting his new technique of clamping blood vessels) and investigates the ties between portraiture, republicanism, masculinity, and the genre of the female nude. It examines how the surgeon was a collector of different forms of realism in paint and in wax. Péan's medical *moulages* of female genitalia are studied in relation to artworks, photographs, and medical models of unconscious and unclothed female bodies in nineteenth-century visual culture in order to explore moments when the assumed objectivity of realist practice is ruptured. Arguing that the oddities of Péan's collection reveal a desire that belies the objective veneer of realist projects, this chapter explores the irrational and fantastical side of realism and the troubles of its truth claims.

Chapter 3 focuses on *Une leçon clinique à la Salpêtrière*, André Brouillet's painting of Jean-Martin Charcot expounding on the hypnotised state of his hysterical female patient. By examining the multiple visualisations of hysteria that Charcot commissioned in wax, plaster, photography, and print, along with the visual and textual works that were influenced by his views, this investigation moves beyond conventional art historical analysis to consider electrotherapy, hypnosis, and other medical procedures and performances used at the Salpêtrière as modern forms of realistic representation. I argue that *Une leçon clinique* – a painting that portrays these modes of visualisation – is ultimately a realist depiction of realist modes of representing hysteria. The painting foregrounds the essential role of visual representations in hysteria studies because they were key to public understanding of the disease and crucial to building Charcot's medical persona. By situating these realist methods in a wider cultural context, I contend that the hysterical female body was a site on which realism 'went mad'.

Conclusion: shared dreams

Chamillac's Salon review, which opened this introduction, exemplifies the intersecting spheres of art and medicine. In his text, paintings become microbes, Salon viewers morph into patients, and viewing art becomes a modern medical procedure. This example demonstrates how art critics, like artists, wished to take part in the emerging culture of scientific medicine, but it also indicates that Chamillac perceived medical men to be equally drawn to the art world. As Chamillac notes, the 'princes of science' were hooked on the 'terrible vaccine' of painting.

Doctors and artists had much in common despite the great differences in their occupations. Both believed that one could know the world through acute observation and meticulous documentation, and that knowledge was produced and skills perfected by examining the human body. Both occupations used powers of observation and relied on the ocular. Artists took on the role of men of scientific medicine: they studied their sitters, examined the environment in which they lived, and portrayed their every inch with microscopic detail. Similarly, many doctors and scientists turned to the visual arts in order to create and commission realistic representations of bodies for their own personal and professional gain, knowledge, and delight – even when such images and objects threatened to fall into the realm of fantasy, madness, and pleasure. The social limitations placed on examining bodies affected both medical and artistic practice.

The close links drawn between art and scientific medicine are not surprising, particularly within the context of 1880s Paris. After all, Pasteur, Péan, and Charcot all expressed with certainty in the popular press that if they had not become men of science, they would have become artists.

Notes

1 Chamillac, 'Le Virus pictural', *La Revue illustrée*, 1 (1887), 337. 'Des jeunes hommes, des vieillards, des femmes blondes ou rouges, brunes ou vertes, des gens décorés, des poètes et des négociants affolés, anémiés, donnant tous les signes du plus profond accablement sortent du Palais de l'Industrie. Courbés et atones, flageoleant sur leurs jambes veules, ils portent à grand'peine un livret rouge, signe distinctif de leur état actuel, destiné à prévenir les personnes saines d'avoir à s'éloigner d'eux au plus vite. Ces malheureux, en effet, viennent de se faire inoculer le microbe de la peinture. Cette vaccine terrible, que certains princes de la science considèrent comme funeste, est à ce point entrée dans leurs mœurs et les moelles de nos plus fiers lapins, qu'ils ne sauraient s'en passer, et que, chaque année, ils en redemandent. Cela et la morphine! Notre race y résistera-t-elle? L'avenir répondra.' All translations from the French are by the author, unless stated otherwise.

2 Nineteenth-century science encompassed various branches of study, including medicine, engineering, and chemistry, but there were great differences between categories. As Ludmilla Jordanova argues, the concept of 'scientist' is a nineteenth-century construction that came into use when laboratory research was just a small activity of those who examined the natural world. Jordanova, *Defining Features: Scientific and Medical Portraits 1660–2000* (London: Reaktion Books, 2000), pp. 13, 61–66.

3 For an overview of portraiture's association with social and economic status, see Joanna Woodall (ed.), *Portraiture: Facing the Subject* (Manchester: Manchester University Press, 1997).

4 Lorraine Daston and H. Otto Sibum, 'Scientific Personae', *Science in Context*, 16:1–2 (2003), 2–3. As they argue, 'Intermediate between individual biography and the social institution lies the persona: a cultural identity that simultaneously shapes the individual in body and mind and creates a collective with a shared and recognizable physiognomy … Personae are creatures of historical circumstance; they emerge and disappear within specific contexts.'

5 For diverse analyses of the influence of medical discourse on French culture, see Douglas P. Mackaman, *Leisure Settings: Bourgeois Culture, Medicine, and the Spa in Modern France* (Chicago: University of Chicago Press, 1998); Anthea Callen, *The Spectacular Body: Science, Method and Meaning in the Work of Degas* (New Haven: Yale University Press, 1995); and Lawrence Rothfield, *Vital Signs: Medical*

Realism in Late Nineteenth-Century Fiction (Princeton: Princeton University Press, 1992).

6 For examinations of the political role of art in the early Third Republic, see Richard Thomson, *The Troubled Republic. Visual Culture and Social Debate in France, 1889–1900* (New Haven: Yale University Press, 2004); Miriam Levin, *Republican Art and Ideology in Late Nineteenth-Century France* (Ann Arbor: UMI Research Press, 1986); Michael Orwicz (ed.), *Art Criticism and its Institutions in Nineteenth-Century France* (Manchester: Manchester University Press, 1994); June Hargrove and Neil McWilliam (eds), *Nationalism and French Visual Culture, 1870–1914* (New Haven: Yale University Press, 2005); and Patricia Mainardi, *The End of the Salon: Art and the State in the Early Third Republic* (Cambridge: Cambridge University Press, 1993).

7 Jack D. Ellis, *The Physician-Legislators of France: Medicine and Politics in the early Third Republic 1870–1914* (Cambridge: Cambridge University Press, 1990); and Philip Nord, *The Republican Moment: Struggles for Democracy in Nineteenth-Century France* (Cambridge, MA: Harvard University Press, 1995).

8 Ellis, *The Physician-Legislators of France*, p. 2.

9 Nord, *The Republican Moment*, pp. 32, 47.

10 Horace Bianchon, *Nos grands médecins d'aujourd'hui* (Paris: Société d'éditions scientifiques, 1891), p. II.

11 For a history of French physicians and medical culture, see: George Weisz, *The Medical Mandarins: the French Academy of Medicine in the Nineteenth and Early Twentieth Centuries* (New York: Oxford University Press, 1995); Ann La Berge and Mordechai Feingold (eds), *French Medical Culture in the Nineteenth Century* (Amsterdam and Atlanta: Rodopi, 1994); and Caroline Hannaway and Ann La Berge (eds), *Constructing Paris Medicine* (Amsterdam and Atlanta: Rodopi, 1998).

12 Key texts on nineteenth-century masculinity include Tamar Garb, *Bodies of Modernity: Figure and Flesh in Fin-de-Siècle France* (New York: Thames and Hudson, 1998), pp. 33–38; Robert Nye, *Masculinity and Male Codes of Honor in Modern France* (New York: Oxford University Press, 1993); Anthea Callen, 'Masculinity and Muscularity: Dr. Paul Richer and Modern Manhood', *Paragraph*, 16:1 (2003), 17–41; Judith Surkis, *Sexing the Citizen: Morality and Masculinity in France, 1870–1920* (Ithaca: Cornell University Press, 2006); Temma Balducci, Heather Belnap Jensen, and Pamela Warner (eds), *Interior Portraiture and Masculine Identity in France, 1789–1914* (Aldershot: Ashgate, 2011).

13 Robert Nye, 'Afterword', in Christopher E. Forth and Bertrand Taithe (eds), *French Masculinities: History, Culture, and Politics* (Basingstoke: Palgrave Macmillan, 2007), p. 239.

14 R.W. Connell and James W. Messerschmidt, 'Hegemonic Masculinity: Rethinking the Concept', *Gender and Society*, 19:6 (2005), 829–859.

15 R.W. Connell, *Masculinities* (Berkeley: University of California Press, 1995).

16 Bridget Alsdorf argues that the notion of collectivity was a contentious idea, particularly as bourgeois society came to terms with the problematic relationship between the individual and the group. Bridget Alsdorf, *Fellow Men: Fantin-Latour*

and the Problem of the Group in Nineteenth-Century French Painting (Princeton: Princeton University Press, 2012), p. 5.

17 Elisabeth Bronfen, *The Knotted Subject: Hysteria and its Discontents* (Princeton: Princeton University Press, 1998); George Didi-Huberman, *Invention of Hysteria: Charcot and the Photographic Iconography of the Salpêtrière,* trans. Alisa Hartz (Cambridge, MA: MIT Press, 2003); Jann Matlock, *Scenes of Seduction: Prostitution, Hysteria, and Reading Difference in Nineteenth-Century France* (New York: Columbia University Press, 1994); Sander Gilman, Helen King, Roy Porter *et al.*, *Hysteria beyond Freud* (Berkeley: University of California Press, 1993); and Janet Beizer, *Ventriloquized Bodies: Narratives of Hysteria in Nineteenth-Century France* (Ithaca: Cornell University Press, 1994).

18 For medical accounts, see Robert Nye, *Crime, Madness and Politics in Modern France: The Medical Concept of National Decline* (Princeton: Princeton University Press, 1984); and Bertrand Taithe, *Defeated Flesh: Welfare, Warfare and the Making of Modern France* (Manchester: Manchester University Press, 1999), pp. 46–96, 130–150.

19 For investigations of the impact of theories of degeneration on late nineteenth-century French art and visual culture, see Fae Brauer and Barbara Larson, *The Art of Evolution: Darwin, Darwinism, and Visual Culture* (Hanover: Dartmouth College Press, 2009); and Barbara Larson, 'Evolution and Degeneration in the Early World of Odilon Redon', *Nineteenth-Century Art Worldwide*, 2 (2003), www.19thc-artworldwide.org, accessed 28 April 2015.

20 Peinard, *La Profession de médecine* (Paris, 1902), p. 138 as cited by Robert Nye, 'Medicine and Science as Masculine "Fields of Honor"', *Osiris*, 2:12 (1997), 60–79.

21 Nye, 'Medicine and Science as Masculine "Fields of Honor"', pp. 60–79.

22 The various conceptions of objectivity within the wide field of science have been examined by Lorraine Daston, who argues that scientific objectivity is not 'monolythic nor immutable' because it is comprised of metaphysical, methodological and moral meanings that are historically specific. Daston, 'Objectivity and the Escape from Perspective', *Social Studies of Medicine*, 22 (1992), 597.

23 See Lorraine Daston and Peter Galison, *Objectivity* (New York: Zone Books, 2007), particularly chapter 4 on 'The Scientific Self', pp. 191–251.

24 For a history of women's acceptance in medical schools in France, see Yvonne Knibiehler and Catherine Fouquet, *La femme et les médecins: analyse historique* (Paris: Hachette, 1983), pp. 193–200; Joy Harvey, 'La Visite: Mary Putnam Jacobi and the Paris Medical Clinics', in La Berge and Feingold (eds), *French Medical Culture in the Nineteenth Century*, pp. 350–371.

25 Knibiehler and Fouquet, *La femme et les médecins*, p. 193. For an account of the debates regarding women artists' access to anatomy and life study during the late eighteenth and early nineteenth centuries in France, see Margaret Oppenheimer, 'The Charming Spectacle of the Cadaver: Anatomical and Life Study by Women Artists in Paris', *Nineteenth-Century Art Worldwide*, 6:1 (2007), www.19thc-artworldwide.org, accessed 28 April 2015.

26 See Nancy Chodorow, *Femininities, Masculinities, Sexualities: Freud and Beyond* (Cambridge: Cambridge University Press, 1991); Donna Harraway, *Simians, Cyborgs, and Women: The Reinvention of Nature* (New York: Routledge, 1991); Catharine MacKinnon, *Women's Lives, Men's Laws* (Cambridge, MA: Belknap Press of Harvard University Press, 2004); Evelyn Fox Keller, *Reflections on Gender and Science* (New Haven: Yale University Press, 1985); Londa Schiebinger, *The Mind Has No Sex? Women and the Origins of Modern Science* (Cambridge, MA: Harvard University Press, 1989).

27 For a more critical historiography of French medicine, see the introduction to Hannaway and La Berge (eds), *Constructing Paris Medicine.*

28 Sarah Betzer, *Ingres and the Studio: Women, Painting, History* (University Park: Pennsylvania State University Press, 2012); Tamar Garb, *The Painted Face: Portraits of Women in France, 1814–1914* (New Haven: Yale University Press, 2007); Melissa McQuillan, *Impressionist Portraits* (London: Thames and Hudson, 1986); Meyer Schapiro, *Impressionism: Reflections and Perceptions* (New York: George Braziller, 1997), pp. 154–178; Roger Cardinal, 'Nadar and the Photographic Portrait in Nineteenth-Century France', in Graham Clarke (ed.), *The Portrait in Photography* (London: Reaktion Books, 1992), pp. 6–24; and Heather McPherson, *The Modern Portrait in Nineteenth-Century France* (Cambridge: Cambridge University Press, 2001), pp. 14–37.

29 Edmond Duranty, *La Nouvelle Peinture, à propos du groupe d'artistes qui exposent dans les Galeries Durand-Ruel* (Paris: E. Dentu, 1876).

30 Maurice Hamel, 'Le Portrait', in Antonin Proust (ed.), *L'art français 1789–1889* (Paris, c.1889), p. 63. 'Tout en obéissant à des tendances diverses, le portrait de nos jours se fait de plus en plus soucieux de vérité intime, dédaigneux des à peu près flatteurs et des mensonges officiels. On veut voir tout l'homme et sa pensée de derrière la tête'.

31 Henri Gervex, *Souvenirs recueillis par Jules Bertaut* (Paris: E. Flammarion, 1924), p. 198: 'le XIXe siècle qui finissait commençait d'appeler l'attention sur cette période de notre histoire. On en remémorait les grandes dates, on en repassait les grands faits, on en peignait les grand hommes.'

32 Robert Rosenblum, 'Portraiture: Fact versus Fiction', in Sébastien Allard and Robert Rosenblum, *Citizens and Kings: Portraits in the Age of Revolution 1760–1830*, exhibition catalogue (London: Royal Academy of Arts, 2007), p. 19.

33 Richard Weisberg, 'The Representation of Doctors at Work in Salon Art of the Early Third Republic in France' (PhD dissertation, New York University, 1995), pp. 57–58. Weisberg argues that scientific advances cannot explain the major shifts in medical portraiture because they had been occurring previously. Rather, he contends that medical portraits changed alongside popular images and understandings of medicine, and that this transformation occurred with the acceptance of Pasteur's theories. Weisberg does not, however, address the major alterations in portraiture that were occurring from the mid-century, such as the fashion for a sense of immediacy and informal portrayals of sitters in everyday environments.

34 Historians of medicine have addressed the complex ties between science and medicine. For a historiographical account of these debates, see John Harley Warner, 'The History of Science and the Sciences of Medicine', *Osiris*, 10:1 (1995), 164–193; and Michael Worboys, 'Practice and the Science of Medicine in the Nineteenth Century', *Isis*, 102:1 (2011), 109–115.

35 William F. Bynum, *Science and the Practice of Medicine in the Nineteenth Century* (Cambridge: Cambridge University Press, 1994); and Anne Marie Moulin, 'Bacteriological Research and Medical Practice in and out of the Pasteurian School', in Hannaway and La Berge (eds), *Constructing Paris Medicine*, pp. 327–349.

36 Philippe Comar (ed.), *Figures du corps: une leçon d'anatomie à l'école des Beaux-Arts* (Paris: Beaux-Arts de Paris les éditions, 2008); and Jean-François Debord, 'De l'anatomie artistique à la morphologie', in Jean Clair (ed.), *L'âme au corps: arts et sciences, 1793–1993* (Paris: Réunions des musées nationaux, Gallimard; Paris: Galeries nationales du Grand Palais, 1993), pp. 102–117.

37 Anthea Callen, 'The Body and Difference: Anatomy Training at the École des Beaux-Arts in the Later Nineteenth Century', *Art History*, 20:1 (1997), 23.

38 The literature on 'the body' and medical culture is extensive. See Michel Foucault, *Naissance de la clinique* (Paris: Presses universitaires de France, 1963) and *History of Sexuality* (New York: Pantheon, 1978); Judith Butler, *Gender Trouble: Feminism and the Subversion of Identity* (New York: Routledge, 1989) and *Bodies that Matter: On the Discursive Limits of 'Sex'* (New York: Routledge, 1993); James Elkins, *Pictures of the Body: Pain and Metamorphosis* (Stanford: Stanford University Press, 1999); Deborah Lupton, *Medicine as Culture: Illness, Disease and the Body in Western Societies* (London: Sage, 1994); Kathleen Adler and Marcia Pointon (eds), *The Body Imagined: The Human Form and Visual Culture Since the Renaissance* (Cambridge: Cambridge University Press, 1993); and Thomas Laqueur, *Making Sex: Body and Gender from the Greeks to Freud* (Cambridge, MA: Harvard University Press, 1990).

39 For investigations of other currently disregarded artists, see Richard Thomson, *Art of the Actual: Naturalism and Style in Early Third Republic France, 1880–1900* (New Haven: Yale University Press, 2012); and Natalie Adamson and Toby Norris (eds), *Academics, Pompiers, Official Artists and the Arrière-garde: Defining Modern and Traditional in France, 1900–1960* (Newcastle-upon-Tyne: Cambridge Scholars Publishing, 2009).

40 For views on visual culture from different disciplinary perspectives, see Svetlana Alpers, Emily Apter, Carol Armstrong *et al.*,'Visual Culture Questionnaire', *October*, 77 (1996), 25–70.

41 For a historiographical account of the methodological problems related to writing about realism in art history, see Richard Shiff, 'Art History and the Nineteenth Century: Realism and Resistance', *The Art Bulletin*, 70:1 (1988), 25–48.

42 For a discussion of realism in relation to other discourses of verisimilitude, such as science, philosophy, and history, see Lawrence Schehr, *Rendering French Realism* (Stanford: Stanford University Press, 1997), pp. 17–18.

43 Abigail Solomon-Godeau, 'Realism Revisited', in Aruna D'Souza (ed.), *Self and History: A Tribute to Linda Nochlin* (London: Thames and Hudson, 2001), p. 71.

44 Pierre Larousse, *Grand dictionnaire universel du XIXe siècle*, vol. 13 (Paris, 1875), p. 755. 'Nous ne saurions avoir la prétention de définir exactement ce qu'il convient d'appeler réalisme, au point de vue de l'art. Le prétendu inventeur du système de peinture auquel on a donné le nom, Courbet, a déclaré ingénument, dans un manifeste publié en 1855, qu'il ne comprenait pas la signification du mot.'

45 Larousse, *Grand dictionnaire universel du XIXe siècle*, vol. 13, p. 757: 'réaliste excentrique'.

46 Pierre Larousse, *Grand dictionnaire universelle du XIXe siècle*, vol. 13, pp. 755–757.

47 Linda Nochlin, *Realism* (Harmondsworth: Penguin Books, 1971); Michael Fried, *Courbet's Realism* (Chicago: University of Chicago Press, 1990); Klaus Herding, *Courbet: To Venture Independence*, trans. John William Gabriel (New Haven: Yale University Press, 1991); Gabriel Weisberg, *The Realist Tradition: French Painting and Drawing 1830–1900* (Cleveland: Cleveland Museum of Art, 1980); Stephen Eisenman, 'The Rhetoric of Realism: Courbet and the Origins of the Avant-Garde', in Stephen Eisenman, Thomas Crow, Brian Lukacher *et al.* (eds), *Nineteenth Century Art*, pp. 212–220 (London: Thames and Hudson, 1994); and Gabriel Weisberg, *The European Realist Tradition* (Bloomington: Indiana University Press, 1982).

48 Fried, *Courbet's Realism*; *Menzel's Realism: Art and Embodiment in Nineteenth-Century Berlin* (New Haven: Yale University Press, 2002); and *Manet's Modernism, or, the Face of Painting in the 1860s* (Chicago: University of Chicago Press, 1996).

49 Thomson, *Art of the Actual.*

50 Edmond and Jules de Goncourt, 'Journal, 10 December 1860', in Charles Harrison and Paul Wood (eds), *Art in Theory, 1815–1900: An Anthology of Changing Ideas* (Oxford: Blackwell, 1998), p. 417.

51 Jules Castagnary, 'Salon review of 1863', in Jules Castagnary, *Salons (1857–1870), avec une préface de Eugène Spuller* (Paris: G. Charpentier et E. Fasquelle, 1892), pp. 104–105. 'L'école naturaliste affirme que l'art est l'expression de la vie sous tous ses modes et à tous ses degrés, et que son unique but est de reproduire la nature en l'amenant à son maximum de puissance et d'intensité: c'est la vérité s'équilibrant avec la science'.

52 Pierre-Joseph Proudon, 'Du Principe de l'art et sa destination sociale', in Harrison and Wood (eds), *Art in Theory*, p. 405.

53 For alternative accounts of the moral status of science in the nineteenth century, see Anne De Witt, *Moral Authority: Men of Science, and the Victorian Novel* (Cambridge: Cambridge University Press, 2013).

54 Daston and Galison, *Objectivity*, pp. 122–124, 185.

55 For examinations of nineteenth-century conceptions of medical progress, see La Berge and Feingold (eds), *French Medical Cultures in the Nineteenth Century*; Andrew Aisenberg, *Contagion: Disease, Government and the 'Social Question' in Nineteenth-Century France* (Stanford: Stanford University Press, 1999); and Robert Fox and George Weisz (eds), *The Organization of Science and Technology in France 1808–1914* (Cambridge: Cambridge University Press, 1980).

56 Paul Lenoir, *Histoire du Réalisme et du Naturalisme dans la poésie et dans l'art depuis l'antiquité jusqu'à nos jours* (Paris: Quantin, 1889), p. I. 'La vérité, la réalité, la nature, sont le terrain commun où ces expressions diverses du sentiment humain doivent coexister. De leur alliance se composent les chefs-d'œuvre.'

57 Lenoir, *Histoire du Réalisme et du Naturalisme*, p. 759. 'La Science, tel est le dernier mot de nos aspirations actuelles. La Science porte en elle le fait, la réalité, la vérité et l'immensité de l'infini.'

58 T.J. Clark, *The Absolute Bourgeois: Artists and Politics in France, 1848–1851* (London: Thames and Hudson, 1973) and *Image of the People: Gustave Courbet and the 1848 Revolution* (London: Thames and Hudson, 1973).

59 Nochlin, *Realism*, pp. 14–17.

60 Peter Brooks, *Realist Vision* (New Haven: Yale University Press, 2005), p. 3.

61 Roland Barthes, *The Rustle of Language*, trans. Richard Howard (Oxford: Basil Blackwell, 1986).

62 James Elkins, *On Pictures and the Words That Fail Them* (Cambridge: Cambridge University Press, 1998), p. 58.

63 Nelson Goodman, *Languages of Art: An Approach to a Theory of Symbols* (Indianapolis: Hackett Publishing Company, 1976), p. 37.

64 Although naturalism was also used to describe these works, the difference between realism and naturalism was dependent upon the critic. While naturalism is understood as a more positivist and scientific form of realism, most current discussions consider them the same thing. As James Elkins states, both should be understood 'indifferently as the practice of making pictures that are said to resemble what they denote'. Elkins, *On Pictures and the Words that Fail Them*, p. 48.

65 Thomson, *Art of the Actual*, p. 9.

66 Gabriel Monod, *Renan, Taine, Michelet: les maîtres de l'histoire* (Paris: Librairie d'art Ludovic Baschet, 1894).

67 Linda Nochlin, 'The Depoliticisation of Gustave Courbet: Transformation and Rehabilitation under the Third Republic', pp. 109–121 and Michael Orwicz, 'Reinventing Édouard Manet: Rewriting the Face of National Art in the early Third Republic', pp. 122–145 in Orwicz (ed.), *Art Criticism and its Institutions in Nineteenth-Century France*.

68 Daston and Galison, *Objectivity*, pp. 37, 135, 246.

69 Natasha Ruiz-Gómez, 'The "Scientific Artworks" of Doctor Paul Richer', *Medical Humanities*, 39:1 (2013), 4–10.

70 For investigation of the troubled ties between photography and science, see Jennifer Tucker, *Nature Exposed: Photography as Eye Witness in Victorian Science* (Baltimore: Johns Hopkins University Press, 2005); and Joel Snyder, 'Visualization and Visibility', in Peter Galison and Caroline Jones (eds), *Picturing Science, Producing Art* (New York: Routledge, 1998), pp. 379–397.

71 Tucker, *Nature Exposed*, p. 4.

72 Tanya Sheehan, *Doctored: The Medicine of Photography in Nineteenth-Century America* (University Park: Pennsylvania University Press, 2011), p. 124.

73 Jonathan Crary, *Techniques of the Observer: On Vision and Modernity in the Nineteenth Century* (Cambridge, MA: MIT Press, 1990), and 'Géricault, the Panorama, and Sites of Reality in the Early Nineteenth Century', *Grey Room*, 9 (2002), 5–25.
74 Kelly Wilder, *Photography and Science* (London: Reaktion Books, 2009); Elizabeth Lunbeck and Lorraine Daston (eds), *Histories of Scientific Observation* (Chicago: University of Chicago Press, 2010); and Jutta Schickore, *The Microscope and the Eye: A History of Reflections*, 1740–1870 (Chicago: University of Chicago Press, 2007).
75 Daston and Galison, *Objectivity*, p. 369.
76 Terry Eagleton, 'Pork Chops and Pineapples', *London Review of Books*, 25:20 (2003), p. 17.
77 Nicholas Green, *The Spectacle of Nature: Landscape and Bourgeois Culture in Nineteenth-Century France* (Manchester: Manchester University Press, 1990), p. 2.
78 Barthes, *The Rustle of Language*.
79 Erich Auerbach, *Mimesis: The Representation of Reality in Western Literature* (Princeton: Princeton University Press, 1953).
80 Gunter Gebauer and Christoph Wulf, *Mimesis: Culture, Art, Society*, trans. Don Reneau (Berkeley: University of California Press, 1992), p. 3.
81 Christopher Prendergast, *The Order of Mimesis: Balzac, Stendhal, Nerval, Flaubert* (Cambridge: Cambridge University Press, 1986), p. 5.
82 Schehr, *Rendering French Realism*, pp. 17–18.
83 Arne Melberg, *Theories of Mimesis* (Cambridge: Cambridge University Press, 1995), p. 2.
84 For examinations of collecting practices within medical museums, see Samuel J.M.M. Alberti and Elizabeth Hallam (eds), *Medical Museums: Past, Present, Future* (London: Royal College of Surgeons, 2013).
85 Crucial investigations of the homosocial include Eve Kosofsky Sedgwick, *Between Men: English Literature and Male Homosocial Desire* (New York: Columbia University Press, 1985); Abigail Solomon-Godeau, *Male Trouble: A Crisis in Representation* (New York: Thames and Hudson, 1997); Anthea Callen, 'Doubles and Desires: Anatomies of Masculinity in the Later Nineteenth Century', *Art History*, 26:5 (2003), 669–699.
86 Georges Didi-Huberman, *Confronting Images: Questioning the Ends of a Certain History of Art*, trans. John Goodman (University Park: Pennsylvania State University Press, 2005), pp. 71–72.
87 For various discussions of the irrational and hidden motives of collecting practices, see Michael Camille and Adrian Rifkin (eds), *Other Objects of Desire: Collectors and Collecting Queerly* (Oxford: Blackwell, 2001).
88 See Jonathan Crary's discussion of Max Klinger's glove cycle in *Suspensions of Perception: Attention, Spectacle and Modern Culture* (Cambridge, MA: MIT Press, 1999), pp. 90–134.
89 Michel Foucault, *The History of Sexuality: The Will to Knowledge, 1* (London: Penguin Books, 1990), pp. 70–71.

90 As Foucault suggests, 'Perhaps this production of truth, intimidated though it was by the scientific model, multiplied, intensified, and even created its own intrinsic pleasures.' Foucault, *The History of Sexuality*, p. 71.

1 The makings of a scientific hero: portraits of Louis Pasteur

Late nineteenth-century Parisian life was infused with science and medicine. Paintings, sculptures, and trinkets celebrated doctors' and scientists' roles in the progress and safety of France, and books, magazines, and newspapers cultivated the public's imagination about these *grands hommes*. Of all the scientific celebrities, Louis Pasteur was one of the most prominent figures.[1] A founder of the study of microbiology, he was known for his vaccines against rabies and anthrax, and for the process of purifying liquids through heat that bears his name. Considered by the 'nation's elite' to be an 'illustrious man, modest in his glory', Pasteur was a heroic model of modern science and manhood.[2] The masculinity of scientific leaders was a crucial component of their identity and power; heterosexual, intelligent, rational, virile, objective, competitive, and white, Pasteur embodied the ideal manliness of a national leader and scientific persona.[3] Significantly, Pasteur's fame was tied to the profusion of visual and textual representations of his body. 'His portrait and his works are universally known', Adrien Marx wrote in *Le Figaro* in 1887. 'Photography, the paint brush and the pen have reproduced his features, recounted his life and published his labours'.[4]

Despite his historical importance, art historians have largely disregarded Pasteur's impact on nineteenth-century French art and visual culture, and overlooked how he came to personify the confluence of art and science in the early Third Republic.[5] Pasteur was an avid collector and producer of images, in addition having his image rendered and distributed by others. He frequented art galleries and Salons, taught science courses at the École des Beaux-Arts in the 1860s, discussed art with friends and colleagues (often through detailed written correspondence), commissioned artworks for his family and workplace, and frequently posed for artists and photographers.[6]

The commemoration of French men – Pasteur in particular – was noted by Georges Olmer, whose book on the 1886 Salon provides a glimpse of this period when the practice of portraying modern scientific men was developing:

> Like the *Revue annuelle de variétés*, the Salon reveres current events and always burns a bit of incense in honour of the men of the day. We were thus expecting to see a portrait of M. Pasteur there. We have two of them, and we have no cause for complaint, for artistic homage to the great man could never be too resounding.[7]

There were, in fact, three paintings of Pasteur on display that year. The first, established academician Léon Bonnat's life-size canvas, represents a mature Pasteur with his young blonde granddaughter against a dark backdrop (Figure 5). Standing erect with one hand under his wool jacket and the other held by Camille, Pasteur exudes power and warmth. Bonnat's technical ability enabled him to produce a highly detailed and intricate painting that captures the minutiae of physiognomies, flesh, and fashion, and represents the chemist as both a national hero and a family man. The second portrait, by Albert Edelfelt, a young and relatively unknown Finnish artist, shows Pasteur as an active scientist, inspecting a glass-enclosed specimen in his laboratory (Figure 6). Bright colours and looser brushwork, along with Pasteur's leaning body and rumpled suit, present an unceremonious glimpse of the chemist at work. The third painting was a small, nearly unnoticed one by Pasteur's close relative, Laurent Lucien Gsell, whose career was just beginning (Figure 7).[8] Here, Pasteur – tucked away in the background – and his colleagues are shown in a busy laboratory. Were it not for the celebrity of Pasteur, Gsell's work might have been dismissed as a still life of thick books and sparkling glass flasks, with bottles and pipettes scattered along diagonal lab benches.

The emergence of new scientific occupations and professional spaces in the 1880s demanded that portraiture adjust to account for modern men and their workplaces. As a genre with strong historical links to royalty and aristocracy, portraiture transferred its status and authority onto its sitters, thus legitimising modern professions. Furthermore, from the mid-1870s, portraiture in France was shedding its image as a low genre and gaining acknowledgement as a new form of history painting – a type of historical document of modern life for future viewers. For example, the novelist and critic Arsène Houssaye redefined history painting in his review of the 1877 Salon by linking painters who portrayed famous modern men with the history painting traditions of Poussin and David.[9] By 1886, portraiture was the *genre du jour* at the Salon. Alfred de Lostalot testified to this new status in his review: 'For the time being, the portrait is the best France has to offer in painting, properly speaking … [P]ortrait painting holds a place in the Salon that one would look for in vain in the other genres.'[10] Portraiture, as primarily commissioned work, allowed artists to display the greatness of their sitters and their own talents, and provided them with relatively stable incomes.[11] That same year, Georges Lafenestre wrote in *Revue des deux mondes* that 'the portrait dominates in both quality and number'[12] and Louis Ganderax pointed out that the celebrity of the sitter – in this case, Pasteur – often overshadowed a painting's aesthetic worth.[13]

The attention granted to Pasteur during the 1886 Salon – in paint and in print – followed a year of debates on Pasteur's newest finding: in July 1885, he enjoyed great success – and subsequent controversy – for his discovery of a rabies vaccine. Word of the vaccine's triumph was made public in October, and over the coming months, newspapers and magazines reported on the increasing number of visitors swarming to Paris to get vaccinated. Two weeks before the opening of the Salon, close to 700 people had sought treatment.[14] Although rabies claimed about fifty lives per year, it was prominent in the public imagination because of its violent symptoms and fatal prognosis. As a disease that infected the central nervous system, rabies victims suffered pain, seizures, paralyses, and hallucinations. Rabies victims were thought to act like animals, violently thrashing about and biting at others.[15] The later stages of the infection often resulted in an inability to swallow and produced a fear of water; for this reason, the term hydrophobia often stood for rabies in contemporary accounts.

The 1886 Salon portraits were the first paintings of Pasteur exhibited after his monumental discovery. More than mere likenesses, these images symbolised an aggregate of modern scientific ideas: the rising social, economic, and cultural status of scientific men; the integration of laboratory science into medical practice; the safety and danger of scientific discovery involving humans; and science's crucial role in France's industrial progress and colonial expansion. Furthermore, the portraits show the multiple layers of Pasteur's public persona, particularly how his identity as a civilised Frenchman was at odds with his extreme professional ambition, ailing health, and association with experimental laboratory science. Pasteur's identity as a modern hero, whose vaccination could ensure the regeneration of a refined French public and protect humanity from a deadly virus, was threatened by his persona as a ruthless scientist who fought for patriotic honour and professional grandeur in a dog-eat-dog world.

Albert Edelfelt: a young Scandinavian in Paris

In April 1885, Edelfelt wrote to his mother, outlining his plans for Pasteur's portrait:

> Next Monday, I shall pay another call on M. Pasteur to see whether there is any possibility of painting his portrait in his laboratory, because it is there alone, in that environment, that I wish to paint him … He must be in his element: his spectacles on his nose, his skullcap on his head, and his microscope before him.[16]

Edelfelt disliked the 'ridiculousness' of official portraits that removed a modern man from his environment. This view was shared by other contemporary

French advocates of modern painting, most famously Edmond Duranty, who stressed in 1876 that a description of the sitter's environment was essential for portraying the essence of the individual.[17] These ideas were echoed a decade later in Salon reviews, when Olmer pleaded for the sitter's everyday surroundings to be the key to his identity:

> The truth! Today we want the whole truth. It must be shown, it must speak ... We expect that the painter will venture into the sitter's home, that he will acquaint himself with not only the figure he must paint, but also the individual's natural milieu. The portrait is developed, embracing both the man and his life. It requires, as props, the instruments of the sitter's glory and fortune or, at the very least, familiar pieces of furniture that reveal the customs of the person represented, his favourite objects that, through cherished routine, have become integral parts of his being.[18]

It was well known that mid-nineteenth-century vanguard painters, such as Manet, portrayed modern identities through an emphasis on surface detail.[19] Manet's much discussed 1868 portrait of Émile Zola evinces the identities of both writer and artist through surrounding objects: a Japanese print, an inkwell, a copy of Manet's *Olympia* and Zola's written defence of the scandalous work. Edelfelt saw the painting of Zola at an exhibition in 1883 and similarly portrayed Pasteur at work, surrounded by the accoutrements of his profession.[20] The scientific props depicted reflect those of earlier portraits of scientists and medical men. For instance, in Joshua Reynolds's 1788 rendering of pioneering surgeon John Hunter, books and anatomical models indicate scholarly pursuits (Figure 9). Still, Edelfelt's portrait differs from older models: Pasteur is depicted working in a modern laboratory rather than posing as a learned man.[21] Edelfelt hoped to rid the painting of artifice by not showing Pasteur posing in official dress, yet Pasteur is nonetheless in the pose of being 'un-posed'. The canvas is almost entirely given over to the energetic tension of his leaning body, his gaze fixed on his experiment in the quest for knowledge. Focused and mentally engaged, Pasteur epitomises intellectual authority and strength.

As a young artist who had come to Paris to study under Jean-Léon Gérôme, Edelfelt became a friend of Pasteur's son, Jean-Baptiste, an aspiring writer and art critic. He made multiple portraits of the Pasteur family, beginning with a portrait of Jean-Baptiste commissioned by his father in 1881. In 1885, Edelfelt asked Louis Pasteur if he could paint his portrait. Pasteur was very willing and the portrait was completed between April and June 1885. Pasteur sat for Edelfelt many times and offered advice. The artist wrote to his mother that 'He was very kind, and he promised me that as a sitter he would not disappoint me. Moreover, he is interested in painting, because at the age of sixteen he absolutely wanted to become a painter, and he thus devoted several summers to that noble art.'[22]

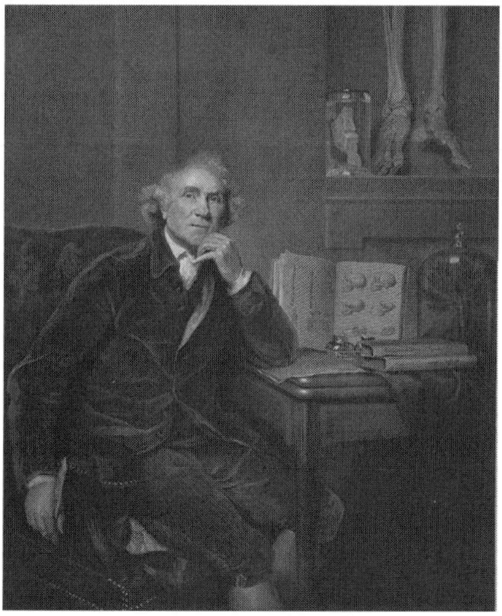

William Sharp after Sir Joshua Reynolds' painting of 1786, *John Hunter* (1788), line engraving, 51 x 38.3cm. 9

Pasteur's familiarity with the arts and previous ambition to become a painter contributed to his opinions about artworks. Letters from a teenage Pasteur to his parents describe portraits he had composed of family members, friends, and teachers – primarily conventional head-and-shoulder compositions against coloured backgrounds. Although Pasteur stopped producing art when he moved to Paris in 1842, many of his pastels hung in his residence (Figure 10).[23] Various nineteenth-century sources demonstrate that these early artworks were no secret from the general public. Art critic Durand-Gréville wrote of a portrait that Pasteur made of his friend Marcou: 'Many of our decorated painters at the Salon have never drawn or modelled a mouth with such accuracy. No one regretted that Pasteur had chosen a career in science. But had he wished, he could have been important among painters.'[24] The *Album Gonnon – iconographie médicale, 1895–1908*, one of the first books to address nineteenth-century medical collections and iconography, also discussed Pasteur's artistic talent.[25] This text explores Pasteur's artistic interests alongside those of Dr Paul Richer, a physician at the Hôpital de la Salpêtrière who later became the chair of anatomy at the École des Beaux-Arts, and Dr Jean-Martin Charcot, head of the Salpêtrière, to explain how men of science influenced artistic production. Napoleon III's appointment of Pasteur as the first professor of geology, physics, and applied chemistry at the École des Beaux-Arts (1863–67) signalled Pasteur's importance to the arts. Pasteur concentrated on finding the chemical compounds in paint to allow for conservation, believing this would preserve French art for future generations. His artistic interests are also apparent in his letters to his wife about visiting museums in Dresden, his friendships with contemporary artists and critics in Paris (including Paul Dubois, Jean-Jacques Henner, and Charles Blanc), and the active role he took in the production of portraits.[26]

Depicting the scientist in the laboratory was a crucial decision for both Pasteur and Edelfelt. It was the locus of Pasteur's discoveries and grandeur: a modern space *par excellence*.[27] Filled with new technologies and tools, its *raison d'être* was discovery. After the loss of the Franco-Prussian war (often attributed to France's inferior scientific position), France's future power and success was in question. Laboratories, as birthplaces of knowledge, promised to keep France a

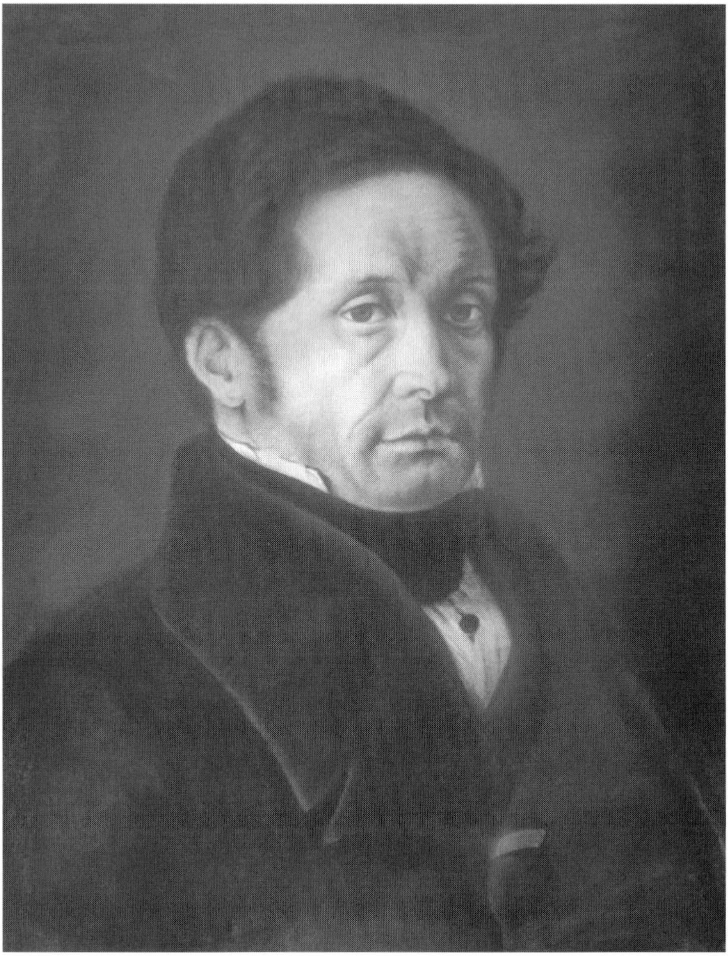

10 Louis Pasteur, *Portrait of M. Pasteur* (1842), pastel.

leading nation. This idea was propagated by Pasteur, who wrote in his speech for his 1892 Jubilee celebrations at the Sorbonne that students should 'live in the serene peace of laboratories and libraries'.[28] Laboratory work, however, needed to be shown as rational and compassionate; scientists could not appear to take too much pleasure in their work, especially in the case of Pasteur's studies, which involved animal experiments. For the most part, Pasteur's relationship with animals was visually documented as curative and humane despite the realities of laboratory experimentation and vivisection. A picture of Pasteur from *Vanity Fair* published in 1887 shows him as a calm and serious man, holding two pure white rabbits in his arms, his right hand stroking a furry back

(Figure 11). A cartoon titled 'The Angel of Innoculation' from 1886 also shows a healing Pasteur: he is a winged-figure hovering over an ugly rabid mutt, preparing to inject the dog with the restorative vaccine.

Edelfelt's portrait of Pasteur served as a record of the artist's time in the laboratory. It was a public announcement of his interactions with the famous scientist and a display of his skills as a painter. When Edelfelt wrote a letter about the portrait's exhibition at the Salon, claiming that '[i]n general, the best portraits are neither commissioned nor paid for, but are made for glory', it is likely that he was addressing both Pasteur's glory and his own.[29] Edelfelt presented himself as young and fashionable by painting Pasteur with identifiable realist tropes: intricate details, smooth brushstrokes, convincingly rendered daylight in a scientific setting, and a recognisable and physiognomically acurate portrayal of the celebrity chemist. By depicting Pasteur alone at work in his laboratory, Edelfelt produced an image that implied that he was privy to the secretive scientist and his experiments. The work also suggested that Edelfelt shared the same company as men like Pasteur and could therefore warrant commissions by prominent individuals and the state.

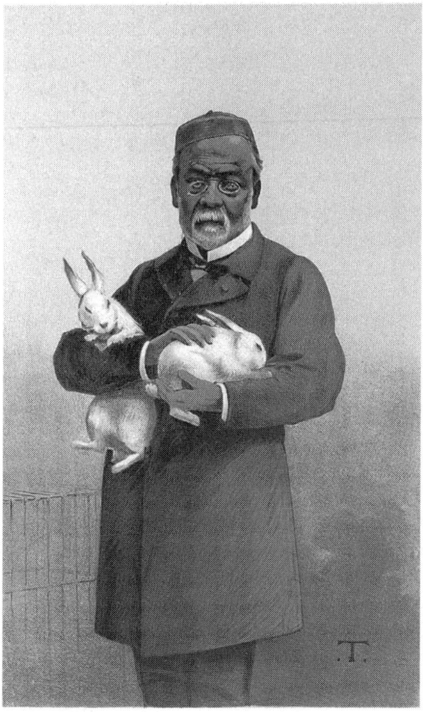

11 'Louis Pasteur', from *Vanity Fair*, 8 January 1887, colour lithograph.

Edelfelt first exhibited his portrait of Pasteur in Helsinki in the summer of 1885 at an exhibition organised for Tsar Alexandre III.[30] Significant social and artistic status was given to young Scandinavian artists who studied in France. 'We went to Paris, learned from the Frenchmen's advanced, logical reasoning; understood that we should stick to nature … With naturalism a national art must result', wrote Erik Werenskiold, a young Norwegian writer. 'If you are still in doubt, go to Paris and see! All French art is permeated with naturalism. You are surely familiar with such names as Corot, Millet, Courbet, Meisonnier and Bonnat?'[31] For Werenskiold, logic, progress, reason, and nationalism were intricately linked to lifelike representations of the visible world. Scandinavian artists were advised to follow the French example in order to produce a modern and nationalist art because they believed that the academies of their native countries were outdated. In turn, a motley mix of French artists, loosely linked by their realist styles, were admired, including the well-established Bonnat whom they regarded as a liberal and modern teacher.[32] Bonnat is often considered a representative of academic art and commercial success, particularly in twentieth-century art history, since he taught at the Académie, was elected to the Salon Jury in 1876, and sold his work for roughly ten times the price of the impressionists, but he also valued public opinion over that of the Académie and voted in support of Courbet at the 1868 Salon, and was praised as the greatest artist since Courbet by Zola in 1878. The inability to categorise Bonnat is evident in Zola's criticism: only a year later, Zola referred to Bonnat as Courbet's slave.[33] These events demonstrate the shifting definitions of realism at the time, as well as the multiple – and often contradictory – characteristics with which it was associated: it was used to describe Bonnat's relatively smooth and detailed paintings of republican leaders *and* Courbet's roughly worked portrayals of peasant life.

Léon Bonnat: portraitist of the Republic

Bonnat's status as a celebrity artist was mentioned in the 1889 book, *Artistes contemporains des pays de Guyenne, Béarn, Saintonge et Languedoc*:

> As you walk through the Salon on a crowded day, following the current where it leads you, that is, before the works that are in fashion, the 'winners', which everyone, from the most naïve of visitors to the most refined connoisseurs, wants to have seen, one of the first paintings toward which the tide will carry you is a portrait by Bonnat.
>
> You will see it, as soon as you enter the room where it hangs, above the swelling sea of heads and hats; you will distinguish some figure that is strongly drawn, solidly painted, with a relief that borders on trompe l'œil, and that, with its robust colours and powerful modelling, dwarfs everything around it. From no matter how far away you see it, and no matter how little you know about the style of the main contemporary artists, you will say without hesitation: 'It is a Bonnat!' And you will not be mistaken, for here the maker's mark leaps to the eye; the workman's signature is apparent in every brushstroke.[34]

The spectacle produced by 'a Bonnat' at the Salon was enhanced by a celebrity sitter. Bonnat had a long waiting list, particularly since his fame conferred status upon the person portrayed. 'Till they have seen themselves on Bonnat's canvas, statesmen doubt their popularity, authors question their genius, actresses tremble for their laurels, millionaires suspect their influence', stated an article in *The Illustrated American* in 1890. 'To have been painted by Bonnat is to have proved yourself somebody; to have had the seal set on your hard-won reputation; to have won, as it were, official recognition of your merit, your weight, your talent, your wealth.'[35]

As a principal portrait painter of the Republic and an ardent nationalist, Bonnat instilled his sitters with historical and national importance. His 1876 portrait of Adolphe Thiers, president of the Third Republic from 1870–73, brought Bonnat national fame. Bonnat's portraits of notable French men and women were very familiar to the public not only because of their display at the annual Salons, but because Bonnat sold the rights to reproduce these works to photographers, etchers, and lithographers.[36] Understandably, the young Edelfelt was nervous about his painting being exhibited at the same Salon as Bonnat's portrait. In a letter to his mother on 30 November 1885, he wrote that Bonnat would give Pasteur a 'proprietary air' and that he would paint 'a frock-coat much better than mine'.[37] Although Bonnat did not include his portrait of Pasteur in the Salon competition, claiming that it would be unfair since he was on the jury, his painting was nonetheless placed in a prominent position while Edelfelt's work was hung in the section for foreign painters.

Bonnat's portraits contributed to the history of France by serving as historical documents for future citizens. Bauzon claimed they were painted with 'the prose of history'.[38] To imbue his works with this power, Bonnat turned to Rembrandt's example. He wrote in his preface to Marcel Nicolle's *Rembrandt aux expositions d'Amsterdam et de Londres*, '[w]hat is striking with Rembrandt is his power, strength and vividness. He represents life, in all its intensity. We see his characters, we converse with them; he resuscitates and revives an entire epoch.'[39] For Bonnat, it was the 'science' of Rembrandt's portraits that could revitalise history. He used the word 'science' to indicate Rembrandt's knowledge of human anatomy ('Rembrandt already masters the science of portraiture. He knows the construction of the human head better than anyone.'), and aligned himself with this scientific approach to art by copying the Dutch master's famous anatomy lesson of Dr Tulp.[40] Léonce Bénédite, the curator at the Musée du Luxembourg during the late nineteenth and early twentieth centuries, also linked scientific and realist approaches. He declared that 'the realist movement is moving in a markedly more democratic and populist direction, following the march of political progress, and with an unprecedented quality of method and objectivity in observation that coincides with the intensive development of the scientific method.'[41] Both Bénédite and Bonnat praised art that followed what they saw as scientific principles and considered it necessary for the production of historically significant work. Realism was considered the best style for authentic representations of France's most important contemporary figures. For Bénédite, it was not only the agent that bound art and science together, but was also the style of democracy and modern French political progress.[42] Was there any other way to portray Pasteur?

Backdrops: debating the quintessential portrait of Pasteur

The majority of Salon criticism concentrated on debating the merits of Bonnat's and Edelfelt's paintings; their very different approaches guided the critics' responses. '[Edelfelt's] portrait is complete', wrote Olmer. 'It speaks about the man and his life's work, and it could easily be the definitive portrait of M. Pasteur.'[43] However, Louis Lafenestre dismissed the painting: 'M. Bonnat's portrait is the historical image; M. Edelfelt's is nothing but an anecdotal image.'[44] The proper way to paint a scientific hero was contested. Lostalot praised the many details of Edelfelt's painting, which inspired meticulous explanations:

> M. Edelfelt's painting shows us M. Pasteur absorbed in his research. His head bowed, he scrutinises a glass bottle in which is suspended a strip of bloody flesh: it is the fearsome spinal cord of a rabid rabbit, which, through the effort of Pasteur's genius, will be converted into a balm that will heal the most horrible of ills. The painting is excellent and exceptionally interesting; the light plays freely over the laboratory equipment, yet no detail detracts from the grandeur of the subject matter.[45]

Ganderax, too, focused on the particularities of modern life, linking contemporary portraiture to the flourishing realist novel.[46] For him, literary realism was considered the perfect model for portraiture; like the novel, it could record contemporary man's interactions with the world. Realism's claim to truth also made it the perfect style for portraying scientific men. As Eugène-Melchior de Vogüé suggested in his 1886 article in *Revue des deux mondes*, the popularity of realism in both genres 'has led to an art more of observation than of imagination', that is, 'Jealous of the rigour of scientific procedures'.[47] In May 1886, *L'art moderne* pushed a similar view when it republished Arthur Stevens's 1868 article 'De la modernité dans l'art': 'To paint a portrait, the artist sums up everything he has contemplated in his life; he puts into play all his knowledge in order to bring the model to life. He is ill at ease with invention or trickery.'[48]

For Lafenestre, the critical success of a portrait at the Salon was guaranteed by the artist's judicious selection of details ('it can be unseemly to submerge this physiognomy under a mass of details that are accurate yet utterly insignificant').[49] He criticised Edelfelt's naturalism for going too far:

> the furnishings speak louder than the figure; the thinker's physiognomy vanishes amidst the sparkling glassware, and despite the 'curiosity appeal' that posterity will certainly attach to the minute and ingenious reportage of the Swedish painter, it is not from him that posterity will ask the definitive image of M. Pasteur.[50]

In Lafenestre's opinion, Bonnat's work, which contained only those elements of the visible world that contributed favourably to the identity of the sitter was the quintessential image of Pasteur.

The ambiguous space of Bonnat's background contrasts with the depth and detail of the laboratory scenes painted by Edelfelt and Gsell. Bonnat's work is relatively devoid of narrative setting: Pasteur and his granddaughter are lit by light and colour, but stand against a painterly backdrop of black, beiges, and reddish-browns. Bonnat rarely portrayed his sitters' homes, possessions, or professions, but his portraits were understood as modern because his figures' gestures were thought to reveal contemporary character.[51] He believed it was difficult to make a portrait that could provide both an accurate representation of a sitter's body and a faithful sense of personality without recourse to scientific methods. Bonnat wrote that 'A work of art and a theory based on experimental research have in common the fact that they both propose a kind of agreement reached between intelligence and nature after bitter combat … ', but he then pointed out that such '[a] manner of truce that will only with difficulty find acceptance within public opinion, especially when the artist takes on the mysteries of human nature with the aim of reproducing both the individual's physical likeness and, at the same time, that within him which is least inconstant and most invisible.'[52] For Bonnat, capturing invisible character and physical likeness were paramount to a successful portrait.

Lafenestre preferred the formal simplicity of Bonnat's more monumental portrait to Edelfelt's laboratory scene:

> The scientist is depicted in isolation so that we can see him better, like a statue on its pedestal. His face, whose brightness above his dark clothing alone commands our gaze, stands out, with an energetic precision, like a crudely struck medallion against a nondescript background, with a power of intellectual expression that is all the greater because there is nothing close by to attenuate it … We may be justified in thinking that whenever there is a face in which intelligence above all, should speak, it is best not to smother this expression of the soul beneath the confused rustling of the murmur of things.[53]

Bonnat's portrait of Pasteur, like the sculptures of prominent Frenchmen exhibited in the public spaces of Paris, became an indicator of status, identity, and professional gain through its simple formal economy of means. And the Salon, like civic squares and academic courtyards, became a venue for the exhibition of prominent male bodies for public pleasure.

Although many critics praised Bonnat's portrait, the artist's detailed depictions, and solid backgrounds, which he used consistently in his work, were also criticised. Bonnat's compositional focus on his sitters and relatively blank backgrounds led many to describe his portraits as dull and photographic.[54] J. Meriem wrote in 1882 that Bonnat's work had 'a cold and photographic precision'.[55] The dullness of Bonnat's portrait of Pasteur was also noted in the 1886 Salon criticism. C. de Beaulieu claimed that 'we can only repeat our admiration of the master's painting whilst begging him to change the backdrops',[56] and Henry Fèvre asserted that '[a]s a portraitist, M. Bonnat is but a passable colourer of deceptive photographs'.[57] Charles Ponsonailhe disparaged the work for its similarities to photographic portraiture in *L'Artiste*, writing that '[t]he illustrious scientist is standing in that stiff pose of a photographer's victim, with one of those copper apparatuses called "a sustainer" that one finds in the photographer's studio stuck down his back'.[58] Bonnat's painting, with its solid background and highlighted figure, is similar to many photographic portraits, including those that Félix Nadar took of professional men, in which they are photographed against a plain backdrop and lit by focused light. However, Bonnat's portrait of Pasteur also counters the populist photographic conventions of the 1880s, since Pasteur is posed in a non-specific space with his granddaughter as his only prop.

By the late nineteenth century, most photographic portraits had appropriated conventions of painted portraiture, particularly the practice of surrounding sitters with objects related to their occupation or social status: ornate materials, classical pillars, and well-stocked bookshelves were all used as a means to construct identity. As more photographic studios opened in Paris and as the cost of portraiture decreased, the public could afford to be photographed in the fancy costumes and elaborate scenes provided by studios. The ease and accessibility of being portrayed above one's station not only contributed to the general belief that portraiture had become the bourgeois genre *par excellence*, but it also decreased its social value, since the objects traditionally associated with nobility were accessible to the masses. Photographic portraiture allowed for the staging of identity and status – it was a performance involving costumes, props, and backdrops. The displayed identity was the product of the photograph.

The similarities between Bonnat's portrait and photography had negative connotations (it was seen as uninspiring, bourgeois, and commercial) that drew parallels to photography's assumed mechanical objectivity. Like a camera, technical and seemingly detached from subjectivity, the artist's painterly skill stood in as a form of mechanical truth. Bonnat measured his sitter's faces before painting them, which aligned the painter with scientific professionals, as phrenologists performed similar tasks. This type of measurement was considered more scientific than artistic, and more objective than subjective, since conventional artistic training promoted the rendering of human proportions based on idealisation rather than individual measurement.

The painting's resemblance to photography connected it to professional photographic portraits of scientific men that illustrated newspaper articles and biographies of French scientific heroes. Reproductions of these photographs were often distributed to friends and family, particularly after the subject's death, and were collected by the public as *cartes de visites*. These portraits were both products and producers of the professionalisation of science and the popular understanding of scientists as celebrities. Pasteur sat for many portraits during his career, most of which were head-and-shoulders shots that showed him seated against a plain backdrop. Pierre Petit took one of the earliest photographs of Pasteur, and the photographer was frequently employed by the chemist for personal and scientific work (Figure 12). In a photograph from the early 1860s, a middle-aged, dark-haired Pasteur leans back in a chair. Dressed in a black wool suit with the chain of his pocket watch visible under his jacket, Pasteur's relaxed posture contradicts the formality of his attire, the rigidity of his closely cropped hair and the seriousness of his steadfast gaze. The young Pasteur exudes confidence and authority. This portrait contrasts with those taken of a mature Pasteur at the height of his scientific reign, particularly those taken by Nadar in 1878.

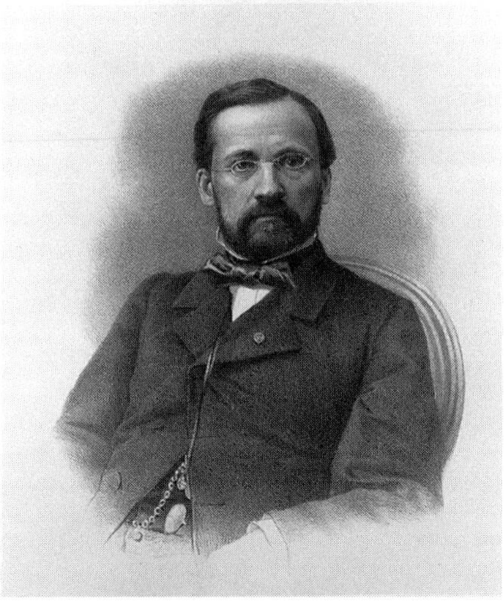

Pierre Petit, *Pasteur* (early 1860s), lithograph on paper. 12

Nadar, a well-known portraitist who photographed the prominent men of France from the mid-century on, had a personal connection to Pasteur through Dr Jacques-Joseph Grancher, Pasteur's neighbour and the first person to inoculate a human patient with the rabies vaccine (Pasteur, a chemist, was not legally qualified to give shots). Nadar took two portraits of Pasteur in 1878. In the first, taken against a plain backdrop from the mid-chest up, a bearded, grey-haired Pasteur stares out at the viewer (Figure 13). He is dressed in a suit, his Légion d'honneur pin aligns with the buttons on his jacket, and a thin chain that runs around his neck and down his chest leads to eyeglasses just outside the frame. The second shows the scientist in profile (Figure 14). Curiously, the two photographs, particularly when examined together, resemble nineteenth-century mug shots. Like institutionally produced photographs of criminals and patients, the up-close and meticulously detailed pictures of Pasteur's face demand a physiognomic reading. Everything is visible: the individual white strands that pepper his hair, the drooping bags under his eyes, the crooked fold of his ear and its fleshy lobe, the slant of his nose, the pattern of wrinkles around his eyes, and the deep line that weaves from his nostril across his cheek only to be lost in a prickly beard.

In fact, many of Nadar's portraits display similarities to the photographs of patients and criminals from nineteenth-century hospitals and police stations, particularly those catalogued by Alphonse Bertillon (Figure 15). These visual parallels show the link between photographic portraiture and science, and between portraiture and art. In his well-known study, Alan Sekula argues that photographic portraiture was a double system of representation that functioned both 'honourifically' and 'repressively': it extended and popularised the

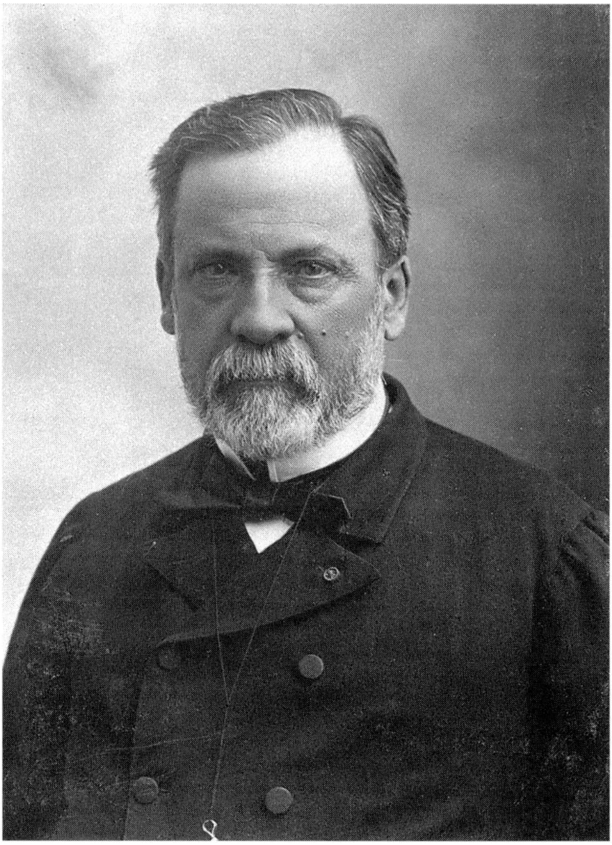

13 Félix Nadar, *Portrait of Louis Pasteur* (c.1878), photograph.

traditional function of portraiture while the medium of photography simultaneously undermined the status inherent to the genre.[59] He claims that the joining of photography with the study of phrenology in 1846 created an archive in which the criminal body was produced in its opposing relationship to the law-abiding bourgeois body. With the emergence of the mug shot and the creation and collection of photographs of criminals by the police in Paris in the 1880s, photographic portraiture became as associated with social deviance, crime, and illness as with heroic healthy bodies.[60] There is no doubt that Nadar's photograph of Pasteur is a portrait rather than a mug shot: the chemist's Légion d'honneur pin, despite being out of focus, indicates his standing as an honourable French citizen. Furthermore, the photograph was taken by Nadar, who was as much a celebrity as those he captured. His signature guarantees its status as a portrait.

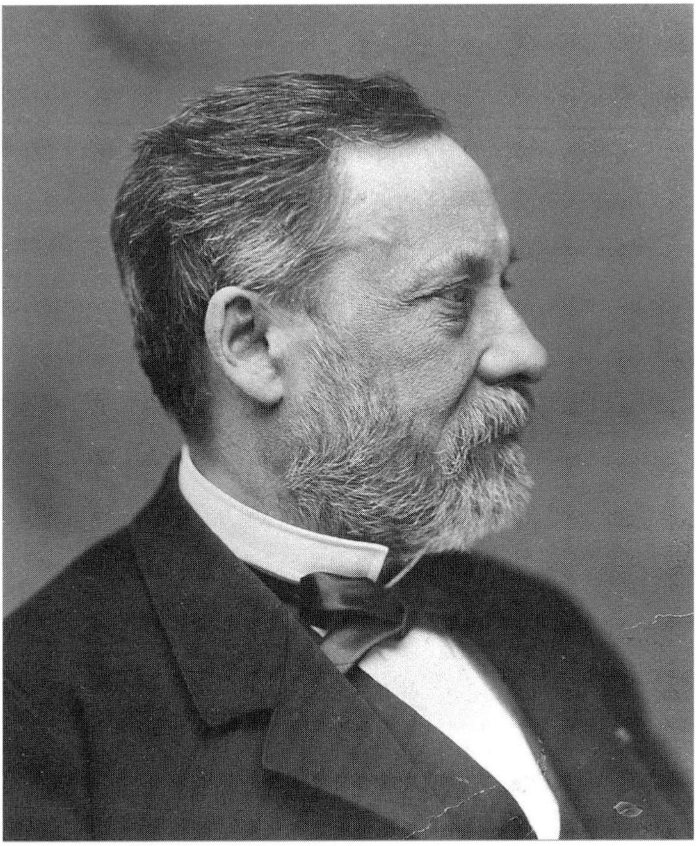

Félix Nadar, *Portrait of Louis Pasteur* (c.1878), photograph. 14

Yet, the visual emphasis on minute bodily detail – accentuated by the simple dark backdrop and highlighted face – invites a physiognomic gaze.

Pasteur's body: ageing, illness, and vision

The representation of celebrities in the press and at the Salon encouraged the public's desire to see and examine famous bodies. Both Edelfelt and Bonnat's portraits of Pasteur provided Salon viewers with convincing images to be studied and scrutinised. The assumed visual accuracy of such portraits armed the public with the ability to inspect every inch of the body portrayed. As was often expressed in medical, pseudo-scientific, and popular texts in the nineteenth century, the study of the body's exterior was considered essential to understanding its interior. The French fascination with classifying bodies based on visual observation evolved from Johan Caspar Lavater's publications

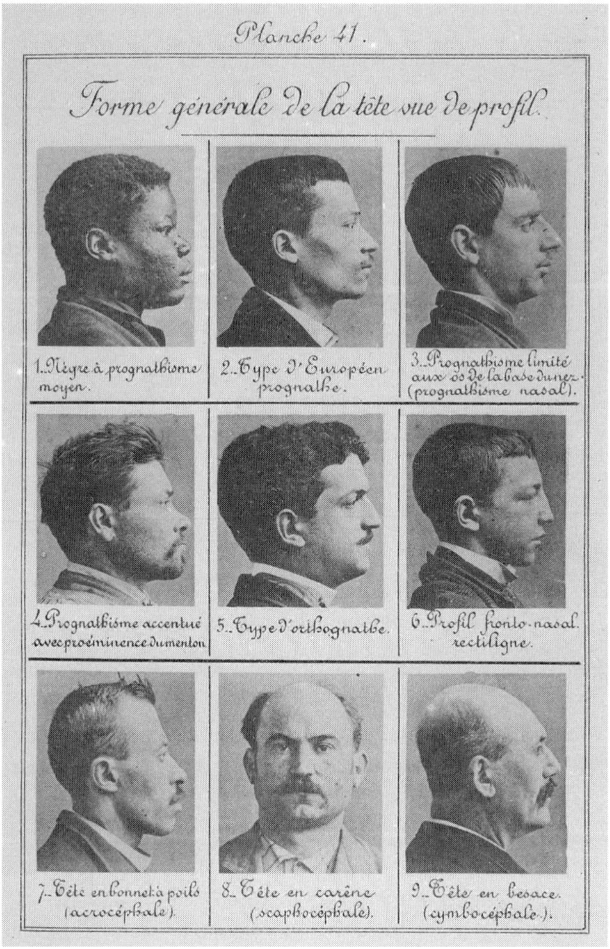

15 Alphonse Bertillon, 'Forme générale de la tête vue de profil' (1893), Bertillon system card.

on physiognomies from the late eighteenth century, and from the considerably augmented French version edited, and in parts authored, by Jacques-Louis Moreau de la Sarthe (translated and first published between 1806 and 1809).[61] By 1831, a phrenology society had been founded in Paris and included established leaders from medicine, law, and philosophy (such as the renowned doctors Casimir Broussais and Philippe Pinel). The publication of Cesare Lombroso Ferrero's *L'uomo delinquente* in 1876, as well as Valentin Magnan and Bertillon's analyses of the relationship between phrenology and criminology, 'confirmed' the belief that intellectual and moral inferiority and superiority could be anatomically explained and justified: exterior physical characteristics were regarded as symbolic of interior states well into the final decades of the century. 'It is science that has as its goal the knowledge of the internal nature of man through knowledge of man's external nature', declared Julien Leclercq in his popular 1896 book, *La Physionomie, visages et caractères*. 'It is science which aims to know man's interior nature through his exterior nature ... No one "masks" himself, no one can take on faculties that he does not possess ... The physiognomy of man does not lie.'[62] The public could take pleasure in Leclercq's pseudo-scientific approach through physiognomic readings of French celebrities. Mixing physiognomy with astrology, the author claimed that Pasteur was a good father, gentle husband, and focused learner. Leclercq's book was typical of those published in the 1890s. As the French literary scholar, Elizabeth Emery shows, these books transformed readers into 'armchair scientists' who could discover the actual identities of celebrities by studying their faces, bodily proportions, signatures, and fingertips.[63] Like these books, the 1886 Salon criticism concentrated on the representation of Pasteur's body since critics believed his painted exterior reflected his inner character.

Salon critics had difficulty coming to terms with how Pasteur should be portrayed. They took distinct positions on Bonnat's and Edelfelt's portraits because they did not see how Pasteur could be justly represented as both a heroic scientist in his laboratory and as an adoring and ageing family man. Although a few condemned Edelfelt's painting for its excessive detail, no one criticised the depiction of Pasteur in a laboratory. In contrast, some critics had a problem with Bonnat's painting because Pasteur was portrayed as a grandfather rather than a scientist. By showing Pasteur's private face in public, Bonnat's painting did not sit comfortably in the heroic republican iconography of the early Third Republic. Perhaps the representation of Pasteur's ageing body contradicted Bonnat's particular realist style, which was frequently described as strong, healthy, masculine, and direct – all characteristics the Republic deemed valuable.[64] Although Bonnat's Pasteur has all the accoutrements of modern male respectability, the addition of his granddaughter appears to have threatened his virility.

The inclusion of Camille altered the traditional single portrait into a painting that displayed a familial bond. Pasteur's role as a family man was often discussed in newspapers, magazines, and books, and was shown in published photographs of the chemist with his grandchildren, children, and wife. In a four-page article for *Revue encyclopédique*, Gsell's brother Paul provides a full account of Pasteur's family: 'The great man has always been an excellent father to his children; his friends remember seeing him bounce a baby on his knees while his wife was undressing another child to put him to bed.'[65] The article was illustrated with family photographs and two pictures of the chemist's childhood homes. American critic, William Walton, proposed that unlike Edelfelt who had 'taken the trouble to paint his sitter in his laboratory, surrounded by the instruments of his researches', Bonnat 'possibly scorning such aids – had chosen to represent the domestic side of the man of science and introduced the little granddaughter to touch our affections.'[66] Although it is possible that Bonnat saw Edelfelt's painting before he began his own, it is unreasonable to suggest that Bonnat would have painted Pasteur in his laboratory, as it was not Bonnat's practice to paint his sitters in elaborate work settings. Furthermore, the decision to include the granddaughter was likely made by J.C. Jacobsen, who commissioned the portrait and followed the wishes of Pasteur's wife, Marie Anne Laurent Pasteur. Critics did not note Mme Pasteur's involvement in the painting, thus attacks on this grandfatherly portrayal were directed at Bonnat. As Olmer wrote, the portrait 'shows us the great scientist in his guise as a loving family man, a doting daddy who is happy to show off his granddaughter. It is also a glory to have beautiful grandchildren; but perhaps it is shared too widely here, and it is not in this guise that posterity will remember the man who lent his name to the cure for rabies.'[67]

Despite the cultural respect given to grandfathers as family leaders – particularly at a time when people feared depopulation and believed children were key to France's future – they also symbolised ageing and inevitably, death.[68] The figure of the grandfather simultaneously exemplified the strength and vulnerability of masculinity: he was the ultimate symbol of wisdom and family dominance (as exemplified by Victor Hugo and the popularity of his 1877 book of poems *L'Art d'être grand-père*), yet his power was threatened by time and bodily deterioration. Significantly, Bonnat painted Hugo's portrait in 1879 and showed him as a focused man, dressed in a black suit, sitting with splayed legs and an inquisitive stare. Like Pasteur, Hugo's hand is tucked into his jacket in a Napoleonic gesture, yet there is no indication of Hugo's role as the sole guardian of his two young grandchildren.

Henry Fèvre questioned Bonnat's rendering of Pasteur in comparison to Edelfelt's:

> M. Bonnat has painted a theatrical Pasteur, his hand on his granddaughter's head, a Pasteur that does not even look like himself … [h]is skin looks oily, and one fears he may have jaundice … M. Pasteur does not possess at all the fatal, pontificating air of a Don Quixote of microbes upon which M. Bonnat has impaled him … M. A. Edelfelt has certainly improved upon M. Bonnat in his own painting of the celebrated vanquisher of rabies. His Pasteur is more good-natured, more detailed, more lively, in his laboratory, sniffing vials, in the midst of scientific investigation; his head stands out as energetically as in the other painting but without the falseness of the shadow or the ridiculous sickly complexion.[69]

For Févre, Bonnat's colour choices left Pasteur appearing yellowed and ill. Perhaps Févre thought that Bonnat's painting Pasteur as a sick man showed a private side of Pasteur that was often denied to the public. Pasteur's health had always been fragile. He had his first stroke, or cerebral haemorrhage, at the age of forty-five, which permanently impaired his speech, gait, and manual dexterity. As a personal friend of Pasteur and his family, Bonnat must have been aware of the scientist's physical ailments. Gerald L. Geison, medical historian and Pasteur specialist, claims that Pasteur's visible age and illness contributed to his public support, since he was seen as a sympathetic man rather than an elitist professional. Geison supports his argument by referencing a contemporary description of Pasteur that emphasises his white hair, wrinkled skin 'seared with the signs of genius' and a mouth affected by paralysis but 'full of kindness'.[70] Although Geison provides textual examples to show how the scientist's ageing and sick body figured Pasteur as a saintly humanitarian, the Salon reviews show that visible representations of a sick Pasteur were not welcome in 1886.

The sickly look described by some Salon critics was attributed to Bonnat's palette; the painting's colours did not create a sense of warmth and robust health. 'If M. Bonnat were to modify his colours – which are dry, dark, perpetually congealed in the sauce whose recipe he proudly transmits to the assistant cooks who are struggling to attain the genius of the head chef – there would no doubt be talk', wrote the the critic of *L'Art moderne*.[71] There is a sense of eerie distance between Pasteur and his granddaughter; they are unsmiling, serious, stiff, and formally dressed. They gaze out at the viewer, their relationship to one another only revealed by the grip of the young girl's white fingers around her grandfather's swollen, purple-ish thumb, by the weight of her small body pressed against his dark uniform, and by his hand resting on her shoulder. The darkness of the background and Pasteur's attire juxtapose the pallor of their skin. Pasteur's solid clothed body makes his flesh appear ephemeral and transparent. One journalist described Pasteur in this painting as 'a bit like a bogeyman'.[72] Paul Lambert was appalled by Bonnat's colours, particularly those used for the granddaughter's skin: 'The poor young girl's face and hands are stained with tobacco juice. Tender colours of childhood!'[73] That the child's depiction was odd was noted in *Journal des arts*: 'There is nothing really childlike about the little girl and the tones of her face have the same harsh accents as her grandfather's face'.[74] Descriptions of the girl's stained and dirty skin seem more appropriate for a picture of a poor child rather than an upper-class girl. Still, she is the most colourful and decorative part of the canvas. In contrast to Pasteur's black suit, which was the universal uniform of the professional elite, Camille's unique attire exhibits social status. The gentle creases of her shiny light blue blouse, the minute lace details of her sleeves, the tiny white flowers that cover her cream skirt, her neatly parted blonde hair and the tiny gold ring on her right hand symbolise the wealth and order of the Pasteur family.

Bonnat's Pasteur does not have an engaging gaze: he is looking to the side. The heavy bags under his eyes make him look tired and worn. In contrast, Camille is attentive and questioning. Despite the frivolity of her puffy dress and the frailty of her fingers and wrists, two large eyes emerge from the shadows of her brow, fixed upon the viewer. Her stare empowers her with an authority that is lacking in this representation of Pasteur. While her body is small, particularly in comparison to her grandfather's, she nonetheless appears to be sheltering the scientist, perhaps, even, as Lambert proposed, leading him. Lambert criticised Bonnat for portraying Pasteur as a blind old man: 'This portrait, which at first glance, looks like a representation of a blind man led by a young girl, is definitely one of the weakest at the Salon'.[75] Pasteur's blindness was further emphasised many pages later when Lambert compared it to M. Landelle's painting *L'Aveugle*.[76] Without the tools of his discoveries and outside of his workspace, Pasteur's body could not easily display the ideal masculinity required of a national hero and man of science. Rather than contributing to Pasteur's grandeur, the inclusion of Camille made the scientist appear vulnerable and weak.

Describing Pasteur as blind underscored the importance of vision in modern science. On the one hand, it revealed the shortcomings of the human body in the face of new optical equipment. On the other, scientific discourse on vision stressed that an expert eye was needed to see, comprehend, and explain the abstracted forms that emerged under a microscope and existed within glass vials.[77] Pasteur's ability to understand how 'invisible' microorganisms function – and his identity as a scientific visionary – is staged in Edelfelt's portrait: only Pasteur sees the curative potential of rabid rabbit spines. New scientific thinking, such as the belief in germ theory, attempted to prove that the invisible existed through laboratory experimentation and clinical practice rather than through visibility alone. Despite technological advancements in vision apparatuses and scientific theories that opened the body and the world to new forms of enquiry, the majority of pseudo-scientific and pseudo-medical discourse remained focused on the body's exterior and stressed what was visible to the unaided eye, since this approach was accessible to those without scientific training or equipment. The ability to see the invisible – to understand microscopic organisms and images – was essential to Pasteur's earlier successes and to his scientific identity.[78] The rabies virus was not discovered until after Pasteur's death, despite Pasteur's and his assistants' efforts to isolate it. Pasteur's early work, particularly on fermentation and anthrax, supported and propagated germ theory. Although John Waller argues that Pasteur's contribution was the product of international scientific debates, the chemist was regarded as the discoverer of germ theory in the French popular imagination.[79] This identity was portrayed and disseminated in visual culture.

Making history in the laboratory: photography and male bonding

Pasteur, like many other men of science, utilised the technological advances and scientific uses of photography. The imaging techniques used at the Pasteur Institute were influenced by the work of pioneering microbiologist, Dr Robert Koch, who introduced microphotography to the study of bacteria. Pasteur began publishing and using photomicrographies in the 1870s. Like the microscope, it was used in scientific pursuits to perform feats impossible for the human eye.[80] Photography appeared to fix this microscopic world into static images: they were both modern scientific apparatuses of sight.[81] In his 1896 thesis, 'Applications de la photographie à la médecine', A. Burais dedicated a few pages to the use of photography at the Pasteur Institute.[82] He argued that photography could improve knowledge because it offered details that went unnoticed by the untrained eye and the microscope. He quoted Dr Emile Roux, Pasteur's chief laboratory assistant (and later rival) to make his point: 'In Microbiology, the best way to write is to put a short text next to a large number of well-executed plates'.[83] Roux's statement emphasises the importance of the visual in scientific study. Text was time-consuming to write, read, and absorb. Unlike photography, it was generally understood as a more subjective record of the writer's experience. However, scientific images were not always legible and needed to be 'translated' by experts through exacting text.

Pasteur's personal and professional use of photography served multiple purposes. It advanced his studies, since photography provided static microscopic images of otherwise invisible organisms that could be referred to at will. It also popularised and spread his discoveries internationally: his photographs of germs and diseases were published in scientific journals, including those produced at the Pasteur Institute (which was founded in June 1887 and inaugurated in November 1888). These photographs presented visible proof of his scientific theories, as well as connected him to technological advances. The building of a photographic studio at the Pasteur Institute contributed to the modernity of science, Pasteur, and his institute. It also located the production and advancements of photography in the scientific realm, as photographic studios were built in the most prominent medical centres in Paris: the Salpêtrière and Hôpital Saint-Louis.

Pasteur had a personal interest in photography that went beyond the representation of microbes. He had specific views on photographic portraiture and how men of science should be portrayed. In October 1881, he thanked Mme Saint-Claire Deville for sending him a photograph of her late husband (Figure 16):

> Dear Madame,
>
> I was very pleased to receive the portrait of my dear friend. My God! Such a likeness! How happy you must be to look at it and thereby read into his soul. I know

> of three admirable photographs: that of M. V. Regnault, that of M. Brongniart, and this one. But this one is even more beautiful and more lifelike than the other two. You would make me most happy, Madame, if you would send me the name of the photographer. Is he always just as inspired? I should like to leave my family something similar when the day comes for me to bid them the last farewell. Infinite thanks, dear Madame, for your gracious memento.
>
> L. Pasteur.[84]

Pasteur praised the portrait for its truthful depiction, pointing out its faithful resemblance. For him, the photograph appeared to replace the body of his close ally, allowing the surviving friends and family constant access to the dead through photographic representation.[85]

Pasteur compared the photograph of Deville with those he owned of other deceased men of science, Henri-Victor Regnault (1810–78) and Adolphe-Théodore Brongniart (1801–76). Regnault, a member of the Académie de sciences, was a physician and chemist at the Collège de France, and was involved in new photographic developments.[86] Brongniart was a professor of botany and physiology who had been president of the Académie de sciences in 1847. Like Regnault and Brongniart, Deville was a scientist, having earned degrees in both science and medicine. The portraits of Regnault and Deville are very similar. Both men are shown dressed in suits and bow ties, sitting on chairs near desks covered with papers, their jackets unbuttoned and legs loosely crossed at the ankle. Each is depicted with one elbow propped up on a table, his head resting on a fist. In her discussion of the pictorial conventions used in portraits of scientists, Ludmilla Jordanova points out how the 'head-on-hand' pose commonly represented learned men. By drawing on portraits from various historical periods, including Robert Walker's portrait of John Evelyn (1648), Mary and Thomas Black's *Messenger Monsey* (1764), and Albrecht Dürer's *Melancholia* (1514), Jordanova claims that this pose, along with the depiction of study-like spaces, books, and the figure in isolation, were conventions employed to construct men of science as pensive and highly educated.[87] For Pasteur, the professionally staged photographic portraits of friends were personal mementoes, material evidence of close friendships and professional alliances among men. His desire to be photographed in the same way shows how portraiture, as a genre, fluctuated between fulfilling personal and professional desires. It also evinces a shared vision of masculinity held and produced by the scientific elite. As is evident in the letter to Mme Deville, Pasteur wished to be photographed in the same way as her husband: dressed in a suit, alone in his workplace, deep in thought, head propped on hand.

Although we do not know if Pasteur was given the name of Deville's photographer, Pasteur was in fact photographed in a similar pose by the photographic studio Dornac et Cie in the late 1880s for the popular series *Nos Contemporains chez eux* (Figure 17).[88] In this portrait, the scientist is shown in his *cabinet de*

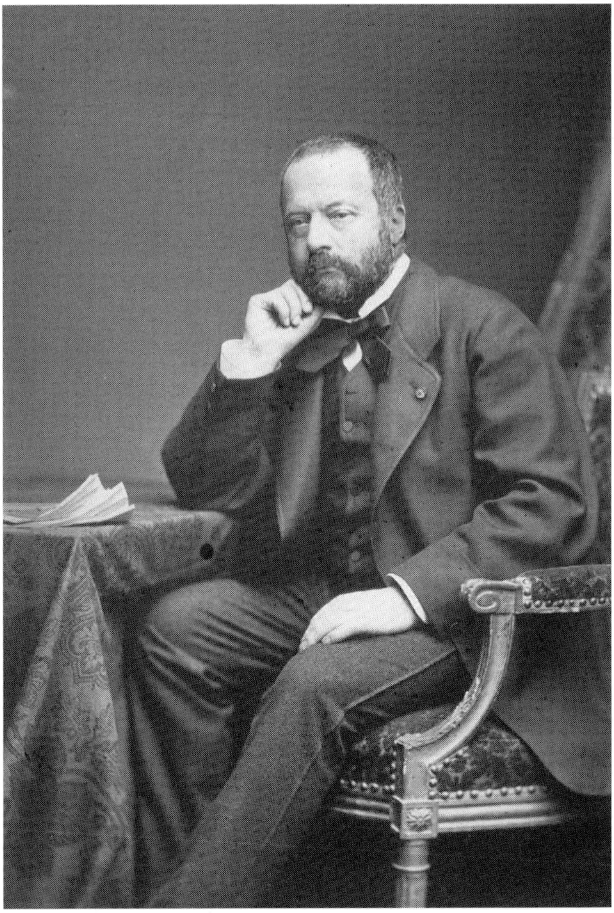

Pasteur's photograph of Henri de Sainte Claire Deville (c.1860–65), photograph. 16

travail, staring out at the viewer, seated near a desk with his ear cradled by his hand. Like Regnault and Deville, he is portrayed as a solitary and serious man, deep in thought. However, this photograph was part of a series that documented the private side of famous people in their homes or workplaces and promised readers insight into their 'real' character. The milieu and objects that surrounded celebrities were as crucial to the sitters' identities in photography as in painted portraiture. Many of these pictures were sold as individual photographs for collecting, and were reproduced in newspapers. Gaston Tissandier published four articles in *La Nature* that focused on the collection's 'scientific' approach. In 1892, he analysed Dornac's portrait of Pasteur, drawing a direct correlation between the objects surrounding Pasteur and the chemist's identity as a *grand*

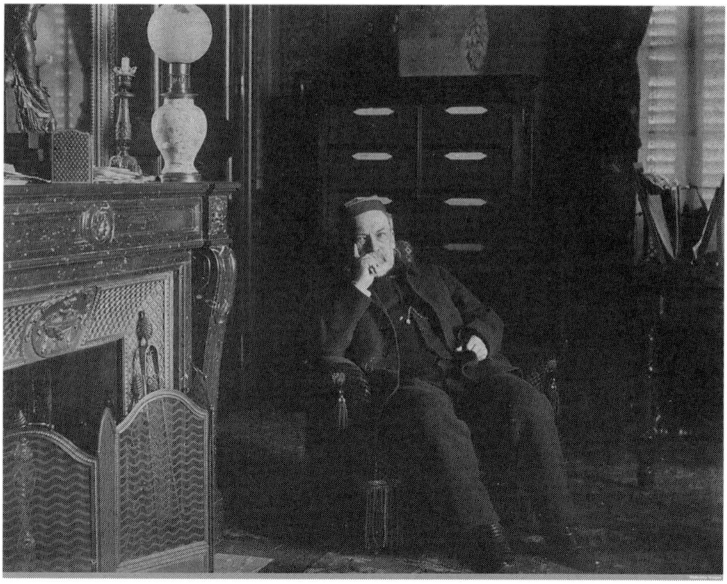

17 Studio Dornac et Cie, *Pasteur* (c.1888), photograph.

homme (in fact, a whole page is used to describe these objects – which includes the portrait of Henri Sainte-Claire Deville and a portrait of Pasteur's teacher J.B. Dumas).[89]

The multiple functions of photographic portraiture for Pasteur are further exemplified by a photograph he owned and exhibited in his home. The photograph, shot in 1847, is a portrait of Pasteur's former teacher, the scientist Jean-Baptiste Biot (Figure 18). The portrait was taken by Louis-Désiré Blanquart-Evrard, a chemist and photographer, in Regnault's laboratory at the Collège de France. Both men helped to found the Société héliographique and the Société française de photographie in 1851, with Regnault serving as president of the latter from 1855 until 1868. Blanquart-Evrard's photograph of Biot was the first collotype in France to be instantly reproduced on paper. He claimed to have improved upon William Henry Fox Talbot's paper negative (calotype) process and propagated his procedure as a new invention.[90] Since advancements in photographic technology were dependent upon chemistry, most early photographers had some scientific knowledge.[91] The rise of photographic studios in medical and scientific institutions, as well as the use of photography in scientific pursuits, made photography both the pastime and the focus of several scientists. Regnault took many photographs, including numerous portraits of his colleagues. Laurie Dahlberg suggests that the scientist's portraits comprise, most likely, the largest nineteenth-century collection of non-commercial portrait photography by one person.[92] Over 150 of his works survive,

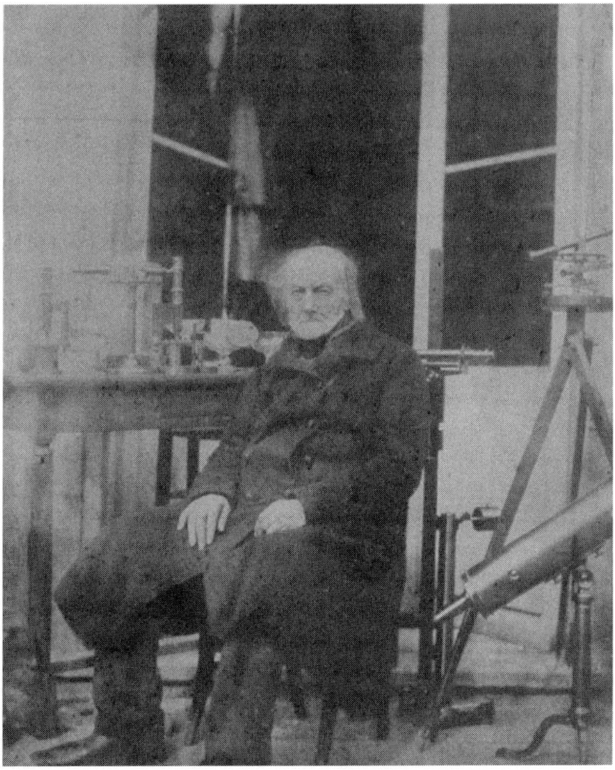

Blanquart-Evrard Louis Désiré, *Portrait de Jean Baptiste Biot* (1847), calotype. 18

of which roughly 50 are portraits of his scientific colleagues. In his portrait of the chemist Thomas Graham (c.1851), Regnault adheres to nineteenth-century artistic conventions of portraying professional men: the dark-suited scientist is seated with scientific accoutrements at his side. Although Regnault depicted men in their workspaces at the Collège de France, surrounded by the tools of science, the same props and rooms were used in numerous portraits, suggesting that the scenes were contrived. Like a photographic studio, Regnault's scientific backdrop was created with carefully placed chairs, books, and kit.

Blanquart-Evrard's portrait of Biot is another example of the intersection between art and science as the handwriting on the bottom left of the image confirms:

> This drawing holds a twofold interest. Not only is it the portrait of one of the great scientific glories of France, it is, moreover, the first successful photographic print taken from life. It was executed in the physics room at the Collège

de France by Blanquart-Evrard, in the presence of a committee composed of members of the Academy of Sciences and the Academy of Fine Arts.[93]

The multiple witnesses to this photographic experimentation attest to the overlap of art and science in the nineteenth century. It is also evidence of men working together, uniting their interests, and pushing towards shared goals. The merging of spheres was reinforced by the genre of portraiture and the medium of photography. Portraiture linked the historical status of an artistic genre and the modernity of a scientific process. Although Blanquart-Evrard located the technological progress of photography in the laboratory by showing Biot in a known and specific scientific space, he adhered to the artistic conventions of painted portraiture: Biot is seated, staring out at the viewer, surrounded by the accessories of his profession. Blanquart-Evrard chose portraiture – rather than still life or landscape – for photographic experimentation. The genre allowed him to display the prominent status of a chemist as well as exhibit his own involvement in scientific experiments. The portrait is the product of this experiment, a record of it, and a portrait of Biot in his laboratory. This constructs Blanquart-Evrard as scientist, witness, and artist.

Significantly, Biot gave this photograph by Blanquart-Evrard to Pasteur, saying, 'If you place this proof alongside a portrait of your father, you will see reunited the images of two people that loved you in about the same way'.[94] For Biot, too, portraiture served professional and familiar bonds. By having his portrait exhibited alongside that of Pasteur's father, he could become Pasteur's professional patriarch. The work proves a personal and professional exchange and records homosocial bonding.

Like Blanquart-Evrard, Pasteur, and Biot, Nadar used portraits for personal and professional purposes. In 1886, Nadar gave a large copy of one of his photographs of Pasteur to Dr Emile Roux.[95] Roux was integral to the discovery of the rabies vaccine – it has even been suggested by scholars, including Geison, that Pasteur's final rabies vaccine was based on Roux's experiments rather than his own. On this copy, now on display at the Pasteur Institute, Nadar wrote: 'To Doctor Roux, Very respectful and admiring homage. Nadar Portrait made in 1886.'[96] By adding the date and dedication, Nadar displayed the connection between Pasteur and Roux at the exact time of the discovery of the rabies vaccine, even though historical evidence dates this picture to 1878. This inscription not only emphasised Nadar's personal connection to the two men, but also highlighted his status as a witness and participant in historical events.

In her examination of Nadar's memoir, *Quand j'étais photographe*, Rosalind Krauss argues that Nadar was more interested in exhibiting his status as witness to history than in displaying his successes as a photographer; Nadar's text is primarily concerned with providing readers with psychological, emotional, and physical accounts of history.[97] Krauss creates flexible positions for Nadar, allowing him to move from photographer to historian or, rather, allowing him to merge the two positions into one. Yet it is not only Nadar's position as witness that is evident in his signed portrait of Pasteur: his role as scientist is also displayed. Nadar's signature and dedication link his name and product (photography) with the scientific leaders Pasteur and Roux; he includes himself in the scientific elite. The 'respectful and admiring homage' is paid to Roux by Nadar through the representation of Pasteur and the photograph itself. Nadar discusses the great innovations of the nineteenth century in *Quand j'étais photographe*, and puts photography in competition with – and ultimately above – other scientific discoveries, including bacteriology, anaesthesiology, steam engines, and the electric light:

> But do not all these miracles pale when compared to the most astonishing and disturbing one of all, the one that seems finally to endow man himself with the divine power of creation: the power to give physical form to the unsubstantial image that vanishes as soon as it is perceived, leaving no shadow in the mirror, no ripple on the surface of the water?[98]

By linking the progress of science with the divinity of creation, Nadar merged the two forces into the figure of the photographer.[99] He empowered himself with the ability to fix bodies and events into print. As a portraitist, Nadar provided representations of bodies that could be documented and studied. He had the power to replace the real with lifelike images.

Competition in the laboratory

Competition was an essential aspect of scientific and artistic communities; it led to both bonding and exclusion in the homosocial spheres. Portraiture was a site of combat and a tool for propaganda for scientists who used it as visual 'proof' of their discoveries, and for artists in need of notice and work. Shown at the Salon, distributed as *cartes de visite,* or reproduced in newspapers, portraits presented, mediated, and consciously manipulated visual records of identities and events. Nowhere is this more evident than in Edelfelt's portrait of Pasteur.

'Pasteur is in the midst of making the biggest discovery of his life: finding a vaccination against rabies', Edelfelt wrote to his mother in April 1885.[100] The chemist was discussing the possibility of a cure for rabies as early as this date, although the first human was not injected with the vaccine until 6 July 1885 and the public announcement was not made to the Académie de Médecine until October 1885. In Edelfelt's portrait, Pasteur's gaze is focused on the spine of a diseased rabbit air-drying in a glass jar: the source of the attenuated rabies virus that was added to a sterile broth in order to make a vaccine. It was this air-drying that led to the discovery of a vaccine, and Pasteur wanted to associate himself with this new scientific procedure.[101] We know from Edelfelt's letters that it was Pasteur's decision to include the glass with the rabid spine. [102]

Although Edelfelt's letter and portrait emphasised Pasteur's key role in creating a vaccine, other historical accounts undermine such declarations and show the vulnerability of the truth claims made by portraiture and realist formal strategies, as well as by esteemed painters and scientists. In fact, it was Roux and not Pasteur who first experimented with rabid spinal cords in this way (ultimately, rabid rabbit spines—not dog spines—were used). According to Adrien Loir, one of Pasteur's assistants, Pasteur came across Roux's experiments and copied them, giving Roux no credit for the discovery.[103] In contrast to Loir's account, Edelfelt presents Pasteur as an independent scientist who is solely responsible for the cure. Portraiture produced convincing histories through mass visibility at the Salon and in reproductions in the popular press. Considering Pasteur's national importance, it is not surprising that it took many decades for his role in the rabies vaccine to be questioned. Why would one ever question the deeds of a 'great man'?

Showing off: portraiture, nationalism, and commerce

Pasteur was a national symbol, particularly after the French defeat in the Franco-Prussian war. He linked science and nationalism by arguing that France had lost the war because its scientific pursuits were underfunded. Although the chemist was sympathetic to republicanism during the Revolution of 1848, he was generally conservative. He openly admired Napoleon Bonaparte and fostered a relationship with Louis Bonaparte, to whom he dedicated his book on wine. In 1868, Louis Bonaparte promoted Pasteur to commander of the Légion d'honneur. In 1875 (after the 1870 abdication of Napoleon III), Pasteur ran for Senate (as a conservative for his hometown of Arbois) on a platform of nationalism and science. Although he lost the election, possibly because he did not fully deny his associations with the Second Empire, Pasteur was nonetheless regarded as a good republican, particularly after 1870 when he avidly supported France in the wake of the war. Pasteur stayed in France after the devastating loss despite many offers to work at foreign universities, expressed anti-Prussian sentiment ('Hatred towards Prussia. Revenge! Revenge!'), returned an honorary doctoral degree from the University of Bonn, and, upon his deathbed, refused the Prussian Order of Merit.[104] A cartoon published in *Le Rire* in 1895 illustrates Pasteur's fervent nationalism, and shows the chemist inoculating himself against the orders of Prussia. Although Pasteur's personal politics shaped his public persona, the majority of visual representations of Pasteur presented him as France's greatest patriot and saviour. As Dr August Lutaud, a critic of Pasteur's work on rabies, wrote in *Pasteur et la rage* in 1887, 'In France, one can be an anarchist, a communist or a nihilist, but not an anti-Pasteurian. A simple question of science has been made into a question of patriotism.'[105]

Science and nationalism were bound through the figure of Pasteur and articulated through renderings of his body. Bonnat's identity as the portraitist of the *grands hommes* of the republic emphasised the national importance of Pasteur, and presented both scientist and artist as patriots. Bonnat's work portrayed a heroic Pasteur, suitably decorated by his Légion d'honneur medal. Unlike Edelfelt's painting, Bonnat's portrait was commissioned. It formed public identities for Bonnat and Pasteur, and exhibited the importance of the man who commissioned the work. Bonnat was hired by J.C. Jacobsen, the owner of the Carlsberg brewing company in Denmark, to make Mme Pasteur a portrait of her husband. Although it is unknown why Jacobsen commissioned Bonnat, it is likely because he was a well-known portraitist of the Third Republic and socialised in the same circles as Pasteur. Pasteur expressed his friendship with Bonnat in a letter to his son about his dismay that Bonnat had not told him that Jacobsen had hired him to paint his portrait.[106]

Pasteur began sitting for Bonnat in early 1886. By March 1886, the portrait was on display in the artist's studio. In a letter from 11 March 1886, Pasteur wrote to Bonnat that Jean-Jacques Henner, a member of their social group (who had also painted portraits of Pasteur and his family), had seen the portrait:

> My Dear Bonnat,
>
> I copy:
>
> 'I have just seen your portrait at Bonnat's. It is magnificent and it is one of his most beautiful works. The little girl is ravishing in her pose and resembles her mother. I am delighted for you and I congratulate you. Sincerely, your devoted Henner'
>
> I have nothing to add, as I concur with Henner and I will send the letter to my son for M. Jacobsen. This man writes that he does not dare request a photograph from Bonnat.
>
> Best Regards, my dear great master.
>
> L. Pasteur[107]

These letters demonstrate a familiarity and warmth between Pasteur, Henner, and Bonnat. Henner was able to see Pasteur's daughter's likeness in the image of Camille, as Pasteur had hired Henner to paint portraits of his family members many years earlier. As a special gift, Henner made a portrait of Pasteur to accompany this commissioned portrait, thus emphasising the chemist's familiar bonds and his own friendship.

Bonnat's portrait was a personal gift, but it had a public function that served the needs of the Jacobsen family. The Jacobsens were a prominent and wealthy Danish family with whom Jean-Baptiste Pasteur became acquainted when he was the secrétaire auprès de l'Ambassade de France in Copenhagen.[108] On 12 April 1885, Jean-Baptiste wrote to his father that J.C. Jacobsen wanted to try the filtering system (*filtre de porcelaine Chamberland*) that Pasteur invented with his colleague Charles Chamberland. The bacterial filter was used in manufacturing and preserving wine, vinegar, and beer. Pasteur sent the Jacobsens a new model of the filter and, shortly thereafter, the Jacobsens commissioned the portrait by Bonnat. The gift, sent in thanks for the filter, reflected Jacobsen's indebtedness to Pasteur's scientific work. Unlike most nineteenth-century brewers who produced beer by visually gauging its readiness, Jacobsen followed Pasteur's example by considering the scientific problems associated with fermentation. In 1875, Jacobsen created a Carlsberg laboratory, divided into a department of chemistry and a department of physiology, in order to produce high-quality, hygienic beer all year round.[109] Pasteur's work ultimately enabled the Carlsberg company to improve production and expand to become the largest brewery in Europe. Bonnat's portrait linked Jacobsen with Pasteur, as a small plaque on the painting displayed the name of the famous brewer. As a form of advertising, this bestowed on Carlsberg beer the safety associated with 'pasturization'. At a time when many doctors and scientists fought against the ads printed in the back of newspapers (they believed these advertisements of quack remedies undermined the status and legitimacy of science), Bonnat's portrait, exhibited at the Salon, provided a subtle yet highly visible endorsement for both Carlsberg and Pasteur.[110]

The relationship between Pasteur and Jacobsen exemplifies the links between republicanism, science, commerce, and art in the capitalist world order of late nineteenth-century Europe. Although France was celebrated for its wine, beer was also understood as a national symbol that reflected the country's industrial strength, scientific knowledge, and wealth. Pasteur used beer to express his anti-Prussian sentiment in his 1876 book *Études sur la bière; ses maladies, causes qui les provoquent, procédé pour la rendre inaltérable, avec une théorie nouvelle de la fermentation.* He wanted all beer made by his methods to be labelled as French in order to help France compete against Prussian breweries.[111] Pasteur believed that through science, commerce, and industry France could achieve greatness and superiority over Prussia. Private business was needed to fund scientific research; in turn, industry could reap the economic gains of scientific discoveries. Although Pasteur was the likely recipient of roughly 10 per cent of France's annual funding for scientific research, he also actively sought out private money, particularly from industrialists.[112] Pasteur's research aided French industry, particularly the silk, farming, wine, and beer trades, and these beneficiaries contributed to his scientific causes. Furthermore, he insisted that the opening and running of the Pasteur Institute be financially supported not only by the money generated by patented vaccines from his laboratory, but also by private and industrial donations.

Bonnat's portrait was not the first image of Pasteur commissioned by the Jacobsens. The family had asked Paul Dubois to make a portrait bust of Pasteur for them, which was displayed in Denmark and at both the 1880 and 1886 Paris Salons. Pasteur's desire to propagate his work and that of his friends is suggested in a letter he wrote his son-in-law before the 1880 Salon:

> I should like M. Jacobsen's name to be glorified, alongside that of Paul Dubois, by an authoritative art critic. You are known at the journal *Le temps,* whose review of the Salon is done by a talented writer, Paul Mantz. It would be highly desirable that in discussing the work of Paul Dubois ... M.P. Mantz would write a few lines recounting the origins of the bust and draw attention to the enlightened generosity of this rich industrialist who invested fifteen hundred thousand francs for the construction of a laboratory devoted to the progress of the brewer.[113]

Pasteur saw the Salon and Salon criticism as sites where scientific, industrial, and artistic identities could be produced and alliances formed. He knew the importance of advertising in the modern age, as well as the value of personal bonds in business. Upon Jacobsen's death, Pasteur asked Jacobsen's son Carl for a cast of Dubois's bust for his home.

The Jacobsen and Pasteur families were further connected by their mutual commitment to the promotion of modern French art. In 1888, Carl Jacobsen organised and funded an exhibition of French painting and sculpture at the Exposition of Industry, Agricultural, and Nordic Arts in Copenhagen.[114] As is depicted in Peder Severin Krøyer's 1889 painting, *Le Comité de l'exposition française à Copenhague 1888, présidé par L. Pasteur*, Jacobsen asked Pasteur to be the honorary president of the exposition. In Krøyer's work, Pasteur is shown sitting at a large meeting table, surrounded by prominent men, including Antonin Proust, the president of the exposition. The exhibition was well advertised in Paris. Pasteur wrote to Jacobsen that '[y]ou are known to all of our artists, who speak highly and with gratitude of your generosity',[115] and Jules Claretie declared in *Le Temps* that the show displayed 'French art, in its most elevated form' and mentioned that Pasteur had given Jacobsen a bas-relief by the sculptor Perraud to honour their friendship, Jacobsen's late father, and his gratitude to Copenhagen.[116] Although this event promoted French art in Denmark and provided Jacobsen with an opportunity to acquire works, it also advertised his family name and company internationally. The donation of artworks to public collections contributed to national strength, as it not only displayed the greatness of national heroes, but also encouraged national culture.[117]

Collecting Pasteur

Unlike Bonnat's portrait, which was hung in Pasteur's home (and remains there as part of the Musée Pasteur), both Edelfelt's and Gsell's paintings were bought for French museums. The ministry of French culture asked Edelfelt for the portrait after the 1886 Salon and claimed that it would be exhibited at the Musée de Luxembourg, then at the Louvre (it ended up at the Sorbonne until 1922 and is now at the Musée d'Orsay).[118] Edelfelt intended to give the painting to Pasteur as a gift, but ultimately, agreed to sell it to the State. With the help of the Finnish artist, Helene Schjerfbeck, he made a copy for Pasteur (this portrait remains on display in Pasteur's 'home' in the house museum of the Pasteur Institute). The acquisition reinforced Pasteur's symbolic importance to the French government and promoted Edelfelt as a prominent Parisian painter. A month after the 1886 Salon, Edelfelt was awarded the Légion d'honneur.[119]

Despite its location 'at the far reaches of room XIX, so high that it is invisible', Gsell's small portrait of his relative was bought by Baron Alphonse de Rothschild during the 1886 Salon,[120] who donated the painting to the Musée des Beaux-Arts de Vannes in 1887 at the request of Paul Leroi, the director of *L'Art*.[121] Yet, unlike Edelfelt's and Bonnat's paintings, Gsell's work received little notice in the press; his portrait was not even considered a candidate in the quest for the quintessential image of Pasteur. The minimal Salon criticism of the painting suggests that its size and location led to invisibility, which was compounded by the fact that compositionally Pasteur is hard to see. Unsurprising, the following year Gsell created a big bold entry for the Salon with Pasteur in the front row (Figure 2).[122]

'Doctor Pasteur': Gsell's portrait of Pasteur at the 1887 Salon

'The number of doctors whose portraits appear in the Salon is unimaginable', wrote Le Roux in his review of the 1887 Salon in *Le Temps*. 'Like M. Charcot and M. Péan, M. Pasteur has been portrayed in his clinic. He watches as a child is inoculated; a tall Arab waits his turn.'[123] Le Roux categorised Gsell's portrait of Pasteur, titled *La Vaccine de la rage au laboratoire de M. Pasteur*, as one of the many portraits of doctors at the Salon. He did not draw a distinction between Charcot and Péan as medical practitioners and Pasteur as a laboratory scientist. The three paintings were regarded as equivalent. The similarities between the works by Gervex, Brouillet, and Gsell were also discussed by Roger Ballu in *L'illustration*: 'perhaps it was by a stroke of bad luck that he delivered to the public a Scene at Pasteur's the year that M. Gervex and M. Brouillet were showing the same scene. Inevitably, there will be comparisons that are detrimental'.[124] That numerous critics commented upon the paintings' similarities is not surprising: the artists relied on similar formal practices and iconographical precedents to portray celebrated men in medical milieux. All three works are large-scale oil paintings of well-known men in their workplaces. In all the portraits, dark-suited, white-haired men command the attention of a crowd, their faces lit by the daylight that falls through large windows. All three men have human beings as their objects of study: Péan is focused on a bare-breasted anaesthetised woman, Charcot on a swooning hysterical woman, and Pasteur on a squirming child and non-French men. Despite the professional differences between Péan and Charcot as physicians and Pasteur as a chemist, the exhibition of these contemporary scenes at the Salon united them and their occupations.

Gsell's *La Vaccine de la rage au laboratoire de M. Pasteur* depicts various people who have come to be inoculated at Pasteur's laboratory. On the right side of the canvas stands a suited Pasteur, holding a piece of paper and staring at a dark-skinned man from Algeria. Described as an 'Arab' in the popular press, this man came from one of France's North African colonies. Numerous sheets of paper clutter the floor, indicating that many people have already received injections (being vaccinated against rabies required multiple jabs at increased levels of potency, and therefore names, dates, and levels of vaccine were diligently recorded). In the centre of the canvas, a well-dressed bourgeois mother holds out her wriggling child, whose bare belly indicates that it was, or is about to be, inoculated by the physician sitting next to Pasteur. Behind the Algerian are Russians and Armenians, their national identities exhibited by long beards and furry hats. *Le Monde illustré* assigned particular nationalities to all the figures depicted, describing this scene at Pasteur's Ulm Street office as 'crammed with people from all over, trusting in the method of the illustrious scientist.'[125]

Unlike the portrait he exhibited in 1886, Gsell's 1887 painting represents Pasteur in a humanitarian, global, and colonial light. The artist replaced the microscopes, books, and pipettes from the earlier portrait with international patients and members of the Parisian public. By excluding scientific tools, Gsell symbolically altered Pasteur's identity as an experimental chemist and portrayed him as a doctor. Pasteur's intense gaze is focused on human beings rather than a virus-filled glass tube. Unlike the 1886 portrait, in which Gsell depicted Pasteur's intellectual endeavours within a private and privileged laboratory, the setting of the 1887 portrait is an accessible place where Pasteur's science is made public and where French colonial power is on display.

La Vaccine de la rage au laboratoire de M. Pasteur conveys Pasteur's international significance and his vaccine's crucial role in the French 'civilizing mission'. The concept of France's 'civilizing mission' is often associated with Prime Minister Jules Ferry's speech to the Chamber of Deputies on 28 July 1885, where he outlined reasons for French colonial expansion.[126] In particular, he claimed that it was not only the right, but also the duty of 'superior races' to civilise 'inferior' ones; colonisation was rationalised by the belief that France could raise its colonies' level of civilisation.[127] Elected as Prime Minister twice (from

1880 to 1883 and 1883 to 1885), Ferry was an ardent republican, and was known for his promotion of colonial expansion and the laicisation of the education system. Significantly, Ferry's financial and political support of scientific learning coincided with Pasteur's professional aims. As Gerald Geison points out, Pasteur was highly skilled at navigating the academic-cum-political system in order to garner support for the expansion of his scientific research.[128]

Despite overwhelming support for his research, the privacy of Pasteur's science was a point of contention between January and June 1887, when Dr Michel Peter attacked the legitimacy and ethics of Pasteur's work on rabies at the Académie de Médecine, claiming, in part, that Pasteur's methods were not purely scientific because he kept them secret.[129] He further claimed that Pasteur's vaccine had killed three people. Pasteur fought back by pointing out that he had allowed both French and international doctors and scientists into his laboratories to check his work and stressed the internationalism of his science and its ability to save all people. The majority of the members of the Académie de Médecine supported Pasteur, including major leaders in the Parisian medical world such as Drs Vulpian and Charcot. Vulpian publicly criticised Peter for denouncing Pasteur, seeing such an attack as equivalent to criticising one's own country: 'I am not afraid to say to him that: as a doctor, academic, philanthropist, [and] patriot, he undertook and continues to pursue a deplorable campaign.'[130]

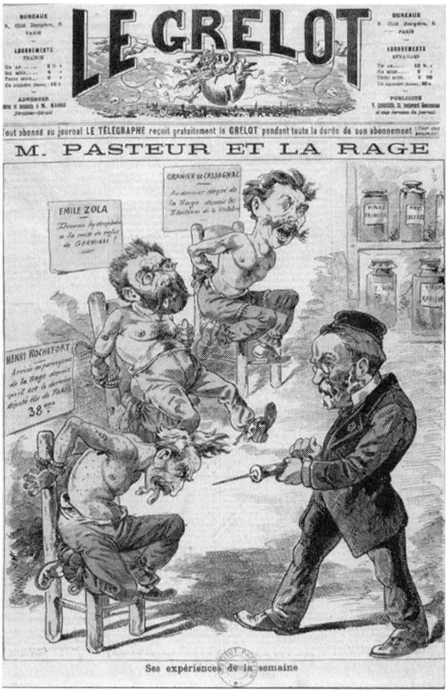

19 'M. Pasteur et la Rage', cover of *Le Grelot*, 8 November 1885.

In the wake of Pasteur's interrogation at the Académie de Médecine, it was crucial that his image at the 1887 Salon show him as the man who brought health and safety to humanity. Pasteur needed to be seen as a man who cured people, not one who experimented on them, in order to maintain public support. In a cartoon of Pasteur published on the cover of *Le Grelot* on 8 November 1885, in which Henri Rochefort, Émile Zola, and Granier de Casagnac are shown tied to chairs, struggling to free themselves in order to flee Pasteur's needle, Pasteur's identity as a cruel experimental scientist competes with his persona as the saviour of humanity (Figure 19). The scandalous identities of the men depicted in the cartoon, however, indicate that Pasteur's science was believed to treat physical ailments *and* cure moral and political ills. This cartoon mocks the popular belief that Pasteur's science could treat anything and anyone by showing him 'curing' the scandalous men in the picture. Gsell must have been familiar with the debates surrounding Pasteur's rabies vaccinations because of his family connections and through the widespread discussions in newspapers and magazines. It is possible that Gsell chose to portray Pasteur as a doctor-like figure, curing bodies, in order to compensate for this bad press.

Gsell's painting showcases Pasteur's integral role in the process of vaccination, even though Pasteur is not physically administering the cure. Although there were debates about whether or not Pasteur deserved an honorary medical degree, he remained a chemist. An article by Mercutio in *La Revue blanche* from April 1886 indicates that the public was well aware of Pasteur's professional status:

> You know that M. Pasteur is not a doctor; he has never studied medicine. Since he is not a doctor, he cannot administer the inoculations himself and must enlist a real doctor to perform these minor procedures ... It does not take away one particle of M. Pasteur's glory not to have personally performed the inoculations whose active ingredients have been prepared using his method.[131]

Pasteur embodied the potential that experimental laboratory science could bring to medicine. As J. Hirschler proclaimed in his book, *Nos docteurs* in 1896: 'Through its admirable experimental methods, and thanks to the genius of a few men like Pasteur, who have opened up a new world for its research and exploitation, medicine has been rejuvenated, it has been transformed.'[132] Hirschler emphasises the dominance of science in all new medical discoveries and technologies when he asks: 'Where is medicine in all these discoveries? Nowhere! Where is Science that must benefit the doctor? Everywhere!'[133] Like the painting by Gsell, many images in the public press showed Pasteur as a scientist, holding a piece of paper in his hand, recording and watching people being inoculated. He was frequently portrayed as the intellectual force behind the physical demands of practising medicine, but was rarely shown touching or puncturing bodies.

Numerous scenes of rabies inoculation, including Gsell's, drew upon renderings of Edward Jenner, the English physician who proved that cowpox provided a vaccination against smallpox during the 1790s.[134] Many pictures of Jenner, including those painted by Ernest Board and Eugène-Ernest Hillemacher, show him vaccinating young children accompanied by their mothers (Figure 20). Similarly, a mother and child occupy the centre of Gsell's 1887 canvas and figure in other portrayals of Pasteur reproduced in the popular press. Yet, unlike the close physical contact depicted in these paintings of Jenner, in which he is shown personally vaccinating children's plump arms, in Gsell's

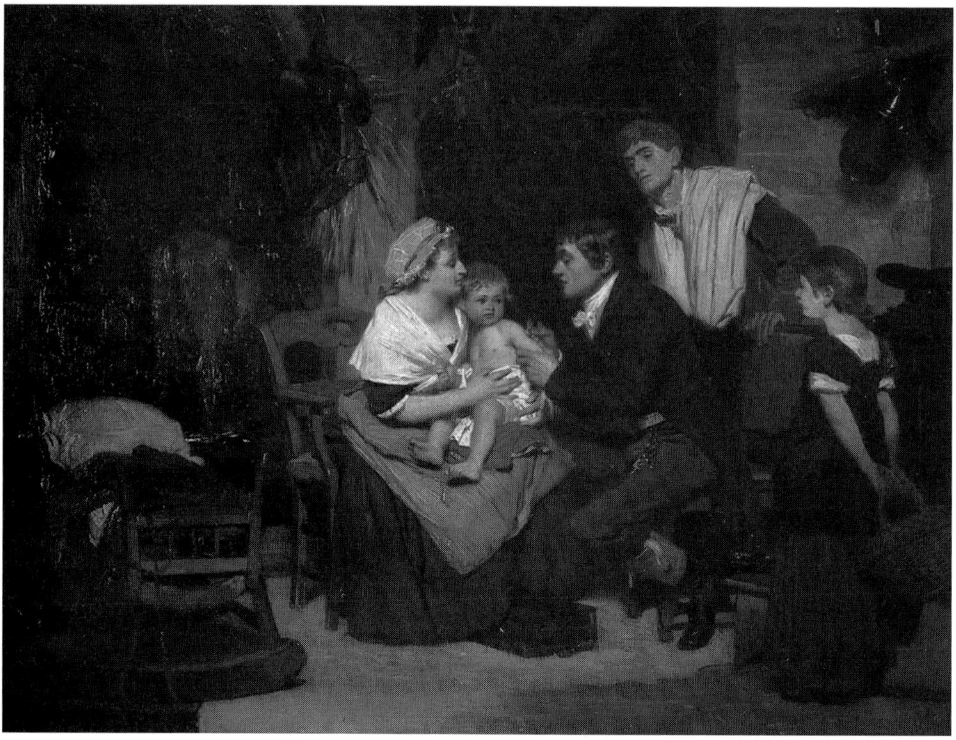

20 Eugène-Ernest Hillemacher, *Edward Jenner vaccinating a boy* (1884), oil on canvas, 73.1 x 92.7cm.

work Pasteur is at a distance from his patients, observing, not touching them. As is evident in Émile Bayard's 1886 gouache, Pasteur was often shown supervising the inoculation (Figure 21). Although many nineteenth-century images show Pasteur overseeing the process – as he is in Bayard's work – many journalists linked the chemist and Dr Jenner. *La Revue blanche* claimed in 1886 that 'Pasteur rose, this year, to the first rank of humanity's benefactors; he is, with Jenner, the propagator of the vaccine, one of the men most deserving of the recognition of his fellow men.'[135] Pasteur's work on rabies gained legitimacy through its connection with Jenner's vaccination, which by the late nineteenth century was fully accepted and practised by the French public and medical establishments. In his 1886 article, Ernest Maindron justified Pasteur's work on rabies by relating it to Jenner's smallpox vaccination, claiming that '[a]lmost all the great discoveries have found obscure detractors … One should have understood that only the future can soundly judge these things.'[136] The link to Jenner solidified Pasteur's identity as both a scientific innovator and a man who cures.

Pasteur's association with medicine and medical men occasionally destabilised his identity as a laboratory scientist, as is evident in a late nineteenth-century

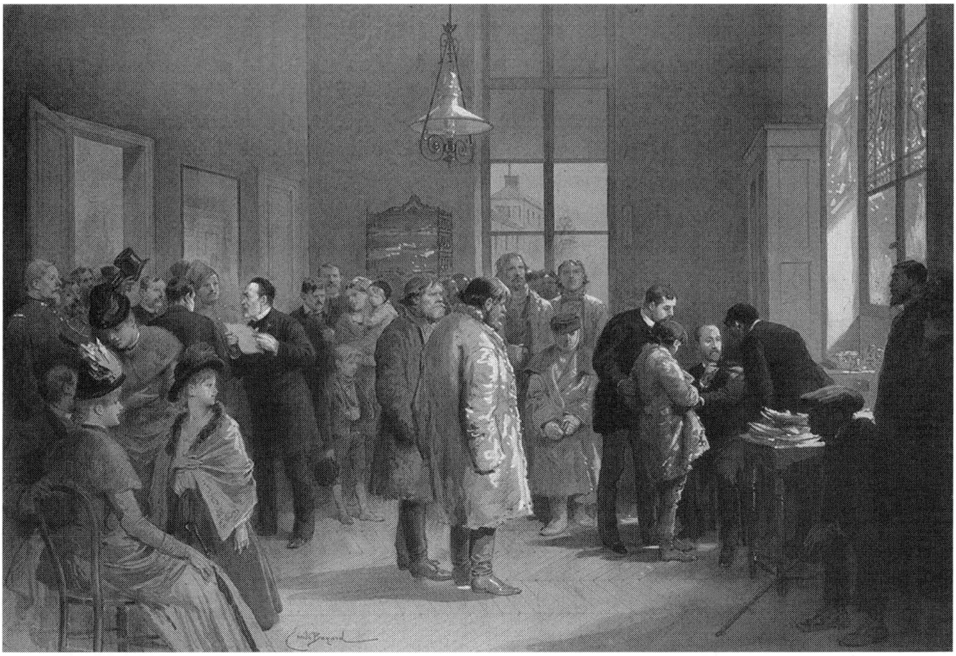

Émile Antoine Bayard, *Séance d'inoculation contre la rage à l'École normale supérieure* (c.1886), gouache. 21

advertisement and collecting card for Chocolat Carpentier, in which he is shown as a doctor injecting patients with the rabies vaccine (Figure 22). In this ad, Pasteur is presented as the seated inoculator, focused on a patient's bare stomach, while his next patient awaits her turn, her bare shoulder symbolising her readiness for the jab. Underneath Pasteur are the words, '*La Médecine*'. By using the figure of Pasteur, symbolic of French strength and well-being, the Chocolat Carpentier company imbued their chocolate with the health and safety associated with the chemist. As an advertisement, the Carpentier image was circulated, and collected, and thus propagated Carpentier's product and the image of Pasteur as a medical doctor who protects humanity. Similarly, Gsell's portrait of Pasteur, seen by thousands of visitors at the 1887 Salon, also exhibited an image of Pasteur as a man who protects and saves. Despite their different mediums and cultural status, both images propagated the importance of Pasteur in modern medicine and the necessity of rabies vaccination.

Representing the vaccinated other: the spectacle of Pasteur's patients

Tales of Pasteur's many patients filled the papers. *L'Évènement* described the scene at the laboratory:

> Everything is going quickly and in the greatest order; I saw a parade in front of me of children of all ages, men and women of all classes and of all nationalities, soldiers from Africa and Tunisia, and finally the famous *moujiks*, of all the most dangerously affected.[137]

La Nature also focused on the diversity of Pasteur's patients:

> From all sides, the victims of rabid dogs were arriving to demand the benefit of Mr Pasteur's treatment. It was the people from Brie, as the master familiarly called them, foreigners, Germans, women, children, etc., a whole world who, every morning, were coming to fill the office adjacent to the large laboratory.[138]

Gsell's painting highlights the spectacle of vaccination, as men and women from around the world are shown in Pasteur's laboratory. Like Gervex's painting of Péan's surgical theatre and Brouillet's portrayal of Charcot's medical stage, Pasteur's laboratory is presented as a popular and fashionable place where the display, scrutiny, and puncturing of bodies is paramount. The act of looking fills Gsell's canvas: Pasteur's eyes are focused on the Algerian. The Algerian watches the twisting child. The mother looks down on her toddler. A crowd of medical men in white coats peek around one another to get a look at the patients and the inoculation procedure, and a young woman leans out from behind Pasteur to stare at the viewer. Gsell's painting stages the importance of seeing in the detection of difference, as bodies of different sexes, ages, races, and cultures are portrayed within the same laboratory. The English physician Dr Alfred J.H. Crespi also noted the entertainment value of Pasteur's procedures:

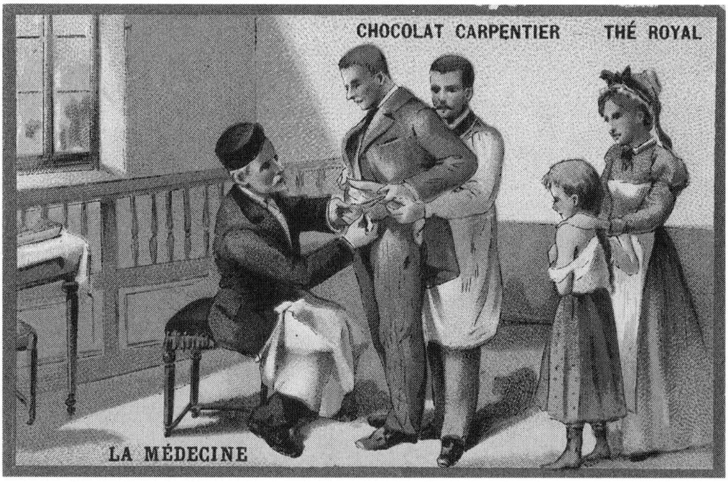

22 'Chocolat Carpentier', advertisement (c.1895–1900), chromolithograph on paper, 6.9 x 10.2cm.

> there was an appearance of something like a show in the proceedings … Many of the aristocratic gentlemen and graceful ladies who passed through the rooms had evidently come to look around, just as they might, later in the day, go for a flower show, or a picture gallery.[139]

The spectacle of inoculation depicted by Gsell drew a crowd at the Salon. As Alexis Martin wrote, we must 'congratulate him sincerely for stopping not only the crowd but connoisseurs in front of his canvas'.[140]

As Michel Foucault argues, the intense scrutiny of bodies was culturally justified as a scientific pursuit, particularly in medical examinations.[141] 'The best doctor … is the one whose gaze penetrates under the mysterious envelope to guess at the mysteries it hides', Adrien Marx wrote in *Le Figaro*.[142] Although looking was required for medical practice, the public viewing of bodies was fraught by the anxieties that arose from the unstable boundaries between scientific observation and public voyeurism. Pasteur's laboratory was a site where medical and public gazes blurred. Doctors, scientists, and Parisian and international publics saw naked stomachs as patients waited their turn, shirts up and bellies bare. A print in *La Nature* shows people who partook in viewing the inoculation procedure while simultaneously exposing themselves (Figure 23). The distinction between professional and public looking is emphasised pictorially: the majority of men on the left are depicted as a group of bodiless heads, their gazes fixed on the patients on the right. In his 1886 article in *Le Soleil*, Jean de Nivelle pokes fun at M. Cattiaux, a critic of Pasteur who was upset that rabies inoculations required bare stomachs. De Nivelle's mocking article quotes Cattiaux's critique in *Bulletin municipal officiel*:

> M. Pasteur administers his inoculations in the stomach. Why there, rather than someplace else? Why not in the arm? M. Pasteur sees women and young girls in his laboratory, and I do not hesitate to describe these inoculations in the stomach as improper.[143]

In response to Cattiaux, Nivelle sarcastically wrote, 'Alas! Why stop there? Why not just say plainly and simply that it was a pornographic institute that was founded?'[144] As Nivelle's article attests, the display of naked bodies and body parts in clinics, laboratories, and hospitals was subject to public criticism, despite the general belief that the medical gaze was rational and objective rather than libidinous. This was not always the case, however, as Chapters 2 and 3 argue.

Unlike the print in *La Nature* that shows a young woman with her stomach exposed, Gsell did not include women's bare bellies in his work. This omission rendered Pasteur's laboratory as a space of curing rather than voyeurism. In contrast to Gervex's and Brouillet's paintings, in which unconscious semi-naked female bodies occupy central positions and point to the salacious side of

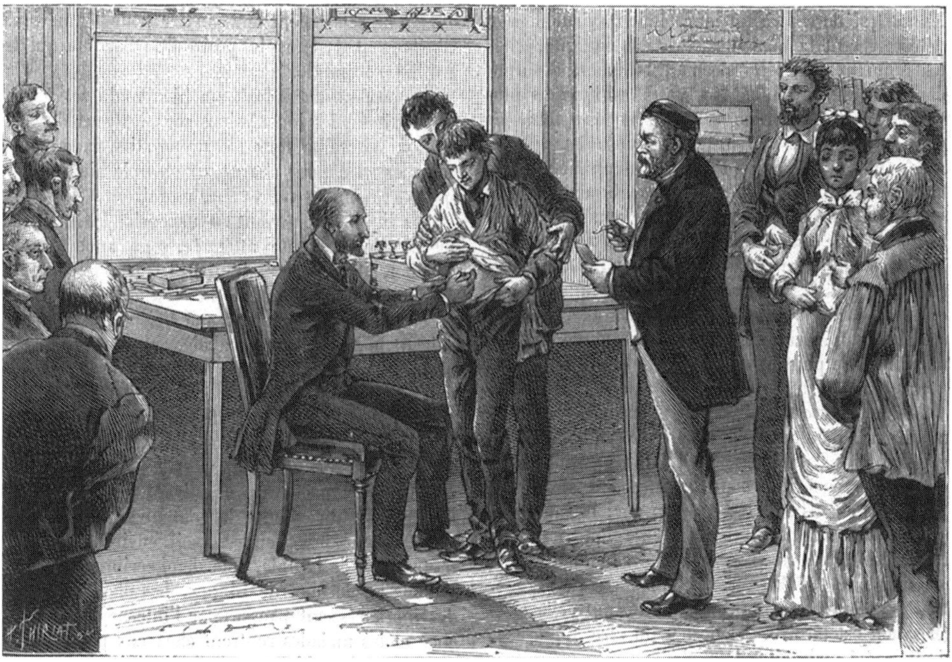

23 'Les opérations de vaccine de la rage au laboratoire de M. Pasteur', from *La Nature*, 14:1 (1886), p. 213, engraving.

medicine, the women in Gsell's canvas are fully dressed, conscious, and engaged. The woman in the centre is a proper bourgeois mother, holding out her child to display the curative power of French science to the Algerian traveller. The expensively dressed child recovering from the jab symbolises the health and wealth of France, as well as the progress of French science, thus serving as a model for the rest of the world to emulate. The bourgeois toddler – like a modern-day baby Jesus – represents the promise of bodily and moral prosperity. By drawing on Christian iconography of the Adoration of the Magi, Gsell transformed the three kings into 'foreign' patients. The well-dressed mother, standing in for the Madonna, symbolises the ideal mother – generous, compassionate, all-giving. By aligning French motherhood with the 'greatest mother of all', Gsell's painting exhibited the new demands of bourgeois motherhood: women were encouraged to protect the health of their children with the help of French science and increased access to education.

The bond between science and family was symbolically on display in Pasteur's laboratory. Two stained-glass panels, which Pasteur commissioned from Gsell's father, Jean-Gaspard Jules Gsell, hung side-by-side in the windows directly above where people were inoculated (Figures 24 a/b). One panel depicts a female figure symbolising Chemistry. She is shown kneeling before a pestle and

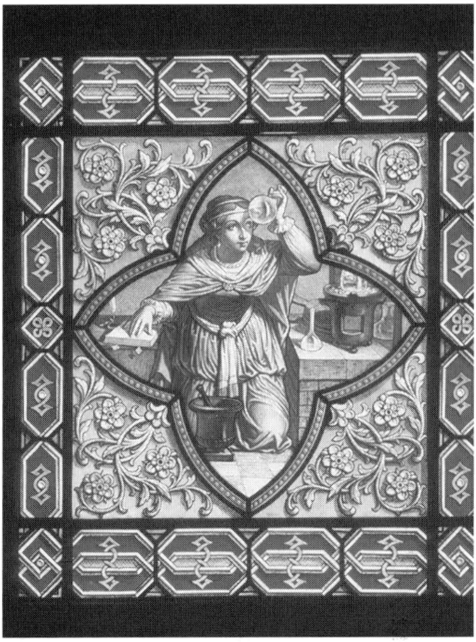
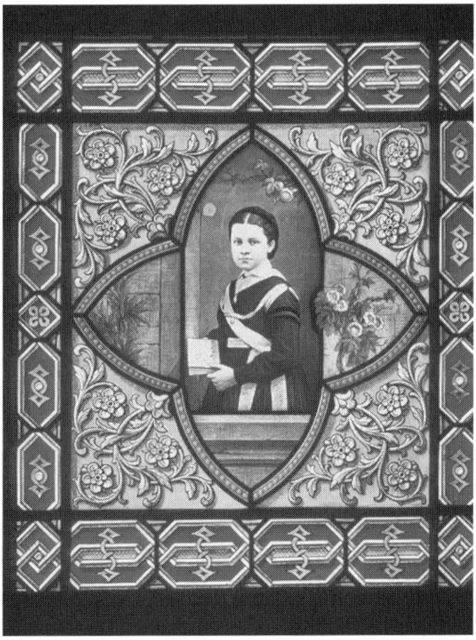

(left) Jean-Gaspard Jules Gsell, *Allégorie de la chimie* (c.1870), stained-glass window. **24a**
(right) Jean-Gaspard Jules Gsell, *Marie-Louise Pasteur* (c.1870), stained-glass window. **24b**

mortar, one hand resting on a book, the other lifting a flask so that she can peer directly at its contents. The glass jar being heated on the burner to her right and the apparently empty flasks refer to Pasteur's work on germ theory and bacteria (Pasteur argued that, despite being invisible to the human eye, bacteria were always present and could be killed off through heating). The second stained-glass panel portrays Pasteur's daughter, Marie-Louise, as a young schoolgirl. Dressed in the uniform of the boarders of the Couvenant des Oiseaux, Marie-Louise is presented as a serious student, her intellectual endeavours emphasised by the book she holds. Placed next to each other, the stained-glass windows represent Chemistry as a female body and a woman's pursuit. Such imagery challenges nineteenth-century gender norms. While idealised female bodies symbolised the general concept of 'Science', showing a recognisable young girl within a scientific sphere was rare. As is evident in the top right-hand corner of the nineteenth-century gouache by Bayard, these images held a prominent place in Pasteur's laboratory. Across from the laboratory door and lit by the sunlight that fell through the windows, the images were seen by all. By exhibiting these works to the public, Pasteur displayed the two most important things in his life, chemistry and family, visually uniting the two and reinforcing science's crucial role in the protection of families and women's role in disseminating scientific knowledge. Under the watchful eye of Chemistry and Pasteur's daughter, the Parisian and international public were inoculated.

Arab/others

Gsell's painting exhibited Pasteur's international significance through the rendering of people from around the world. Despite the cultural differences highlighted in *La Vaccine de la rage*, the painting shows rabies vaccination as indiscriminate. Pasteur is portrayed as a man who protected and insured the health of France and all humanity. By showing Pasteur's science as tolerant and universally accessible, Gsell's Pasteur fitted comfortably within textual accounts that stressed the chemist's humanitarianism. Raymond Poincaré, who would later become President of France, eulogised Pasteur using the same terms: 'Humanity, which you have helped, will surround your glory in a unanimous and imperishable cult wherever national rivalries dissolve, and wherever the common faith in unlimited progress is kept alive and strong.'[145] Science simultaneously unified and divided nations. Scientific discourse forged unity as it showed that scientific medicine could cure humans regardless of sex, class, race, or gender, but it also provided 'scientific proof' that differences existed and not all were considered equal. The close contact of different cultures in Pasteur's laboratory led to national comparisons and exposed prejudices, as Crespi's quoting from an article in *Fortnightly Review* attests: 'French and Belgian peasants are clean and neat, but lower order Spanish, Portuguese and Russians are dirty and loathsome to a degree.'[146] Pasteur's science was regularly promoted as egalitarian and objective despite its political and economic motivations. Great scientific battles between European countries took place in non-European territories because these nations offered French scientists ample specimens and unstudied diseases. Science could 'progress' quickly in places where human experimentation was permitted. Although French doctors and scientists wrote about wanting to improve the lives of all people, spreading French science was crucial for consolidating the French 'civilising mission' and for projecting France as a world power. The French military, for example, required protection from diseases – including malaria – that weakened armies.[147] The expansion of French scientific medicine in non-European nations functioned as a colonising tool.[148] Through public health initiatives and disease prevention, promoted by the opening of Pasteur Institutes overseas (starting with one in Indochina in 1891), Pasteurian medical science promised to reduce mortality rates, strengthen labour forces, and transform colonial subjects into defenders of French values. Futhermore, French medicine 'scientifically' justified the take-over of lands and people. By constructing colonised people as barbaric and sick, French intervention was believed to humanise and civilise.[149] Colonised subjects were often presented as innocent and naive, and 'needed' medical intervention, as were French children. In Gsell's work, the Arab man and young child are linked pictorially as both are shown as the main recipients of inoculation.

La Vaccine de la rage shows rabies vaccination as a trustworthy procedure. The representation of European patients and doctors next to a North African man displays the significant role of French medical procedures in colonial expansion. The French regarded the rabies inoculation as progressive compared to non-European medicine, which was frequently considered tribal, rural, archaic, and non-scientific. In order to construct the modern superiority of French medicine, Gsell included a North African man, draped in cloth, to symbolise the figure's 'backwards', 'primitive', and 'childlike' ways. He is shown as the recipient and beneficiary of French knowledge; here, scientific colonisation is curative and generous. Although Arabs were deemed worthy of saving from diseases, they were nonetheless understood (popularly and medically) as inferior and sick. Despite the humanitarian guise of scientific medicine – exemplified here by Gsell's painting – the French desire to control and dominate their colonised subjects remains. Gsell glossed over the realities of colonisation to offer Salon viewers the spectacle of a colonised subject – a spectacle that they were familiar with through the various North African displays at the *Expositions Universelles*, as well as chance sightings of Pasteur's foreign patients in Paris.

On 29 May 1886, *La Nature* published an article by Gaston Tissandier, accompanied by a photograph of 'Arabs' standing in the Jardin du Luxembourg (Figure 25). In the print, eight men and women are shown in cultural dress, surrounded by French onlookers. As described in *La Nature*, the photograph was taken by an amateur photographer who happened to come across this crowd in the park:

> His attention was drawn to a number of passers-by gathered around a group of Arabs. These were 'Pasteur's Arabs', as his assistants called them, or rather, Arabs who had been bitten by rabid dogs and were being treated by M. Pasteur. The camera was pointed at the Arabs, who had agreed to follow the directive 'don't move!' And voilà! Here we have the positive image obtained, reproduced in *La Nature*.[150]

In the photograph, the spectacle of the Arabs was produced by their difference from the French.[151] Dressed head-to-toe in white, their heads covered with layers of cloth, the Arab bodies contrast against the varied, but uniformly dark, Parisian garb.

Crespi's textual description of Pasteur's laboratory demonstrates how non-European bodies heightened the spectacle of vaccination, and shows how cultures were misidentified through prejudice. Crespi describes a meeting at the laboratory:

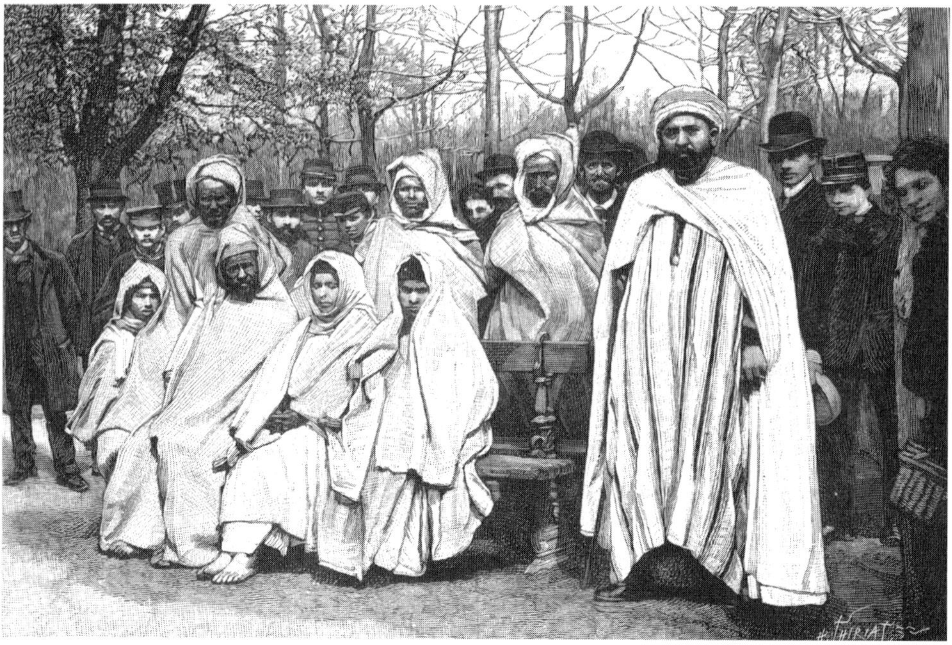

25 'Groupe des Arabes mordus par des chiens enragés, venus à Paris pour subir le traitement prophylactique de M. Pasteur', from *La Nature*, 29 May 1886, p. 401, engraving after an amateur photograph.

> I noticed a dark man of fifty, whom I cross-examined. He was a physician from Cairo, sent to Paris to investigate the matter … Among the patients were two foreign women – one tall, the other short, both singularly handsome. 'What are these people?' I enquired. 'One', he replied, 'is an Arab; the other, I don't know.' The short woman whom he had called an Arab heard him, and politely begged his pardon, disclaiming any Arab blood.[152]

As Crespi's commentary attests, Arab bodies, be they physicians or patients, were a source of speculation: their presence was as spectacular as Pasteur's scientific feats. Such comments also question the trustworthiness of sight and its role in the categorisation of bodies. Crespi's account forces us to reconsider the reading of 'Pasteur's Arabs' in Gsell's work – could this draped stranger be a doctor or a learned man?

Gsell's Salon painting, like the amateur's photograph in *La Nature* and Crespi's detailed description, were understood as accurate accounts of Pasteur's Arab patients. In all works, the patients' cultural identities are prominent due to their difference from the French. Despite its humanitarian message, Gsell compositionally grouped the figures by nationality. The Russians and Armenians talk behind the lone Arab while the large group of French men and women form a cluster that dominates the canvas. Unlike the foreign men, who are portrayed as patients and linked to children, the French men are medical or scientific professionals; they comprise the dominant group. Like the educated and powerful male audience painted by Brouillet, the faces and bodies of the French men blur into one another, forming a uniformity in which only subtle facial characteristics differentiate one man from the other. The masculinity of scientific practitioners is shown as collective and inquisitive – they look, judge, and administer modern discoveries. In contrast, the Arab man stands alone. The folded white drapery of his attire and his slip-on shoes differs from the contemporary Parisian dress of Pasteur and the group of people depicted on the right: the French men are shown in dark suits while the women wear fashionable Parisian dresses and fancy hats. His gnarled wooden stick contrasts with the thin and delicate cane held by a *parisienne*. French modernity is symbolised by the intricate and voguish store-bought clothing – even the young child is adorned with high socks, layered undergarments, leather shoes, and a jacket with cuffs. In contrast, the Arab, in a simple sheet-like garb, is shown as 'primitive', secured in a past untouched by the advances of science and fleeting fashion. Even compared to the hand-made patterned clothing of the Russians, he appears to be from a previous time. This juxtaposition helped justify and proselytise the French 'civilising mission' as a peaceful and necessary project.

Wolf bites: the Russians

Behind the Arab on the 'foreign' side of the painting are three Russian peasants. Known as *moujiks*, these men were identified by their furry hats and long beards, as well as their likeness to representations of Pasteur's Russian patients in newspapers and published photographs.[153] The most recognisable were a group from Smolensk. Gaston Tissandier described their visit to Pasteur in his article about the Arabs in *La Nature*:

> The case of the nineteen Russians who were bitten by a rabid wolf must be discussed separately. There are profound differences between the repercussions from wolf bites and the bites of a rabid dog. Wolves, in the relentless fury of their attack, introduce a greater quantity of the rabies virus. If the preventive treatment is delayed for a few days, it is likely that the disease will already have spread throughout the entire system.
>
> We reproduce on page 401 a photograph of one these Russians to show the enormous size of the tear from the wolf's bite. Another Russian had had his lips ripped off; yet another had been bitten in the forehead with such fury that one of the animal's teeth remained lodged in his skull. They all suffered serious injuries, and three of them died. But had the usual mortality statistics for rabid wolf bites been applied to the nineteen Russians from Smolensk, the

> proportion would have been the reverse: out of the nineteen, sixteen would have succumbed.[154]

The Russians were widely known as the most severely infected of all Pasteur's patients. Therefore, saving them from wolf bites was a great feat for the chemist. The personal significance for Pasteur is evidenced by the dedicated photograph of the group of Russians on their trip to Paris that he gave to his granddaughter, Camille. Russians were included in many images of Pasteur with patients – for example, in the engraving published in the English publication *The Graphic* in 1886, Pasteur is surrounded by children and Russians. Pasteur had a great respect for Russians: he invited Russian scientists to work at his institute and established seven rabies inoculation centres in Russia. Pasteur also encouraged a Franco-Russian alliance as a means to strengthen France's position against Prussia.[155] By including them in his painting, Gsell exhibited the prominent role of Russian scientists in Pasteur's laboratory and the acceptance of Pasteurian principles in Russian hospitals, but, more importantly, one of Pasteur's greatest triumphs in his work on rabies.

Pasteur's boys: heroism and sacrifice

Gsell relied on the exoticism of Pasteur's foreign patients to draw a crowd to his work at the Salon. Significantly, he chose these 'exotic' patients rather than the first person to benefit from Pasteur's rabies vaccine: the young French boy, Joseph Meister. On 6 July 1885, Pasteur treated a nine-year-old Alsatian child who had been severely bitten by a rabid dog. Meister was given a cumulative treatment of twelve injections of the rabies vaccine progressing from the least to the most virulent. Before beginning the process, Pasteur discussed the case with Dr Vulpian, who was a colleague at the Académie des sciences and a member of the French rabies commission, and Dr Grancher, who was the clinical professor of children's diseases at the Paris Faculté de médecine. They decided that Meister should be vaccinated because the child had nothing to lose. A few months after Meister's successful treatment, the mayor of Vilers-Farlay asked Pasteur to try his vaccine on a fifteen-year-old boy, Jean-Baptiste Jupille, who had been bitten by a rabid dog while saving other children. Pasteur used Jupille's heroic and dramatic story to gain public support in the speech he gave to the Académie des sciences on 26 October 1886, in which he announced the great successes of his rabies treatment on humans:

> The Academy will perhaps not hear without emotion the story of the courageous actions and presence of mind of a child whose treatment I undertook last Tuesday. He is a shepherd, fifteen years old, by the name of Jean-Baptiste Jupille, from Villers-Farlay (Jura), who, upon seeing a large, suspicious-looking dog rush at a group of his little friends, all younger than he, armed

with a whip, threw himself in front of the animal. The dog seizes Jupille's left hand. Jupille then throws the dog to the ground and holds him down, and with his right hand opens its mouth to free his left hand, not without being bitten several more times, and then, with the light of his whip, binds its muzzle and, grabbing one of his wooden clogs, knocks it unconscious.

I will hasten to keep the Academy abreast of developments in this most recent case.[156]

Jupille was an ideal patient: an innocent and selfless boy whom science could save. Pasteur symbolically aligned himself with Jupille and used him as a surrogate of sorts. Firstly, Jupille and Pasteur came from the same part of France. Pasteur had publicly recounted how he had witnessed the effects of rabies at close range during his childhood, when a rabid dog attacked villagers from a nearby town. Secondly, Jupille's identity as a selfless shepherd tied him to Pasteur, whose name, modest manners, and noble contributions to humanity often led to Pasteur being called, and portrayed as, 'the good shepherd'. Although Pasteur's first patient, Meister, came to signify the nationalism of science, embodying and justifying France's right to Alsace after the Franco-Prussian war, it was Jupille's story that visually represented the violence of rabies and the human battle against it, and symbolised Pasteur as strong and altruistic.

Pasteur chose the image of Jupille as the public face of the Pasteur Institute (Figure 26). The chemist commissioned Emile-Louis Truffot to make a sculpture of Jupille for the front lawn of the Pasteur Institute. The sculpture represents the boy battling a rabid dog, who glares with crazed eyes and bared teeth. Jupille is portrayed in the moment of overpowering the animal: he has a grip on the dog's neck and a rope tied around its snout. Truffot's sculpture was the only artwork on the Pasteur Institute's grounds. It set the tone of the institute and its purpose. 'This group that recalls an act of heroism is placed in front of the staircase of honour of the main entrance. It prepares, as it were, the visitor for the feelings that a visit to the Pasteur Institute will not fail to inspire', Gaston Tissandier wrote in *La Nature*. 'This establishment, singular in this world, is not only, in fact, a temple of science, it is also the sanctuary of charity and devotion. And one knows not what we should most admire in the one who was the founder, or of the discoverer of new and fertile doctrines, or of the benefactor of humankind.'[157]

Tissandier's article was published alongside four images of the institute: two were plans of the buildings and their rooms, another was an outside shot of the building and the last was a picture of Truffot's sculpture. The sculpture is also present in most nineteenth-century images of the institute that filled the newspapers on the occasion of its opening in 1888. The inclusion of this sculpture is significant because the Pasteur Institute was devoid of ornament. As described in *L'Univers illustré*: 'No rich ornamentation appears, no unnecessary

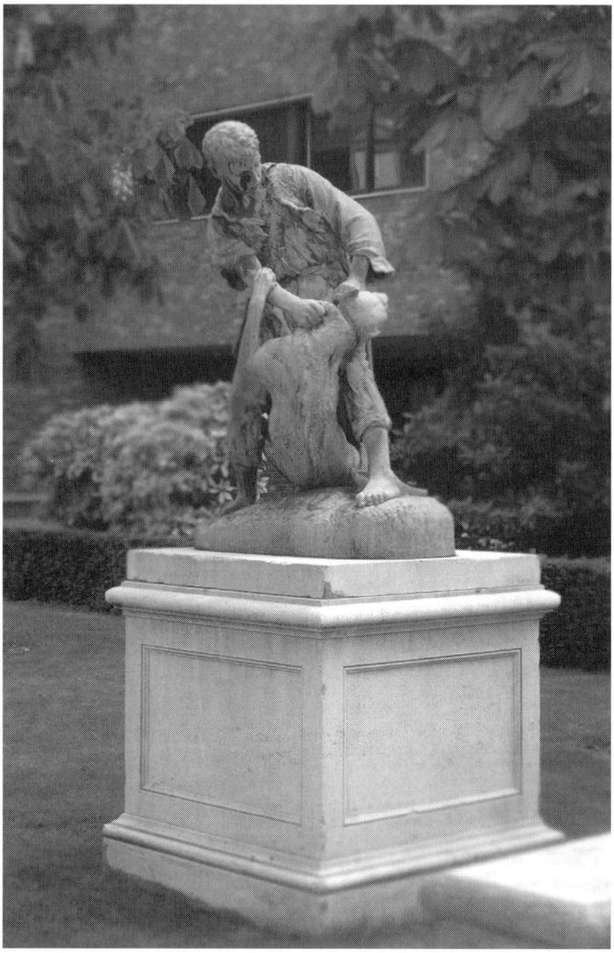

26 Truffot, *Jean-Baptiste Jupille* (1887), bronze.

decoration: at first one has the impression of being in a house solely devoted to science, to the search for the solace of humanity's sickness.'[158] The sculpture of Jupille was an integral part of the institute rather than a frivolous decoration.

Although Truffot's sculpture depicts the story of one of Pasteur's first patients, it exemplifies the characteristics with which Pasteur and the institute wished to be associated: courage, strength, and selflessness. Pasteur, often regarded as a saintly or Christ-like figure, was frequently surrounded by Christian symbols of innocence: haloes, flowing white robes, and lambs (Figure 27). The sculpture's portrayal of Jupille's physical strength and fight against rabies signifies Pasteur's intellectual and scientific struggle against the virus. It also symbolises the battles fought by laboratory science against Nature, which was understood as wild and uncontrollable, embodied in Truffot's work by the snarling mad dog. Jupille's selfless act emphasised Pasteur's role, and science more generally, in the protection of children and families. The sculpture showed that rabies was dangerously real, had a source, and had to be destroyed. This was important as some of Pasteur's critics argued that it was hard to prove someone had rabies when the rabid animal could not be found; it was even suggested by some that Pasteur gave his patients rabies rather than cured them.

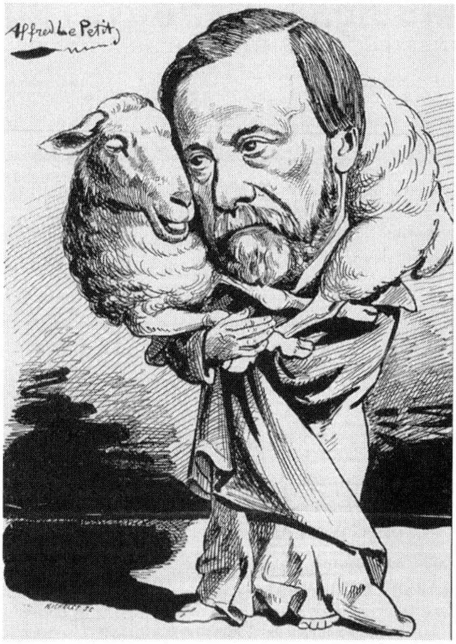

27 Alfred Le Petit, 'The Good Shepherd', from *Le Charivari*, 27 April 1882.

The public's familiarity with – and fear of – rabies was frequently manifested in the acting out of rabies symptoms. Like other sensational nineteenth-century ailments, such as hysteria, rabies fascinated the public with its assortment of astonishing and highly sexualised symptoms (during an attack of rabies, patient would often tear off clothing, salivate profusely, bite others, and contort into orgasmic poses). Members of the bourgeoisie – well versed in hyperbolic accounts of rabies symptoms and various evolutionary theories – feared that an animal within themselves could break through bourgeois manners, customs, and clothing. Cases of hysterical rabies – where patients acted out rabies symptoms without having been bitten – point to the extreme pathological fear of this virus. Pasteur himself was fooled by a case of hysterical rabies.[159] 'In the phobic imagination of the nineteenth century, the semiotics of rabies centred on violence and sexuality, and its etiology on repression', Kathleen Kete argues. 'The fear of rabies lies at the intersection of the organising themes of bourgeois life and can be read as an expression of uneasiness about modern civilisation and its tolls, about the uncertain conquest of culture over nature.'[160] These anxieties were based on the belief that civilised life could alter one's natural disposition and caused illness. People feared that rabies was a product of modernity. The increased popularity of keeping dogs as domestic pets was thought to spontaneously cause rabies because pets were not allowed to fulfil their natural mating urges in cramped city apartments. As Kete points out, rabies was linked to sex, as ostensibly unhealthy sexual behaviours were tied to spontaneous rabies in dogs.[161] As rabies threatened to upset the controlled and rational lives of middle- and upper-class Parisians, it also promised the spectacle of the bourgeoisie gone mad. Like the images of hysterics at the Salpêtrière that showed convulsing semi-clothed women, photographs of rabies patients showed bodies out of control, tongues exposed, eyes half shut, and muscles contracted. The bodies of rabies victims, like those of hysterics, were defined as sick by their difference from the controlled and clothed bodies of the bourgeoisie who exemplified the rules of proper social comportment. Yet, this surface civility could not be trusted to erase or contain the beast within.

Gsell's painting does not depict people suffering from rabies, nor does it represent the sexualised spectacle of uncontrolled bodies on display. Such a portrayal would have threatened Pasteur's scientific persona even if it did attract more Salon viewers (certainly the paintings of Péan and Charcot relied upon the potentially salacious contact of clothed male bodies with semi-nude women to entice the crowd). Nonetheless, it did draw upon the spectacle of Pasteur's patients, as did Truffot's sculpture. Many of Pasteur's patients acquired celebrity status. Papers published stories about them, with emphasis on those who travelled to be cured in Paris. The tales of the Newark Boys, six young Americans from New Jersey who were bitten by a rabid dog and sent to Paris, filled the American and Parisian press. As Bert Hansen argues, the sustained American interest in this story changed popular expectations of medicine by showing that medical news was thrilling to the general public.[162] As exemplified by the Newark Boys – who were on display to the American public at the Globe Museum in New York – the spectacle of inoculated bodies drew a crowd.[163]

Funding the Pasteur Institute

Pasteur's science spread his reputation and France's fame internationally, and raised funds for the Pasteur Institute. Although the Pasteur Institute received money from the French government, it was primarily funded by private donations and the Pasteur laboratory's patented discoveries. Monetary contributions became a form of public entertainment: newspapers listed all those who had donated, from the poorest of Parisians to international royals and wealthy industrialists.[164] Pasteur emphasised the importance of public sponsorship: 'Institut Pasteur – Souscription publique, 1888' was exhibited prominently above the grand entrance.

International contributions were crucial to funding the institute. Pasteur actively sought international financial support, acquiring major donations from Alexander III, tsar of Russia, and Pedro II, emperor of Brazil. Other major donors were heads of state, wealthy wives of industrial leaders, and upper-class Frenchmen. The chemist publicly displayed his thanks to those who gave by commissioning busts of the largest benefactors.[165] The number of busts of French women demonstrates the active role that they had in philanthropic projects, including supporting scientific medicine. Mme Boucicaut, the widow of the founder of the supermarket chain Bon Marché, not only gave

250,000 francs to the Pasteur Institute, but also founded a new hospital in Paris that adhered to Pasteurian concepts: patients were no longer separated by sex, but were divided based on their medical or surgical needs, and those without infectious diseases were separated from those who were contagious. Exhibited in the Salle des bustes, the location of the inauguration ceremony of the Pasteur Institute, these sculptures provided the donors with cultural and historical status.[166] The visibility of those who donated portrayed the Pasteur Institute as an international organisation where science and industry met for the greater good of humanity.

Considering the timing of Gsell's painting's exhibition at the Salon (a year and a half before the Institute's opening), it is clear that the work advertised the Pasteur Institute and encouraged public donations. By portraying Pasteur as an active and healthy figure, despite the physical ailments that plagued the chemist, Gsell built public confidence in the ageing man's abilities to lead. Furthermore, in being described by critics as realistic, the painting was understood as an accurate rendering of the scientist, and therefore its political and economic aims appear to have gone unnoticed. Although Gsell could not show Pasteur in his institute, as it was still under construction, the image exhibited laboratory science as Pasteur wished it to be understood:

> I appeal to you on behalf of these sacred places that are known by the expressive name of *laboratory*. Demand that they be multiplied and enriched. These are the temples of the future, of wealth and well-being. It is here that humanity grows, becomes stronger and better. It is here that humankind learns to read in nature's works, works of progress and universal harmony, while its own works are too often those of barbarism, fanaticism and destruction.[167]

The laboratory, like the institute, signified Pasteur. Science, laboratories, the institute, and Pasteur became symbolically intertwined, as each one represented the ideal characteristics of the other. Gsell's portrait stood in for what the Pasteur Institute was soon to symbolise. As Dr Janicot wrote in 1888 on the occasion of the inauguration, this 'establishment recalls a scientific and humanitarian conquest that will do more for the honour of our country than a large bloody victory'.[168]

Conclusion: a final portrait

When Pasteur died on 28 September 1895, newspapers celebrated his life and scientific discoveries, and printed letters of condolence from foreign leaders, scientists, and celebrities. A state funeral was planned, and Pasteur's body was brought through the streets of Paris from the Pasteur Institute to Notre Dame, accompanied by 1,400 gardiens de la paix, 600 members of the infantry of the republican guard, and 200 cavalry men.[169] A photograph of the procession

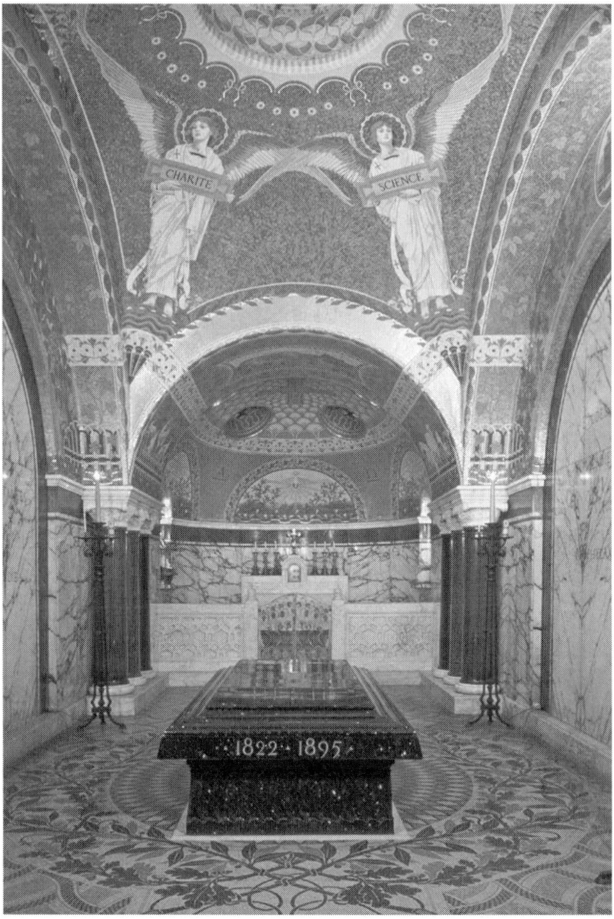

28 Pasteur's mausoleum (1896).

shows the Parisian public lining the streets to watch the funeral carriage, adorned with flags, make its way towards the grand cathedral. Although the French government offered to inter Pasteur's body at the Pantheon, his family wanted him buried at the Pasteur Institute, and built a private funeral chapel on the ground floor to house his body.[170]

Influenced by the late Roman Mausoleum of Galla Placidia in Ravenna, Italy, Pasteur's chapel is an example of nineteenth-century symbolist architecture and design. The brightly coloured mosaic tiles and stylised decorative murals in the chapel are the antitheses of the realistic portraits commissioned by and for the scientist during his lifetime (Figure 28). Gsell, Bonnat, and Edelfelt portrayed Pasteur as a valiant modern man through heroic narratives and realistic portrayals. Realism, as the naturalising agent *par excellence* during the

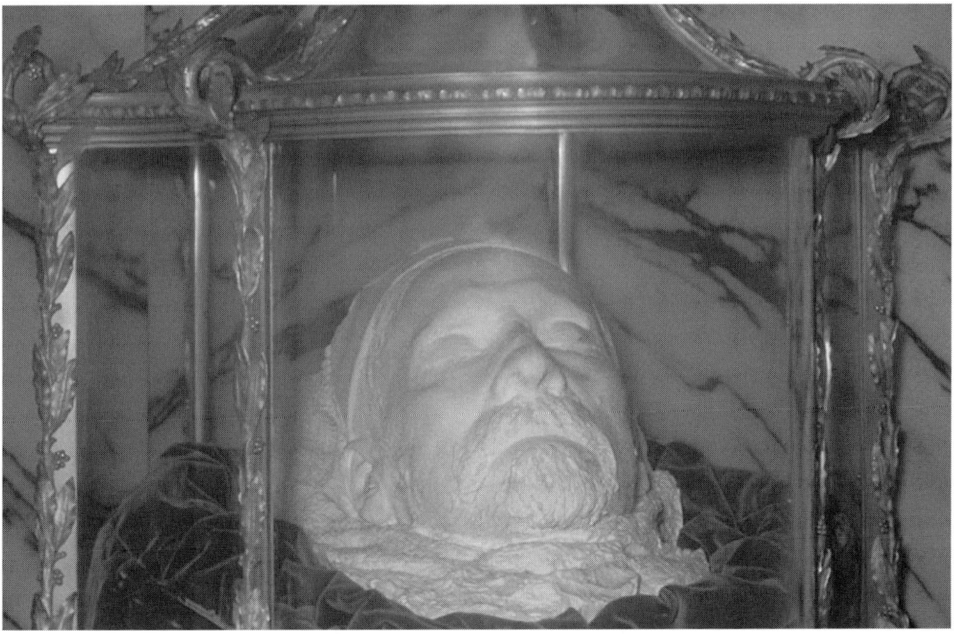

Plaster death mask of Pasteur in Pasteur's mausoleum. 29

nineteenth century, was seemingly able to depoliticise and neutralise contemporary events and people through its verisimilitude. As a style that was understood to symbolise truth and objectivity, it was considered ideal for representations of scientific culture and historical documentation. Despite the stylistic differences between the Salon portraits and the mosaic murals, the rhetoric and symbolism of Pasteur remains, as images of laboratory instruments, dogs, rabbits, and Jupille decorate the vaulted ceiling, along with the words 'Charité', 'Science', 'Foi', and 'Esperance'.[171]

Within Pasteur's highly ornate and symbolist tomb is the final realistic portrait executed in his presence: his death mask (Figure 29).[172] This effigy is intimately connected to the chemist's physical body: it constantly evokes Pasteur's corporal presence through the imprint left from his minute skin creases, the fleshiness of his earlobes, the prominent curve of his nose, and the tiny eyelashes and whiskers that emerge from the plaster surface. Since the death mask is an indexical mould that supplies evidence of Pasteur's body, it provides a truth claim unavailable to painted portraiture. Yet, the mask is unable to give a record of the chemist's achievements, politics, relationships, and desires.[173] Pasteur's chapel, death mask, and portraits show the impossibility of distinct boundaries between the real and the ideal Pasteur, the symbolic and the actual, as much as they reveal the inability of any one style or medium to claim a monopoly over truth. Pasteur's identity was produced by multiple representations of himself and others. Salon paintings, crude cartoons, photographic portraits, stained-glass windows, amateur photographs, newspaper illustrations, mosaic tiles, and portrait busts all contributed to his reputation as a modern chemist, humanitarian, father, experimental scientist, doctor, and blind old man. The multiple realistic portrayals of Pasteur at the 1886 and 1887 Salons helped construct his history and his identity, yet historical identities, like the characteristics given to styles and mediums, are unstable, putting pressure on the true and the untrue, reality and fantasy, the factual and the fictive.

Notes

1 Many histories have been written on Pasteur and his discoveries. The main primary sources are René Vallery-Radot, *Pasteur, histoire d'un savant* (Paris: J. Hetzel, 1883) and *La vie de Pasteur* (Paris: Hachette et cie, 1900). The most thorough secondary sources are: Gerald L. Geison, *The Private Science of Louis Pasteur* (Princeton: Princeton University Press, 1995); Bruno Latour, *The Pasteurization of France* (Cambridge, MA: Harvard University Press, 1988); René Dubos and Thomas D. Brock, *Pasteur and Modern Science* (Madison: Science Tech Publishers, 1988); and Patrice Debré, *Louis Pasteur* (Paris: Flammarion, 1994).

2 'Inauguration de l'Institut Pasteur', *Le Soir*, 19 November 1888, n.p. 'Un vrai grand homme, acclamé par toutes les élites du pays, un savant français, salué par tous les représentants des grandes puissances, un illustre, modeste dans sa gloire.' (A truly great man, acclaimed by the nation's elite, a French man of science, hailed by all the representatives of the great powers, an illustrious man, modest in his glory.)

3 For an account of masculinity within the medical context of nineteenth-century France see Robert Nye, 'Honor, Impotence, and Male Sexuality in Nineteenth-Century French Medicine', *French Historical Studies*, 16 (1989), 48–71, and 'Medicine and Science as Masculine "Fields of Honor"', *Osiris*, 12 (1997), 60–79. For a discussion of scientific personas and the role of biography and portraiture, see Daston and Galison, 'The Scientific Self', in *Objectivity*, pp. 191–251.

4 Adrien Marx, 'M. Pasteur et le Docteur Peter', *Le Figaro*, 23 January 1887, n.p. 'Son portrait et son œuvre sont universellement connus. La photographie, le pinceau et la plume ont reproduit ses traits, raconté sa vie et publié ses labeurs.'

5 Barbara Larson's focused look at Odilon Redon's fascination with Pasteur's work, particularly Pasteur's studies of germ theory, is an exception. As she notes, Redon and Pasteur corresponded with one another, and Redon sent Pasteur a set of his lithographic prints titled *Origins*. See Larson, *The Dark Side of Nature: Science, Society, and the Fantastic in the Work of Odilon Redon* (University Park: Pennsylvania State University Press, 2005), pp. 85–106.

6 Bert Hansen has built upon Richard Weisberg's research to examine Pasteur's close friendships with artists. See Bert Hansen and Richard E. Weisberg, 'Louis Pasteur's Three Artist Compartriots – Henner, Pointelin, and Perraud: a Story of Friendship, Science, and Art in the 1870s and 1880s', and 'Louis Pasteur (1822–1895),

his Friendship with the Artists Max Claudet (1840–1893) and Paul Dubois (1829–1905), and his Public Image in the 1870s and 1880s', *Journal of Medical Biography*, forthcoming.

7 Georges Olmer, *Salon de 1886* (Paris: L. Baschet, 1886), p. 76. 'Comme la Revue annuelle de Variétés, le Salon sacrifie aux actualités et brûle toujours un peu d'encens en l'honneur des hommes du jour. Nous nous attendions donc à y voir figurer un portrait de M. Pasteur; nous en avons deux, et nous sommes loin de nous en plaindre, car l'hommage artistique rendu au grand savant ne saurait être trop éclatant.'

8 Aug. Dalligny, 'Le Salon de peinture', *Le Journal des arts* (11 May 1886), n.p.: 'une petite toile dans les tons gris, placée trop haut pour qu'on puisse bien saisir les détails qui semblent très justes' (a small canvas painted in shades of grey, hung too high for one to really see the details, which seem very accurate).

9 Arsène Houssaye 'Le Salon de 1877', *L'Artiste* (June 1877), p. 420.

10 Alfred de Lostalot, 'Le Salon de 1886: la peinture', *Gazette des beaux-arts* (1886), p. 456. 'Le portrait est ce que nous avons de mieux en France, pour le moment, dans la peinture proprement dite. … [L]a peinture de portrait a une tenue, au Salon, que l'on chercherait vainement dans les autres genres.'

11 For general discussions of portraiture in nineteenth-century France, see McPherson, *The Modern Portrait in Nineteenth-Century France*; McQuillan, *Impressionist Portraits*; and Pierre Vaisse, 'Between Convention and Innovation: the Portrait in France in the Nineteenth Century', in Félix Baumann, Maurianne Karabelnik, and Jean Sutherland Boggs (eds), *Degas Portraits* (London: Merrell Publishers, 1994), pp. 118–127.

12 Georges Lafenestre, 'Le Salon', *Revue des deux mondes* (May–June 1886), p. 590: 'le portrait seul y domine par la qualité comme par le nombre.'

13 Louis Ganderax, 'Causerie sur le Salon', *La République française,* 2 May 1886: 's'occupe plus volontiers de savoir qui est le modèle d'un portrait que d'en juger la valeur. S'il fallait juger de la popularité des personages par l'empressement qu'apportent les beaux-arts à reproduire leurs traits, on devrait supposer … que les contemporains prééminants sont: M. Pasteur, qui a deux portraits en pied, l'un comme grand-père et l'autre comme cultivateur de virus … Les portraits de personnages connus de tout genre abondent et peuvent satisfaire bien des curiosités.' ([The Salon viewer] is more preoccupied with knowing who is the sitter of a portrait than judging its value. If one had to judge the popularity of the figures by the overzealousness with which the fine arts attempt to replicate their features, we should suppose … that the pre-eminent contemporaries are: M. Pasteur, who has two full-length portraits, one as a grandfather and the other as a virus cultivator … Portraits of all types of well-known people are abundant and can satisfy much curiosity.)

14 Richard E. Weisberg and Bert Hansen, 'Collaboration of Art and Science in Albert Edelft's Portrait of Louis Pasteur: the Making of an Enduring Icon', *Bulletin of the History of Medicine*, 89:1 (2015), 74.

15 For a discussion of public understandings of rabies, see Kathleen Kete, '*La Rage* and the Bourgeoisie: The Cultural Context of Rabies in the French Nineteenth

Century', *Representations*, 22 (1988), 89–107; and Bert Hansen, 'America's First Medical Breakthrough: How Popular Excitement about a French Rabies Cure in 1885 Raised New Expectations for Medical Progress', *The American Historical Review*, 103:2 (1998), 373–418.

16 Letter from Edelfelt to his mother, 18 April 1885, cited in Association Arbois-Pasteur, *Rappelez-vous Pasteur l'Arboisien: L'artiste et ses amis artistes* (Arbois: Association Arbois-Pasteur, 1995), p. 50. 'Lundi prochain, j'irai à nouveau chez le vieux Pasteur pour voir s'il y a une possibilité de faire son portrait dans le laboratoire, parce que c'est seulement là, dans cet environnement, que je veux le peindre ... [C]'est dans son élément qu'il doit être: les lunettes sur le nez, la calotte sur la tête et le microscope devant lui.'

17 Duranty, *La Nouvelle Peinture.*

18 Olmer, *Salon de 1886*, p. 76. 'La vérité! On la veut tout entière aujourd'hui. Il faut qu'elle se montre, il faut qu'elle parle ... On attend du peintre qu'il transporte à domicile, qu'il apprenne à connaître non seulement la figure qu'il doit peindre, mais le milieu ou cette figure se meut naturellement. Le portrait se développe, il embrasse l'homme et sa vie. Il exige pour accessoires les instruments de sa gloire et de sa fortune, où tout au moins les meubles familiers, qui trahissent les mœurs du personnage représenté, ses objets préférés, devenus, par une chère habitude, des parties intégrantes de son être.'

19 Linda Nochlin, 'Impressionist Portraits and the Construction of Modern Identity', in Colin B. Bailey, John Bruce Collins, Linda Nochlin *et al.* (eds), *Renoir's Portraits: Impressions of an Age* (New Haven: Yale University Press, 1997), p. 66.

20 *L'Horizon inconnu: L'art en Finlande 1870–1920*, exhibition catalogue, Musées de Strasbourg, Galerie de l'Ancienne douane (Strasbourg: Helsinki Musée des beaux-arts Ateneum, 1999).

21 For a worthy discussion of the artistic conventions used in eighteenth- and nineteenth-century portraits of doctors and scientists, see Jordanova, *Defining Features.*

22 Letter from Edelfelt to his mother, 27 April 1885, in Association Arbois-Pasteur, *Rappelez-vous l'arboisien*, p. 51. 'Il était très gentil et m'a promis qu'en tant que modèle, il n'allait pas me décevoir, de plus il s'intéresse à la peinture parce qu'à l'âge de seize ans, il voulait absolument devenir peintre et que pour cela il se consacra durant plusieurs étés à cet art noble.'

23 For further information about Pasteur's artistic interests, see Denise Wrotnowska, 'Pasteur et l'art', *Médecine de France*, 66 (1955), 9–16; Maurice Vallery-Radot, *Pasteur: savant et artiste* (Paris: Éd. Hervas, 1995); and René Vallery-Radot, *Pasteur dessinateur et pastelliste (1836–1842)* (Paris: Publications André Marty, É. Paul, 1912).

24 Durand-Gréville's article on Pasteur in *L'Intermédiaire des chercheurs et des curieux*, 10 September 1888, as cited in M. Vallery-Radot, *Pasteur: savant et artiste*, p. 26. 'Beaucoup de nos peintre médaillés au Salon n'ont jamais dessiné ni modelé une bouche avec autant de justesse. Personne ne regretta que Pasteur ait choisi la carrière scientifique. Mais s'il avait voulu, il serait devenu quelqu'un parmi les peintres et, qui sait? Peut-être un très grand peintre.'

25 A. Gonnon, *Album Gonnon – iconographie médicale, 1895–1908* (Lyon: Protat Frère, 1909), p. VII: 'vers l'âge de 16 ans, Pasteur avait songé à se faire peintre. On possède de lui des pastels si remarquables par la précision du coup d'œil, qu'on a peine à croire qu'ils sont sortis de la main d'un adolescent.' (At around the age of sixteen, Pasteur had considered becoming a painter. Some of his pastels are so remarkable in terms of precision of the eye that is it hard to believe that they come from the hand of an adolescent.)

26 For a discussion of Pasteur's personal relationships with men in the art world, see Weisberg, 'The Representation of Doctors at Work in Salon Art of the Early Third Republic in France', pp. 584–586.

27 *Grand Festival au profit de l'Institut Pasteur, organisé par la Conférence 'Scientia', Palais du Trocadéro, 11 Mai 1886* (Paris: Impr. de Motteroz, n.d. [1886]). Eugène Manuel's poem (read publicly at a soirée celebrating Pasteur at the Trocadero on 11 May 1886) intricately links Pasteur to the laboratory. 'Où donc est sa grandeur? / Où se fait son histoire? / Elle se fait là-bas, dans ce laboratoire, / Où l'univers est suspendu; / Où, grave et simple, un homme, acharné sur sa tâche, / Engage avec nos maux un duel sans relâche, / Et nous rend tout l'honneur perdu!' (Where, then, is his grandeur? / Where is his history made? / It is there, in that laboratory, / Where the universe is suspended; / Where, simple and grave, a man struggles at his task, / Engages in a relentless duel with our ills, / And restores to us all the lost honour.)

28 Louis Pasteur, *Jubilée de M. Pasteur* (Paris: Gauthier-Villars et fils, 1893), as cited in Geison, *The Private Science of Louis Pasteur*, p. 262.

29 Edelfelt letter, 1887, in Association Arbois-Pasteur, *Rappelez-vous Pasteur l'Arboisien*. 'Les meilleurs portraits qu'on fait, ne sont en général jamais commandés ni payés, mais sont faits pour la gloire.'

30 Bertel Hintze, 'Albert Edelfelt', unpublished manuscript in Musée Pasteur archives, Edelfelt Dossier, c.1935, pp. 184–189. Bertel Hintze has claimed that Edelfelt's painting became a cultural weapon for the Finnish public because it was believed to exhibit the strength and sophistication of Finland as an independent nation.

31 Erik Werenskiold, *Aftenposten*, 8 November 1886, Oslo, as cited in Siulolovao Challons-Lipton, *The Scandinavian Pupils of the Atelier Bonnat 1867–1894* (Lewiston: Edwin Mellen Press, 2001), pp. 127–128.

32 Challons-Lipton, *The Scandinavian Pupils*, pp. 127–129.

33 Challons-Lipton, *The Scandinavian Pupils*, pp. 17–23. For Zola's criticism of Bonnat, see Émile Zola, *Documents littéraires, études et portraits* (Paris: G. Charpentier, 1881), which contains his reviews of the 1878 and 1879 Salons.

34 Louis Bauzon, Paul Berthelot, Paul Bonnefon *et al.*, *Artistes contemporains des pays de Guyenne, Béarn, Laintonge et Languedox* (Bordeaux: G. Gounouilhou, 1889), p. 8. 'Quand vous parcourez le Salon, aux jours de foule, et que vous suivez le courant où il vous mène, c'est-à-dire devant les œuvres qui ont la vogue, qui "font recette", et que tout le monde, depuis le plus naïf des visiteurs jusqu'aux connaisseurs les plus raffinés, veut avoir vues, un des premiers tableaux devant lequel le flot vous poussera sera un portrait de Bonnat. Vous l'apercevrez, tout en entrant, dans la salle où il se trouve; par-dessus la mer houleuse des têtes et des chapeaux, vous

distinguerez quelque figure fortement dessinée, solidement peinte, se présentant avec un relief à friser le trompe-l'œil, et écrasant autour d'elle, de ses tons robustes et de son modelé puissant, tout ce qui l'entoure; du plus loin que vous la verrez, pour peu que la manière des principaux artistes contemporains vous soit connue, vous n'hésiterez pas, vous direz: "C'est un Bonnat!" et vous ne vous tromperez point, car ici la marque de fabrique saute aux yeux, la griffe de l'ouvrier se traduit à chaque touche.'

35 'French Painters "Chez Eux" III', *The Illustrated American*, III (27 September 1890), 609–613, as cited in Alisa Luxenberg, 'Léon Bonnat (1833–1922)', PhD dissertation, New York University, 1990, p. 188.

36 Luxenberg, 'Léon Bonnat', p. 182.

37 Letter from Edelfelt to his mother, 30 November 1885, in Association Arbois-Pasteur, *Rappelez-vous Pasteur l'Arboisien*, p. 54: 'une redingote bien meilleure que la mienne'.

38 Bauzon *et al.*, *Artistes contemporains des pays de Guyenne*, p. 12. 'On a dit de M. Bonnat, pour atténuer l'éloge et la gloire qui lui sont dus, que son art tenait de la prose. Ne chicanons pas sur les termes: acceptons le mot de prose, puisque prose il y a; mais croyons bien au moins, pour nous en tenir à son admirable et magistrale galerie de portraits contemporains, que la postérité ne s'en plaindra point, car cette prose est singulièrment énergique et virile, nette, expressive et sonore: elle a le parler haut, ferme et clair; elle a l'autorité, elle s'impose. Prose donc, enfin, si l'on veut; mais c'est la prose de l'histoire.' (It is said of M. Bonnat, to attenuate the praises and glory that are his due, that there is something prosaic about his work. Let us not quibble over terminology: let us accept the word *prose,* since prose there is. But at very least let us believe, limiting ourselves to his admirable and masterly gallery of contemporary portraits, that posterity will find no cause for complaint, for this prose is singularly energetic and virile, clean, expressive and resounding: it speaks loudly, decisively and clearly; it has authority, it is imposing. Prose, therefore, if one wishes; but it is the prose of history.)

39 Léon Bonnat, 'Préface', in Marcel Nicolle, *Rembrandt aux exposition d'Amsterdam et de Londres* (Paris: Ollendorff, 1899), p. I. 'Ce qui frappe chez Rembrandt, c'est la puissance, la force et l'éclat. Il représente la vie dans toute son intensité. On voit ses personnages, on cause avec eux, il ressuscite et ranime toute une époque.'

40 Bonnat, 'Préface', p. III. 'Rembrandt possède déjà à fond la science du portrait. Il connaît la construction de la tête humaine mieux que personne.'

41 Léonce Bénédite, *La Peinture au XIXe siècle d'après les chefs-d'œuvres des maîtres et les meilleurs tableaux des principaux artistes* (Paris: E. Flammarion, n.d. [c.1906]), pp. xi–xii. '[L]e mouvement réaliste s'accentue dans un sens démocratique et populaire, qui suit la marche des progrès politiques et avec un caractère inédit de méthode et l'objectivité dans l'observation, qui est en concordance avec le développement intense de l'esprit scientifique.'

42 For a discussion of the relationship between realism, republicanism, and science, see Levin, *Republican Art and Ideology in Late Nineteenth-Century France,* pp. 37–41.

43 Olmer, *Salon de 1866*, p. 76. 'Ce portrait est complet. Il dit l'homme et le labeur de sa vie, et il pourrait bien être le portrait definitif de M. Pasteur.'

44 Lafenestre, 'Le Salon', p. 581. 'Le portrait de M. Bonnat est l'image historique; celui de M. Edelfelt n'est qu'une image anecdotique.'

45 Lostalot, 'Le Salon de 1886: la peinture', p. 459. 'La peinture de M. Edelfelt nous montre M. Pasteur absorbé dans ses recherches; la tête penchée, il consulte du regard un bocal de verre où pend un lambeau de chair sanglante: c'est la terrible moelle de lapin rabique qui, par l'effort de son génie, se convertira en baume guérisseur du plus horrible mal. Le tableau est excellent et rempli d'intérêt; la lumière joue librement sur les ustensiles du laboratoire, et cependant aucun détail ne vient distraire de la grandeur du sujet.'

46 Louis Ganderax, 'Causerie sur Le Salon', *La République française*, 10 June 1886, n.p. 'Le principal, aujourd'hui, pour la peinture de genre ou plutôt pour la peinture, c'est l'homme; j'entends l'homme contemporain, saisi dans son milieu habituel: à la campagne, à la ville ou à la maison … Quoi d'étonnant? Vers la fin de ce siècle, où la science des religions et l'histoire des peuples ont commencé de se bien établir, ne voyons-nous pas la vogue triomphale du roman? Et de quelle sorte de roman? De celui qui se fonde sur l'observation de la réalité pour représenter à notre esprit un groupe de personnes contemporaines ou une seule. En s'adressant à nos yeux, la peinture à l'heure qu'il est, ne fait guère autre chose.' (The main thing today in genre painting, or rather, painting in general, is man, by which I mean contemporary man, captured in his habitual surroundings: in the countryside, in town, at home … Why should that surprise us? Towards the end of this century, when the science of religions and the history of nations have begun to be well established, are we not seeing the triumph of the novel? And what sort of novel? One that is grounded the observation of reality in order to represent to our minds an individual or a group of contemporary people. Today's painting, addressing itself to our eyes, is scarcely doing anything else.)

47 Eugène-Melchior de Vogüé, 'De la littérature réalistes – à propos du roman russe', *Revue des deux mondes* (May–June 1886), 289: 'ont abouti à un art d'observation plus que d'imagination … Jaloux de la rigueur des procédés scientifiques.'

48 Arthur Stevens, 'De la modernité dans l'art', *L'art moderne* (10 May 1886). 'Pour faire un portrait, l'artiste résume toute ce qu'il a médité dans sa vie; il met en jeu toute sa science, afin de faire vivre le modèle. Il est mal à l'aise pour inventer et pour tricher.'

49 Lafenestre, 'Le Salon', p. 597. 'Autant il peut être utile d'expliquer une physionomie par l'accompagnement choisi de quelques accessoires révélant ses habitudes intellectuelles ou physiques, autant il pourrait être inconvenant de noyer cette physionomie sous l'amas de détails exacts, mais parfaitement insignifians [sic]. Le naturalisme, tel que peuvent le pratiquer les portraitistes … n'est point du tout l'acception en bloc de tous les détails qu'offre pêle-mêle la nature, mais seulement le choix intelligent, parmi les détails, de ceux qui peuvent communiquer plus de clarté, plus d'éclat, plus de force, plus de charme au sujet traité.' (To the same extent that it can be useful to explain a subject's physiognomy by way of a select group of props that reveal his intellectual or physical habits, it can be unseemly to

submerge this physiognomy under a mass of details that are accurate yet utterly insignificant. Naturalism, as it can be practised by portraitists … does not at all imply the wholesale acceptance of all the details that nature offers pell mell, but rather an intelligent selection, among all the details, of those which can lend the most clarity, the most brilliance, the most strength and the most charm to the subject portrayed.)

50 Lafenestre, 'Le Salon', p. 597: 'le mobilier parle aussi haut que la figure, la physionomie du penseur s'efface au milieu des verreries qui scintillent, et, malgré l'intérêt de curiosité que la postérité attachera certainement au reportage minutieux et ingénieux du peintre suédois, ce n'est pas à lui qu'elle demandera l'image définitive de M. Pasteur'.

51 Luxenberg, 'Léon Bonnat (1833–1922)', pp. 138–139.

52 As cited in Vincent Ducourau, 'Introduction', in *Léon Bonnat, 1833–1922: portraits d'apogée* (Bayonne: Musée Bonnat, 1998), n.p. 'Une œuvre d'art et une théorie fondée sur des recherches expérimentales ont ceci de commun qu'elles nous proposent l'une et l'autre comme un arrangement conclu entre l'intelligence et la nature après d'âpres combats … [u]ne manière d'armistice difficile à faire accepter par le jugement du public, surtout quand l'artiste s'attaque au mystères de la nature humaine dans le but de restituer en même temps que la ressemblance physique d'un individu, ce qu'il y a en lui de moins inconstant et de plus invisible.'

53 Lafenestre, 'Le Salon', p. 598. 'Le savant est isolé, bien isolé, pour qu'on le voie mieux, comme une statue sur son piédestal. Son visage, dont la clarté, au-dessus des vêtemens [sic] noirs, saisit seul le regard, s'enlève, avec une précision énergique, comme une médaille rudiment frappée, sur le fond indifférent, avec une force d'expression intellectuelle d'autant plus entière que rien alentour ne peut l'atténuer … Il est permis de croire que, chaque fois qu'il s'agira d'un visage où l'intelligence surtout doit parler, il sera convenable d'user de discrétion et de ne pas étouffer cette parole de l'âme sous le bruissement confus du murmure des choses.'

54 Luxenberg points out that Bonnat was familiar with and surrounded by photographs. Although there is no evidence to explain his use of photography, or that his use differed from that of other artists, it is most likely that he used them in order to create physical likeness. Interestingly, Luxenberg notes that Bonnat's artistic development ran counter to photography's. Luxenberg, 'Léon Bonnat (1833–1922)', p. 159.

55 J. Meriem, 'Tableaux et statues (Salon de 1882)', in Olivier Lépine, *Équivoques: peintures françaises du XIXe siècle*, exhibition catalogue, Musée des Arts Décoratifs, 9 March–14 May 1973 (Paris: Union central des arts décoratifs, 1973), p. 31: 'une précision froide et photographique.'

56 C. de Beaulieu *Le Salon de 1886*, supplement to *La gazette du dimanche* (Paris: Blond et Barral, 1886), pp. 24–25: 'on ne peut que se répéter en admirant la peinture du maître et en le priant d'en changer les fonds.'

57 Henry Fèvre, *Études sur le Salon de 1886 et sur l'exposition des impressionistes* (Paris: Tresse et Stock, 1886), p. 33. 'Comme portraitiste, M. Bonnat ne fait l'effet que d'un passable coloriste de fallacieuses photographies.'

58 Charles Ponsonailhe, 'Salon de 1886', *L'Artiste* (June 1886), 440–441, as translated in Weisberg, 'The Representation of Doctors at Work in Salon Art of the Early Third Republic in France', p. 605.
59 Alan Sekula, 'The Body and the Archive', *October*, 39 (1986), 7.
60 For an informative discussion of how photography functioned as a tool of social discipline, see John Tagg, 'Power and Photography: Part One, A Means of Surveillance: The Photograph as Evidence in Law', *Screen Education*, 36 (1980), 17–55, and Tagg, *The Burden of Representation: Essays on Photographies and Histories* (Basingstoke: Palgrave Macmillan, 1988).
61 The literature on eighteenth- and nineteenth-century physiognomy and phrenology is extensive. For discussions related to art and medicine, see Martin Kemp and Marina Wallace, *Spectacular Bodies: The Art and Science of the Human Body from Leonardo to Now* (London: Hayward Gallery, 2000), pp. 95–146; Clair (ed.), *L'âme au corps: arts et sciences 1793–1993*, particularly essays in 'Le temps de la phrénologie', pp. 196–299; Barbara Maria Stafford, *Body Criticism: Imagining the Unseen in Enlightenment Art and Medicine* (Cambridge, MA: MIT Press, 1991), pp. 84–129.
62 Julien Leclerq, *La Physionomie, visages et caractères* (Paris: Chez tous les librairies, 1896), pp. 5–6. 'C'est la science qui a pour but la connaissance de la nature intérieure de l'homme par sa nature extérieure … Personne ne 'masque', personne ne peut s'arroger des facultés qu'il ne possède pas … la physionomie de l'homme ne ment pas.'
63 Elizabeth Emery, 'Dornac's "At Home" Photographs', *Proceedings of the Western Society for French History*, 36 (2008), 221.
64 For a discussion of how nineteenth-century art critics believed Bonnat's realism fulfilled Republican aims, see Luxenberg, 'Léon Bonnat', pp. 130–131.
65 Paul Gsell, 'Pasteur intime', *La Revue encyclopédique* (14 January 1895), p. 20. 'Pour ses enfants le grand homme a toujours été un excellent père: ses amis se souviennent de l'avoir vu faisant danser un bébé sur ses genoux pendant que sa femme en déshabillait un autre pour le mettre au lit.'
66 William Walton, *Chefs-d'œuvre de l'exposition universelle de Paris, 1889* (Philadelphia: George Barrie, 1889), p. 102.
67 Olmer, *Salon de 1886*, p. 76: 'nous montre le grand savant sous l'aspect aimable et familial d'un papa gâteau, heureux de montrer sa petite-fille. C'est une gloire aussi d'avoir de beaux petits-enfants; mais elle est peut-être un peu trop partagée, et ce n'est pas sous cet aspect que la postérité se représentera l'homme qui a attaché son nom à la guérison de la rage.'
68 For an account of medical beliefs that contributed to public fears of depopulation, see Nye, *Crime, Madness and Politics in Modern France*.
69 Fèvre, *Études sur le Salon de 1886,* p. 33. 'M. Bonnat a peint un Pasteur théâtral, la main sur la tête de sa petite fille, un Pasteur qui ne se ressemble même pas; sa peau est comme huilée, et on redoute pour lui la jaunisse … M. Pasteur n'a pas du tout cet air fatal et pontifiant de don Quichotte du microbe dont M. Bonnat l'a empalé … M. A. Edelfelt a certainement enfoncé M. Bonnat dans la peinture du célèbre désenrageur. Son Pasteur est plus bonhomme, plus fouillé, plus animé,

dans son laboratoire, flairant des fioles, en pleine investigation scientifique; la tête ressort aussi énergiquement que celle du premier sans la fausseté d'ombre ni tous ses ridicules de teintes maladives.'

70 Percy F. Frankland and Grace C. Frankland, *Pasteur* (New York: Macmillan, 1898), pp. 209–210, as cited in Geison, *The Private Science of Louis Pasteur*, p. 271.

71 'Si M. Bonnat modifiait sa couleur sèche, noire, immuablement figée dans la sauce dont il transmit orgueilleusement la recette aux marmitons qui s'efforcent d'atteindre au génie du cuisinier chef, il y aurait sans doute des murmures.' 'Le Salon de 1886', *L'Art moderne* (23 May 1886), p. 163.

72 Gsell, 'Pasteur intime', p. 20. 'un peu croquemitaine.'

73 Paul Lambert, *Le Salon de 1886* (Paris: C. Marpon, E. Flammarion, 1886), p. 18. 'La pauvre jeune fille a la figure et les mains passées au jus de tabac. Tendres couleurs de l'enfance!'

74 'Le Salon de 1886', *Journal des arts* (26 May 1886). 'La petite fille n'a rien de bien enfantin et les tons de sa figure ont le même accent accusé que ceux du visage de son grand-père.'

75 Lambert, *Le Salon de 1886*, p. 18. 'Ce portrait qui, à première vue, a l'air d'être celui d'un aveugle conduit par une jeune fille, est certainement un des plus faibles du Salon.'

76 Lambert, *Le Salon de 1886*, p. 45. '*L'Aveugle* de M. Landelle, me fait l'effet d'une seconde édition du portrait de M. Pasteur par M. Bonnat, avec la différence que l'aveugle de M. Landelle a l'air d'y voir clair, tandis que le portrait de M. Bonnat ressemble à un aveugle.' (M. Landelle's *L'Aveugle* feels to me like a second edition of M. Bonnat's portrait of M. Pasteur, with the difference that M. Landelle's blind man looks like he sees clearly, whereas M. Bonnat's portrait looks like a blind man.)

77 Schickore, *The Microscope and the Eye*.

78 Schickore's history of the microscope aptly explores how theories of vision and understandings of the retina informed ideas about the restrictions and possibilities of microscopy, and vice versa. *The Microscope and the Eye*, pp. 25, 238–239.

79 For a general account of the history of germ theory, see John Waller, *The Discovery of the Germ: Twenty Years that Transformed the Way we Think About Disease* (Cambridge: Icon Books, 2002).

80 For an account of the use of photomicrographs and their relationship to scientific photograph and objectivity, see Daston and Galison, *Objectivity*, pp. 115–190.

81 For an analysis of how conceptions of sight changed with the emergence of new technologies of vision, see Crary, *Techniques of the Observer* and Schickore, *The Microscope and the Eye*.

82 A. Burais, 'Applications de la photographie à la médecine', PhD dissertation, Paris, Faculté de medecine, 22 July 1896, pp. 27–28. 'Dès l'origine de la Photographie, on a compris les services que cette nouvelle conquête scientifique pourrait rendre aux savants utilisant le microscope. Non seulement elle fixe d'une façon durable l'image d'une préparation qui peut être modifiée au bout de peu de temps, mais encore, par son caractère d'indiscutable authenticité, elle permet de mieux faire

comprendre les descriptions et parfois montre des particularités ou des détails qui, au microscope, peuvent échapper à l'œil le plus exercé.

Comme le disait, en 1887, M. le Dr Roux, chef du service de Microbiologie technique à l'Institut Pasteur: "En Microbiologie, la meilleur manière d'écrire est de mettre un texte court à côté d'un grand nombre de planches bien faites."' (From the inception of photography, we have understood the benefits this new scientific triumph could bring to scientists using the microscope. Not only does a photograph durably fix the image of a specimen that may later be modified, but also, through its quality of undisputable authenticity, it allows for a better understanding of verbal descriptions and sometimes shows particularities or details that, through the microscope, might escape even the most practised eye.)

83 Roux, as quoted in Burais, 'Applications de la Photographie'. 'En Microbiologie, la meilleure manière d'écrire est de mettre un texte court à côté d'un grand nombre de planches bien faites'.

84 Letter from Pasteur to Mme Sainte-Claire Deville, 5 October 1881, in Louis Pasteur, *Correspondance, 1840–1895, réunie et annotée par Vallery-Radot* (Paris: Flammarion, 1940), p. 259. 'Chère Madame, J'ai été bien heureux de recevoir le portrait de mon cher ami. Mon Dieu! Qu'il est ressemblant! Que vous devez être heureuse de le regarder et de lire dans son âme en le voyant! Je connais trois photographies admirables, celle de M. V. Regnault, celle de M. Brongniart et celle-ci. Mais celle-ci est plus belle et plus vraie encore que les deux autres. Vous me feriez le plus grand plaisir, chère Madame, de me donner le nom du photographe. Est-il toujours aussi bien inspiré? J'aimerais laisser à ma famille quelque chose d'approchant, le jour où il faudra lui dire le dernier adieu. Merci donc, et mille fois, chère Madame, de votre gracieux souvenir. L. Pasteur.'

85 Photography was often associated with death in the nineteenth century: Balzac's belief that he lost a layer of himself when photographed and the use of photography in mortuary portraiture evidence the association of the medium with death. More recently, Roland Barthes conceptualised photography as a medium of death, seeing death in every photograph as a statement of 'that-has-been'. Barthes, *Camera Lucida: Reflections on Photography*, trans. Richard Howard (New York: Hill and Wang, 1981).

86 For an informative account of Regnault's role in photography, see Laurie Dahlberg, *Victor Regnault and the Advance of Photography: the Art of Avoiding Errors* (Princeton: Princeton University Press, 2004).

87 Jordanova, *Defining Features*, pp. 41–43.

88 Emery, 'Dornac's "At Home" Photographs', 209–224.

89 Gaston Tissandier, 'Nos savants chez eux', *La Nature*, 20 (13 February 1892), 168–170.

90 For the discovery of this invention and its controversy, see André Jammes, 'A Glaring Act of Scientific Privacy?', in *Photography: Discovery and Invention, Papers Delivered at a Symposium Celebrating the Invention of Photography* (Malibu: J. Paul Getty Museum, 1990), pp. 63–70; and Dahlberg, *Victor Regnault and the Advance of Photography*, pp. 10, 17, 26–28.

91 Between 1839 and 1850, the Académie de Sciences heard over 230 reports on photography. Dahlberg, *Victor Regnault and the Advance of Photography*, p. 24.
92 Dahlberg, *Victor Regnault and the Advance of Photography*, p. 79.
93 'Ce dessin offre un double intérêt. Non seulement il est le portrait de l'une des grandes gloires scientifiques de la France: il est en outre la première épreuve photographique réussie d'après nature. Exécuté dans le cabinet de physique du Collège de France par Blanquart-Evrard, en présence d'une commission de membres de l'Académie des sciences et de l'Académie des Beaux-Arts.'
94 Vallery-Radot, *La Vie de Pasteur*, p. 95. 'Si vous placez cette épreuve à côté du portrait de votre père, vous pourrez voir réunies les images de deux personnes qui vous ont aimé à peu près d'une même façon.'
95 For examinations of how photographic portraits were used for personal and professional propaganda, see Donald E. English, *Political Uses of Photography in the Third French Republic, 1871–1914* (Ann Arbor: University of Michigan Press, 1984).
96 'A M. le Docteur Roux, très respectueux et admiratif hommage, Nadar, portrait exécuté en 1886'.
97 Rosalind Krauss, 'Tracing Nadar', *October*, 5 (1978), 29–47.
98 Cited in Krauss, 'Tracing Nadar', 30.
99 Krauss sees the trace in photography standing between science and spiritualism. See Krauss, 'Tracing Nadar', 35.
100 Letter from Edelfelt to his mother, 23 April 1885, in Association Arbois-Pasteur, *Rappelez-vous Pasteur l'Arboisien*, p. 50. 'Pasteur est en train de faire la plus grande découverte de sa vie: trouver le vaccin contre la rage.'
101 Weisberg and Hansen have argued that while Edelfelt's portrait of Pasteur became a celebrated image of the scientist as the saviour against rabies, at the time the painting was made, neither Edelfelt nor Pasteur could have known that the vaccine would be successful. See Weisberg and Hansen, 'Collaboration of Art and Science in Albert Edelft's Portrait of Louis Pasteur: The Making of an Enduring Icon', p. 73.
102 Letter from Edelfelt to his mother, 17 June 1885, in *Rappelez-vous Pasteur l'Arboisien*, pp. 52–53. It is likely that Edelfelt mistakenly claimed that the spine belonged to a dog rather than a rabbit as these experiments were not performed on dog spines. 'Pasteur se dit très satisfait. Le vieil original est très intéressé, propose des changements etc. … Comme il a peint lui-même, il sait parler d'art. Il m'a fait enlever la bouteille de microbes et à la place mettre dans sa main un grand ballon de verre avec à l'intérieur un morceau de la moelle épinière d'un chien suspendue à un fil. Le vieux dit que c'est quelque chose dont on n'a pas encore connaissance, mais qui va avoir une grande importance plus tard.' (Pasteur says he is very satisfied. The old eccentric is very interested; he proposes changes, etc. … Since he has done some painting himself, he knows how to speak about art. He had me remove the bottle of microbes and instead have him hold in his hand a round-bottomed flask containing the spinal cord of a dog, suspended by a thread. The old man says that this is something that is not yet known, but that will be of great importance later on.)

103 Adrien Loir, *À l'Ombre de Pasteur* (Paris: Le Mouvement sanitaire, 1938), p. 66.
104 Pasteur, *Correspondance, 1840–1895*, pp. 491–492. For an account of Pasteur's political work, see Geison, *The Private Science of Louis Pasteur*, pp. 43–45.
105 Doctor August Lutaud, *M. Pasteur et la rage: Exposé de la méthode Pasteur – fréquence de la rage – insuccès du nouveau traitement – la rage du chien et du loup – statistiques complètes, etc.* (Paris: J. Lévy, 1887), as translated in Geison, *The Private Science of Louis Pasteur*, p. vi.
106 Pasteur, letter from Pasteur to his son Jean-Baptiste, 25 September 1885, in Pasteur, *Correspondance, 1840–1895*, p. 41.
107 Pasteur, Letter from Pasteur to Bonnat, 11 March 1886, in *Correspondance 1840–1895*, p. 62. 'Mon Cher Bonnat, Je copie: "Je viens de voir votre portrait chez Bonnat. Il est magnifique et c'est une de ses plus belles œuvres. La petite fille est ravissante comme pose et ressemble à sa mère. Je suis bien heureux pour vous et je vous en félicite. De tout cœur votre tout dévoué, Henner" Je n'ajoute rien sinon que j'ose penser comme Henner et que je vais envoyer la lettre à mon fils pour M. Jacobsen. Cet homme bien écrit qu'il n'ose pas réclamer à Bonnat une photographie. Bien à vous, mon cher grand maître. L. Pasteur.'
108 For a discussion of the close relationship between the Pasteurs and the Jacobsens, as well as an account of the commissioning of Bonnat's portrait, see Denise Wrotnowska, 'Une amitié de savants, Pasteur et Jacobsen', *Histoires des sciences médicales* (July–December 1970), 137–139.
109 Most beer in northern Europe was only available seasonally, as hot weather affected the bacteria in beer. See E.M. Sigsworth, 'Science and the Brewing Industry, 1850–1900', *The Economic History Review*, 17:3 (1965), 536–550.
110 For a discussion of nineteenth-century French advertising, see Marc Martin, *Trois siècles de publicité en France* (Paris: Editions Odile Jacob, 1992).
111 Louis Pasteur, *Études sur la bière; ses maladies, causes qui les provoquent, procédé pour la rendre inaltérable, avec une théorie nouvelle de la fermentation* (Paris: Gauthier-Villars, 1876), p. vii. 'L'idée de ces recherches m'a été inspirée par nos malheurs. Je les ai entreprises aussitôt après la guerre de 1870 et poursuivies sans relâche depuis cette époque, avec la résolution de les mener assez loin pour marquer d'un progrès durable une industrie dans laquelle l'Allemagne nous est supérieure.' (This research has been inspired by our hardships. I undertook it immediately after the 1870 war and have continued relentlessly since that time, with the determination to carry it far enough to make headway and a lasting progress in an industry in which Germany is superior to us.)
112 For an account of Pasteur's funding, see Geison, *The Private Science of Louis Pasteur*, pp. 40–42.
113 Pasteur, letter to Vallery-Radot on 21 May 1880, in *Correspondance, 1840–1895*, pp. 135–136. 'Je voudrais que le nom de M. Jacobsen fût glorifié à côté de celui de Paul Dubois par un critique d'art authorisé. Vous êtes connu au journal *Le temps* dont la revue du Salon est faite par un écrivain de talent, Paul Mantz. Il serait très désirable qu'en parlant de l'œuvre de Paul Dubois … M. P. Mantz voulût bien raconter en quelques lignes l'origine du buste, signaler la générosité éclairée

de ce riche industriel qui a consacré quinze cent mille francs à l'érection d'un laboratoire destiné aux progrès du brasseur.'

114 For a discussion of this exhibition, see Anne-Birgitte Fonsmark, *Manet, Gauguin, Rodin … Chefs-d'œuvre de la Ny Carlsberg Glyptotek de Copenhague*, exhibition catalogue, Musée d'Orsay (Paris: Réunions des musées nationaux, 1995), pp. 2–3.

115 Pasteur, 1 January 1888, in Pasteur, *Correspondance, 1840–1895*, IV, p. 235: 'tous nos artistes vous connaissent et parlent de vos libéralités avec de grands éloges et toutes sortes de sentiments reconnaissants.'

116 Jules Claretie, *Le Temps*, 1 July 1890, as cited in Wrotnowska 'Une amitié de savants', pp. 137–139: 'l'art français le plus élevé qui soit.'

117 For a range of examinations of the relationship between French nationalism and the arts, see Hargrove and McWilliam (eds), *Nationalism and French Visual Culture 1870–1914*.

118 Hintze, 'Albert Edelfelt', p. 4.

119 Weisberg, 'The Representation of Doctors at Work in Salon Art of the Early Third Republic in France', p. 620.

120 'Salon de 1886', *L'Art* (14 June 1886), p. 251: 'toute au dernier rang de la salle XIX, si haut qu'elle est invisible.'

121 Yvonne Le Garrec, 'Le "Laboratoire de Pasteur" par L. L Gsell au Musée de Vannes', *Association des anciens élèves de l'Institut Pasteur*, newsletter 2001, p. 57.

122 Walton described Gsell's and Brouillet's works: 'These are very large canvases, with many figures the size of life or near it.' Walton, *Chefs-d'œuvre*, p. 88.

123 Hugues le Roux, 'La Vie à Paris: A travers le Salon', *Le Temps*, 30 April 1887. 'On n'imagine pas le nombre des médecins dont le portrait figure au Salon. Comme M. Charcot, comme M. Péan, M. Pasteur a été peint dans sa clinique. On inocule sous ses yeux un petit enfant; un grand Arabe attend son tour.'

124 Roger Ballu, 'Salon de 1887', supplement to *L'illustration* (30 April 1887), n. 2305, n.p.: 'peut-être a-t-il joué de Malheur en livrant au public une Scène chez M. Pasteur l'année où M. Gervex et M. Brouillet exposaient des scènes analogues. Il est des comparaisons fatales qui sont préjudiciables.'

125 Olivier Merson, 'Le Salon de 1887', *Le Monde illustré* (14 May 1887), n.p. 'M. Pasteur dans son cabinet de la rue d'Ulm, cabinet encombré de gens accourus de partout, confiants dans la méthode de l'illustre savant. A gauche, un Arabe, des Arméniens, des Russes; à droite, une foule; au centre, une jeune mère tenant dans les bras son enfant auquel l'opérateur s'apprête à inoculer le virus sauveur. Debout, au premier plan, de profil, M. Pasteur lit une lettre que lui a remis l'Arabe.'

126 For a discussion of France's 'civilizing mission' over the course of the nineteenth century, see Margaret A. Majumdar, *Postcoloniality: The French Dimension* (New York: Berghahn Books, 2007), 23.

127 Jules Ferry, 'Madagascar, le devoir et le refus du "recueillement," Chambre des députés (28 juillet 1885)', in Odile Rudelle (ed.), *La République des citoyens. Tome II* (Paris: Imprimerie Nationale, 1996), p. 318.

128 Gerald Geison, 'Organizations, Products, and Marketing in Pasteur's Scientific Enterprise', *History and Philosophy of the Life Sciences*, 24:1 (2002), 42–44.

129 Marx, 'M. Pasteur et le Dr Peter', n.p.

130 'Séance du 18 janvier 1886', in *Bulletin de l'Académie de médecine,* vol. 17 (Paris: G. Masson, 1887), 112. 'Aussi je ne crains pas de lui dire: comme médecin, comme académicien, comme philanthrope, comme patriote, il a entrepris et il poursuit une campagne déplorable.'

131 Mercutio, 'Causerie', *La Revue blanche* (15 April 1886), n.p. 'Vous savez que M. Pasteur n'est pas médecin, il n'a jamais étudié la médecine. Or, n'étant pas docteur il ne peut faire lui-même ses inoculations et est obligé de s'adjoindre un vrai médecin pour pratiquer ces petites opérations. … Cela n'enlèvera pas une parcelle de gloire à M. Pasteur de n'avoir pas fait lui-même les inoculations dont les agents actifs ont été préparés par sa méthode.'

132 J. Hirschler, *Nos docteurs* (Paris: J. Hirschler, 1896), p. 12. '[L]a médecine actuelle s'est lancée dans ce mouvement de découverte. Grâce à ses admirables méthodes expérimentales, grâce au génie de quelques hommes comme Pasteur, qui ont ouvert à ses investigations, à ses exploitations, un monde nouveau, elle s'est rajeunie, elle s'est transformée.'

133 Hirschler, *Nos docteurs*, p. 17. 'Où est la médecine dans toutes ces découvertes? Nulle part! Où est la Science qui doit profiter au médecin? Partout!'

134 Jordanova points out that although Jenner was well known for his work on smallpox, he was also a surgeon, country squire, and natural historian. Therefore, his social and professional positions were never simple. Jordanova, *Defining Features*, p. 24.

135 A.P., 'Echos de la Science', *La Revue blanche* (15 January 1886), 5. 'Pasteur s'est élevé, cette année, au premier rang des bienfaiteurs de l'humanité; il est, avec Jenner, le propagateur de la vaccine, un des hommes ayant le plus mérité la reconnaissance de ses semblables.'

136 Ernest Maindron, 'Une Caricature sur la découverte de la Vaccine – Jenner – M. Pasteur', *La Nature*, 14:2 (1886), 679–704, 160. 'Presque toutes les grandes découvertes ont trouvé d'obscurs détracteurs … On aurait dû comprendre que c'est à l'avenir seul qu'il appartient de juger sainement de ces choses.'

137 'M. Pasteur et les Conseillers Municipaux', *L'Évènement*, 30 March 1886, n.p. 'Tout se passe rapidement et dans le plus grand ordre; j'ai vu défiler devant moi des enfants de tous âges, des hommes et des femmes de toutes classes et de toutes les nationalités, des soldats d'Afrique et de Tunisie, et enfin les fameux moujiks, de tous les plus dangereusement atteints.'

138 A. Cartaz, 'La rage: traitement prophylactique de M. Pasteur', *La Nature*, 14:1 (27 February 1886), 214. 'De tous côtés, des victimes des chiens enragés arrivaient réclamer le bénéfice du traitement de M. Pasteur. C'étaient les gens de Brie, comme les appelait familièrement le maître, des étrangers, des Allemands, des femmes, des enfants etc., tout un monde qui, chaque matin, venaient remplir le cabinet attenant au grand laboratoire.'

139 J.H. Crespi, 'Pasteur at Home', *Gentleman's Magazine* (March 1890), 266–273.

140 Alexis Martin, 'Guide du visiteur – la peinture et la sculpture au Salon de 1887', supplement to *La Gazettte des femmes* (10 May 1887), 54: 'félicitons-le sincèrement d'arrêter non seulement la foule, mais encore les connaisseurs devant sa toile.'

141 Foucault, *Naissance de la Clinique*.

142 Marx, 'M. Pasteur et le Docteur Peter', n.p. 'Le meilleur docteur … est celui dont le regard pénètre sous la mystérieuse enveloppe pour deviner les mystères qu'elle cache.'

143 Jean de Nivelle, 'Haute-comique', *Le Soleil*, 31 March 1886, n.p. 'M. Pasteur pratique ses inoculations au ventre. Pourquoi là plutôt qu'ailleurs? Pourquoi pas au bras? M. Pasteur reçoit dans son laboratoire, des femmes et des jeunes filles, et je n'hésiste pas à qualifier d'inconvenante cette inoculation au ventre.'

144 de Nivelle, 'Haute-comique', n.p. 'Hélas! Pourquoi s'être arrêté en chemin? Pourquoi n'avoir pas déclaré tout nettement qu'il s'agissait de la fondation d'un Institut pornographique?'

145 Louis Lumet, *Pasteur, sa vie, son œuvre: ouvrage orné de 121 gravures* (Paris: Hachette, 1923), pp. 168–170, as translated in Geison, *The Private Science of Louis Pasteur*, p. 259.

146 Crespi, 'Pasteur at Home', p. 271.

147 For an account of the impact of diseases on European colonisation, see Philip D. Curtin, *Disease and Empire: The Health of European Troops in the Conquest of Africa* (Cambridge: Cambridge University Press, 1998); and Curtin, *Death by Migration: Europe's Encounter with the Tropical World in the Nineteenth Century* (Cambridge: Cambridge University Press, 1989); Laurence Monnais, 'Preventing Medicine and "mission civilisatrice": Uses of the BCG Vaccine in French Colonial Vietnam Between the Two World Wars', *IJAPS*, 2:1 (2006), 40; Anne-Marie Moulin, 'Patriarchal Science: The Network of the Overseas Pasteur Institutes', in P. Petitjean, Catherine Jami and A.M. Moulin (eds), *Science and Empires: Historical Studies about Scientific Development and European Expansion* (Dordrecht: Kluwer Academic Publishers, 1992), pp. 307–322. For a discussion of malaria and the expansion of French colonies, see William B. Cohen, 'Malaria and French Imperialism', *The Journal of African History*, 24:1 (1983), 23–36.

148 John Farley argues that the study of tropical medicine was fundamentally imperialist. For his examination of late nineteenth- and early twentieth-century tropical medicine, see *Bilharzia: A History of Imperial Tropical Medicine* (Cambridge: Cambridge University Press, 1990).

149 See James R. Lehning for an examination of how French colonial subjects were turned into 'good' republicans. Lehning, *To Be a Citizen: The Political Cutlure of the Early French Third Republic* (Ithaca: Cornell University Press, 2001).

150 Gaston Tissandier, 'M. Pasteur et le traitement de la rage', *La Nature*, 14:1 (29 May 1886), p. 401. 'Son attention fut attirée par un rassemblement de promeneurs qui entouraient un groupe d'Arabes. C'étaient "les Arabes de Pasteur", suivant l'expression des assistants, ou plutôt les Arabes mordus par les chiens enragés et traités par M. Pasteur. Voici l'appareil braqué sur les Arabes, qui consentent à obéir au 'ne bougeons plus', et voilà le positif obtenu reproduit dans *La Nature*.'

151 See Gen Doy for a discussion of French photographs of North Africans, particularly Arab women. Gen Doy, *Women and Visual Culture in Nineteenth-Century France, 1800–1852* (New York: Leicester University Press, 1998), pp. 220–248.

152 Crespi, 'Pasteur at Home', pp. 266–273.

153 For a discussion of *moujiks*, see A.E. Cazalet, 'The Moujik', *The Economic Journal*, 11:44 (1901), 575–581.

154 Tissandier, 'M. Pasteur et le traitement de la rage', p. 402. 'Il faut mentionner à part les dix-neuf Russes qui ont été mordus par un loup enragé. Il existe de profondes différences entre les suites de morsures par les loups ou par les chiens enragés. Le loup, en s'acharnant sur ses victimes, introduit en plus grande quantité le virus rabique. Si l'on retarde de quelques jours le traitement préventif, on risque d'arriver quand l'économie tout entière est déjà envahie par le mal.

'Nous reproduisons, page 401, la photographie de l'un de ces Russes pour montrer quelle énorme déchirure la morsure du loup enragé avait pratiquée. Un autre Russe avait eu les lèvres arrachées; un autre avait été mordu au front avec tant de fureur qu'une des dents de la bête était restée incrustée dans le crâne; tous avaient été soumis à des blessures graves, trois d'entre eux sont morts. Mais si l'on appliquait aux dix-neuf russes de Smolensk les statistiques de mortalité établies à la suite des morsures par les loups enragés, la proportion serait renversée; sur les dix-neuf, seize auraient succombés.'

155 Drs Metchnikoff and Gamaleïa were two Russians who worked at the Pasteur Institute. The importance of Russia and Russians was addressed in the speeches given at the Pasteur Institute inauguration in 1888. See *Inauguration de l'Institut Pasteur* (Sceaux: Charaire, 1888).

156 Louis Pasteur, 'Communications faites à l'Académie de sciences', 19 May 1884, in *Le Traitement de la rage* (Paris: Marpon et flammarion, 1886), pp. 26–27. 'L'Académie n'entendra peut-être pas sans émotion le récit de l'acte de courage et de présence d'esprit de l'enfant dont j'ai entrepris le traitement mardi dernier. C'est un berger, âgé de quinze ans, du nom de Jean-Baptiste Jupille, de Villers-Farlay (Jura), qui, voyant un chien à l'allure suspecte, de forte taille, se précipiter sur un groupe de six de ses petits camarades, tous plus jeunes que lui, s'est élancé, armé de son fouet, au-devant de l'animal. Le chien saisit Jupille à la main gauche. Jupille alors terrasse le chien, le maintient sous lui, lui ouvre la geule avec sa main droite pour dégager sa main gauche, non sans recevoir plusieurs morsures nouvelles, puis, avec la lumière de son fouet, il lui lie le museau, et, saisissant l'un de ses sabots, il l'assomme.

'Je m'empresserai de faire connaître à l'Académie ce qui adviendra de cette nouvelle tentative.'

157 Gaston Tissandier, 'L'Institut Pasteur', *La Nature* (17 November 1888), 406. 'Cet établissement, unique dans le monde, n'est pas seulement, en effet, un temple de la science, c'est aussi le sanctuaire de la charité et du dévouement. Et l'on ne sait ce que l'on doit le plus admirer chez celui qui en a été le fondateur, ou du découvreur de nouvelles et fécondes doctrines, ou du bienfaiteur de l'humanité.'

158 'Inauguration de l'Institut Pasteur', p. 742. 'Aucune ornamentation riche n'apparaît, aucune décoration superflue: on a, dès le premier abord, l'impression de se trouver dans une maison uniquement consacrée à la science, à la recherche du soulagement des maux de l'humanité.'

159 Kete, '*La Rage* and the Bourgeoisie', pp. 89–90.

160 Kete, '*La Rage* and the Bourgeoisie', p. 90.

161 Kete, '*La Rage* and the Bourgeoisie', p. 94.
162 Hansen, 'America's First Medical Breakthrough: How Popular Excitement about a French Rabies Cure in 1885 Raised New Expectations for Medical Progress', p. 374.
163 Bert Hansen, *Picturing Medical Progress from Pasteur to Polio: A History of Mass Media Images and Popular Attitudes in America* (New Brunswick: Rutgers University Press, 2009), p. 66.
164 Doctor J. Janicot, 'Inauguration de l'Institut Pasteur', *Le Figaro*, 15 November 1888, n.p.
165 Pasteur's correspondence, particularly a letter written to Dr Grancher on 18 October 1887, evinces his involvement in the creation of these portrait busts. 'S.M. Don Pedro m'a dit hier qu'il allait m'écrire pour me donner rendez-vous rue Vauquelin. Ne pensez-vous pas qu'il aurait lieu de lui conter cette affaire des bustes, lui demander le sien, demander ultérieurement celui du Sultan? Leur royauté peut bien compter pour une somme d'argent et nous aurions mieux le caractère international.' (S.M. Don Pedro told me yesterday that he was going to write to me to arrange a meeting in the rue Vauquelin. Don't you think it would be appropriate to tell him about the busts, ask for one of him, and later ask for one of the Sultan? Their royalty might bring in a sum of money, and we would have a better international representation.) Letter from Pasteur, *Correspondance 1840–1895*, 18 October 1887, pp. 221–222.
166 For a nineteenth-century discussion of these busts, see Janicot, 'Inauguration de l'Institut Pasteur'.
167 Louis Pasteur, *Quelques réflexions sur la science en France* (Paris: Gauthier-Villars, 1871), p. 6: 'prenez intérêt je vous en conjure à ces demeures sacrées que l'on désigne du nom expressif de *laboratoire*. Demandez qu'on les multiple et qu'on les orne: ce sont les temples de l'avenir, de la richesses et du bien-être. C'est là que l'humanité grandit, se fortifie et devient meilleure. Elle y apprend à lire dans les œuvres de la nature, œuvres de progrès et d'harmonie universelle, tandis que ses œuvres à elle sont trop souvent celles de la barbarie, du fanatisme et de la destruction.'
168 Janicot, 'Inauguration de l'Institut Pasteur', n.p.: 'établissement rappellera une conquête scientifique et humanitaire qui aura plus fait pour l'honneur de notre pays qu'une grande victoire sanglante'.
169 Most nineteenth-century newspapers between 29 September and 7 October 1895 provide accounts of the funeral. See 'Les Obsèques de Pasteur', *La République Française*, 6 October 1895. For a discussion of the state funerals of men of science and medicine, see Christiane Sinding, 'Claude Bernard and Louis Pasteur: Constructing Images through Public Commemorations', *Osiris*, 2:14 (1999), 61–85.
170 The architect Charles-Louis Girault, winner of the Grand Prix de Rome, designed the chapel, Auguste Guilbert-Martin provided mosaics, and Luc-Olivier Merson painted the chapel. For a discussion of the chapel, see Albert Delaunay and Hilda Benichou, *Pasteur Institute: the Museum, the Main Library, the Chapel* (Paris: Institute Pasteur, 1972), pp. 21–24.
171 'Charity', 'Science', 'Faith', and 'Hope'.
172 For analyses of death masks, see Marcia Pointon, 'Casts, Imprints and the Deathliness of Things: Artefacts at the Edge', *Art Bulletin*, 96:2 (2014), 170–195;

Emmanuelle Héran, 'Le dernier portrait ou la belle mort', in Héran (ed.), *Le Dernier Portrait* (Paris: Réunion des musées nationaux, 2002), pp. 25–101; and Édouard Papet, 'A fleur de peau: le moulage sur nature au XIXe siècle', in Édouard Papet (ed.), *À fleur de peau: Le moulage sur nature au XIXe siècle*, Musée d'Orsay (Paris: Réunion des musées nationaux, 2001), pp. 17–25.

173 See Marc Gotlieb's discussion of Henri Regnault's death mask in 'Legends of the Painter Hero: Remembering Henri Regnault', in Hargrove and McWilliam (eds), *Nationalism and French Visual Culture*, pp. 101–128.

2 The sleep of reason: Dr Péan's collection of bodies in paint and in wax

In Henri Blaze de Bury's 1863 story, *Les Bonshommes de cire*, the narrator discusses the feeling of being in a room surrounded by wax bodies:

> You know the strange and mysterious sensation that comes over you in the presence of these bizarre figures, so vividly realistic, and to which a certain sense of dread prevents you from speaking because you are not entirely certain that their lips would not reply. You draw back and you draw closer; it is like a hysterical, morbid curiosity, a sort of repulsive attraction.[1]

In this passage, the realism of the wax figures lures the spectator into the realm of the unknown and inexplicable. The lifelike quality of the wax appears to have erased the medium to produce a seemingly 'real' body. Confronted with such mimetic representations, the viewer loses all sense of reason. De Bury's curiosity takes over: his eyes move over the smooth surface of the wax, absorbing the intricacies and details of the body. Seconds later he recoils in fear and disgust, only to be drawn back towards this human-like body. Here, the spectacle of realism produces insanity, compulsion, and hysteria. This differs from the 1886 and 1887 paintings of Pasteur, where subject matter, sitter, and stylistic strategies produced realisms that were understood primarily as rational and documentary, and induced feelings of pride in French science.

In contrast to the majority of late nineteenth-century discourses on realism that associated it with truth, logic, and neutrality, de Bury's text exposes realism's other side: the unknown, the irrational, the excessive, and the veiled. This chapter will explore how the façade of realism reveals as much by what it conceals as by what it actively displays. Realism's often contradictory characteristics will not only be considered evidence of its obvious inability to produce reality, but will be understood as an essential part of its drive to do so. Concentrating on Henri Gervex's oil painting *Avant l'opération* (Figure 3), this chapter will explore how the main protagonist of this work, Dr Jules Émile Péan, was a collector of different forms of realism – waxworks included – and will argue that the oddities of his commissions reveal a fascination with female bodies and diseases that belies the rational veneer of realist projects. By focusing on the moments when realism's assumed stability, objectivity, and rationality are ruptured, it will explore the pathological, the hysterical, and the repulsive attraction of the real as it falls beyond the category of reason.

Gervex's realist portrait at the 1887 Salon

Péan, a surgeon of great celebrity and controversy, commissioned Gervex to paint his portrait to celebrate and memorialise his acceptance into the Académie de Médecine in 1887. Hung in room 13, *Avant l'opération* initiated the series of medical images shown at the 1887 Salon. Paul Desjardin described the painting as 'a sensational work'[2] and Charles Darcours claimed it 'captures almost all the sounds in room'.[3] As implied by the painting's longer title, *Avant l'opération: le Docteur Péan enseignant à l'hôpital Saint-Louis sa découverte du pincement des vaisseaux* (Before the operation: Dr Péan at the Hôpital Saint-Louis, presenting his new technique of clamping blood vessels), this painting stages the doctor lecturing at the Hôpital Saint-Louis, a hospital in Paris that specialised in venereal and skin diseases. Péan is standing at the helm of the operating table, surrounded by assistants, colleagues, and nurses. In one hand, he holds his celebrated invention, clamps designed to attach to blood vessels to reduce the amount of blood leaving the body during surgery. With the other hand, he gestures to the attentive crowd. Of equal importance to the picture, Gervex painted a medical still life to Péan's right: surgical instruments are scattered around the table top, a spiky metal tool pierces a fleshy yellow sponge and other sponges rest safely in a labelled jar. Droplets of blood stain the white tablecloth and, closer to Péan, thin surgical utensils lie used in bloody water, while other instruments are placed with their shiny handles facing out, ready for use. The immediacy of this medical still life contributed to establishing this painting as a realist work since still life was traditionally a realist genre *par excellence* that prioritised the close observation of objects. On the operating table, Gervex painted a pale young woman, bare to the waist, the white of her naked flesh and enveloping sheets contrasting with the black cloth of the tailored suits and hospital uniforms. The minute details of the still life, the rendering of daylight through the windows, and the depiction of a modern medical scene prompted contemporary critics to remark that Gervex's work was a painting of utmost realism.

Critics used rhetoric of non-intervention often associated with mechanical objectivity, and usually attributed to scientific images, to describe Gervex's approach. Georges Lafenestre, for example, praised Gervex for 'no personal invention whatsoever – not in the lighting of the room, nor in the disposition of the figures, nor in the grouping of the accessories; this is to remain, in a word, a copyist of reality, pure and simple'.[4] Maurice Hamel also commended the artist for painting a work without 'any tragic or tearful intention' that kept 'the eloquence of the truth … everything is said simply, with the certainty of a scientific claim'.[5] For these critics, Gervex's realism equated scientific neutrality. Through his attention to detail and depiction of a contemporary scene, Gervex fabricated an image whose painted surface was considered as clinical as its subject matter. He replaced the idealism of academic painting through a style that signalled a more precise and objective understanding of the visible world.

Louis de Fourcaud argued in his lengthy account of the 1887 Salon in *La Revue illustré* that the only two essential laws of art are 'honesty in the observation and, logic in the execution'.[6] De Fourcaud described Gervex as a realist painter, and commended *Avant l'opération* for having an 'accurate sense of the situation, natural poses, sober harmony in the colours, an effect that is straightforward, in no way melodramatic'.[7] De Fourcaud's comments reflect the prominent nineteenth-century assumption that rationality and logic took form in subtle colouration, subdued light effects, intricate details, and lack of dramatisation. The aestheticisation of scientific principles within the artistic sphere demonstrates the ways in which scientific language and metaphors were used to described medically themed paintings and empower artistic discourse. The appropriation of scientific principles, and the desire to observe and record the visible world meticulously, replaced art's connection with subjectivity, mythology, and creativity with the seemingly more concrete contemporary world in which calculation, documentation, and innovation reigned.

The role of subjectivity in producing objectivity is complex. It is not simply that science was objective and art subjective, and consequently that physicians eschewed subjectivity and artists embraced it. Rather both fields and occupations required a certain amount of personal involvement to craft what were understood as objective images. Daston and Galison skilfully tease out some of these problems with respect to 'scientific pictures', and argue that by the second half of the nineteenth century, the subjective involvement of doctors was seemingly removed from scientific images by having the viewer take on the role of expert interpreter of mechanically produced images, such as photography. This differed from earlier models of image production, when the expert was actively – and knowingly – involved in their production. However, as Josh Ellenbogen argues, not all photographs had to appear devoid of human agency to have scientific authority. Étienne-Jules Marey, for example, was not completely opposed to mediated picture making; photographers had to intervene in the process to produce the desired scientific image and data.[8] Yet, as Salon criticism demonstrates, the drive to rid visual representations of subjectivity was sought by many in the art world, particularly when the subject matter was scientific.

De Fourcaud's insistence on the superiority of realistic images in the modern age is evident in his article on contemporary art at the *Exposition Universelle* of 1889, where Gervex's work was displayed. De Fourcaud wrote that he would accept any subject in painting as long as artists portrayed 'real people engaged in real actions, lit with the same light that surrounds us, breathing the same air that we breathe. Give us the truth.'[9] Gervex created this sense of reality pictorially through the use of style and narrative, and thus produced a painting that was accepted as a truthful account of an actual event. The medical scene as staged within the painting gave the viewers seemingly unproblematic access to this 'actual' event, while the smooth brushstrokes, delineated figures, and naturalistic lighting gave the painting an easy 'readability' and apparent equivalence to the visible world. Many viewers were convinced of the reality of this scene. Roger Ballu claimed that it felt as if one was a part of the depicted scene:

> It is impossible to better render the impression of interior light, of that impalpable atmosphere, illuminated by the window with its raised white drapes, casting cool highlights onto the faces and moving over the bare walls of the hospital room. The sense of air in this restrained perspective, in sum, is unimaginable. We enter into it, we are there inside it, we breathe it.[10]

The ease with which Ballu accepted Gervex's painting as a stand-in for reality reflects the tendency to believe that detailed images are trustworthy depictions of lived events, even when we know that the only evidence of the original situation or point of view is the painting itself.[11]

Gervex promoted the historical importance and truthfulness of his work in order to advance his career, secure his reputation, and attract new clients. He wrote in his memoirs:

> This was the era when the discovery of the hemostat was revolutionising the old methods. Dr Péan, standing before the unconscious body of a young woman on whom he was about to operate, was speaking, holding between his fingers the famous instrument. In the blink of an eye I saw the painting to be made. I did a few sketches and abandoned once and for all the banal profile of the classic portrait.[12]

Gervex referred to the act of sketching from life in order to cultivate his experience of watching Péan as immediate and unmediated. Sketching, unlike painting, was more closely aligned with experiencing reality since it was executed in the presence of the model. The lines and brisk marks of a drawn sketch implied an immediacy not associated with the smoothly painted surface and modelled figures of a time-consuming 'finished' Salon painting. Gervex positioned himself as part of modernity's progress by linking his artistic innovations in portraiture with Péan's medical invention. This portrayed the artist as both a witness to, and participant in modern scientific and artistic advancement. Gervex cultivated his identity as a modern realist painter not only through a rejection of certain artistic conventions – the 'banal profile of the classic portrait' – but also by emphasising the contemporaneity of events that he himself witnessed and sketched.

Scientific medicine was a key element of modernity. Baudelaire had already invoked the anatomy theatre as an appropriate pretext for modern nudes in his essay on the 1846 Salon.[13] Medical scenes were ideal subjects for realist paintings. In 1887, Darcours praised the medical theme of *Avant l'opération*: 'It is an interesting painting whose realist theme is preferable to the romantic subjects that have too often been treated by an artist of great talent.'[14] Like the laboratory in Gsell's portrait of Pasteur and the clinic in Brouillet's *Une leçon clinique*, the operating theatre was a quintessential modern location: a venue of innovative surgical experimentation and a place where discoveries were made and implemented.

The increased use of antisepsis and anaesthetics during the 1880s greatly increased the survival rates of patients who went under the knife, and transformed surgery into a more humane and painless procedure. Although Gervex painted a few speckles of blood on the white tablecloth in the foreground

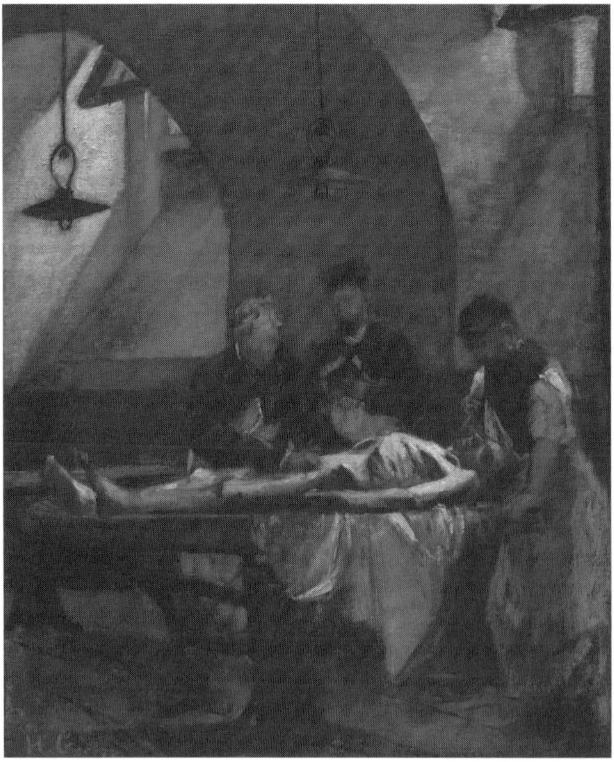

30 Henri Gervex, Study for *L'Autopsie à l'Hôtel-Dieu* (1876), oil on canvas, 53.3 x 43.2cm.

of *Avant l'opération*, there is blood on neither the sheets covering the operating table, nor the medical men's clothing. Rather, the operating theatre is shown as a clean and ordered space filled with up-to-date technologies and hygienic advancements: a chloroform-covered cloth is held near the patient's face, newly invented tools are being sanitized in water, a patient lies on a contemporary operating table and Péan holds his ground-breaking scientific instrument. Although Péan did not fully adhere to Joseph Lister's conception of antisepsis (he did not use carbolic acid during surgery), he insisted on the common practice of washing hands and instruments before surgery.[15] Gervex's detailed rendering of this scene exhibited his familiarity with the operating theatre, Péan's modern methods, and the advances of scientific medicine.

Gervex's attempt to be associated with cutting-edge medical progress began when he painted a medical theme in *Autopsie à l'Hôtel-Dieu* (Figure 30).[16] His strategy was successful. Larousse's *Grand dictionnaire universel du XIXe siècle* noted that this work established Gervex's identity as a modern painter: 'In 1876, with *Autopsie à l'Hôtel-Dieu*, Monsieur Gervex tackled the modern subjects that were to establish his reputation and place him among the ranks of the most prominent artists of the young school.'[17] This painting depicts three men standing around a cadaver in a cavernous dissection room in Paris: a working-class orderly with a bushy moustache looks down on the dead body and holds the slab steady, a bearded medical intern grips the specimen's thigh to make an incision, and a junior doctor watches the procedure while rolling a cigarette. Salon critics praised the accuracy of the painting. 'We ought to appreciate the candour of his execution and the sincerity that dominates his work', wrote M. Charles Yriarte. 'The light outlines the objects and penetrates the bodies, his poses are accurate, his drawing is honest and his means are straightforward.'[18] In his memoirs, Gervex claimed to have come across this realist subject by chance, while on a '*flânerie*'.[19] By aligning himself with Baudelaire's *flâneur* – an exemplar of heroic masculinity in modern Paris – he stressed the immediacy of his personal experience, the reality of the scene, and his identity as a painter of modern life. He also cultivated his identity as a modern artist by claiming that he had applied '[his] theory of modern art the most completely' to *Autopsie à l'Hôtel-Dieu*.[20] Significantly, Gervex won a second place medal for *Autopsie à l'Hôtel-Dieu* at the 1876 Salon and his painting was purchased by the State for the Musée de Limoges.[21] In the coming years, Gervex was introduced to Manet and Puis de Chavanne as the painter of *Autopsie*. Returning to a medical theme in 1887, Gervex built on his past success by creating another painting that was considered modern in subject matter, style, and approach.

Front row seats: identity, republicanism, and spectatorship in group portraiture

In his 1887 Salon review in *Le Témoin*, Victorien Maubry commented that portraits should be primarily 'a source of glory and of gain'.[22] Clearly, this was the goal of *Avant l'opération*. Gervex's portrayal of Péan, which highlights his surgical skills and signatory invention, staged modern medical masculinity as powerful and intelligent. Gervex drew on the genre of portraiture to emphasise status and authority. Some Salon reviewers, however, criticised the work for publicising Péan's skills so obviously. *L'Univers illustré* noted that it should have been titled *Portrait de Docteur Péan* and published a cartoon that depicted the surgeon's head as twice the size of all the other figures' (Figure 31).[23] An article in *Paris illustré* suggested that the real purpose of the painting was to 'preserve the memory of the invention of Dr Péan's famous surgical method',[24] a comment of particular importance since Péan's identity as the inventor of the hemostatic clamp was controversial. The question of who invented this particular clamp was discussed in both the popular and medical press during the 1880s, as well as in Péan's obituaries in 1898, even though Péan's arterial clamp was one of many such instruments invented before and during this period.[25] The controversy arose when a certain Dr Verneuil claimed that his discovery of *forcipressure* – applying pressure to blood vessels in order to restrict blood flow – preceded Péan's invention. Péan, who referred to his own invention as *pincement des vaisseaux* (clamping of the blood vessels), dismissed Verneuil's claim by insisting that his clamping came before Verneuil's pressure. Although the controversy continued in medical circles until his death, Péan's identification with hemostatic clamps, like Pasteur's with the cure for rabies and Charcot's with hysteria, was secured historically with the help of a Salon portrait. By commissioning a painting, particularly one made by a popular member of the Academy who no longer had to put his works before the jury, Péan exploited the authority and tradition of the Salon to display himself as the unquestioned inventor. This was furthered by the painting's exhibition at the *Exposition Universelle* of 1889, where it exemplified the progress of French advances, both artistic and medical.[26] The promotion of Péan as an inventor was accentuated because he is the only one holding the clamps even though a study for the work shows Monsieur Mathieu, the manufacturer of the surgical instrument, with them in his hand. In the finished painting, Mathieu is empty-handed, though his left hand remains poised as it is in the sketch.

Péan's unrelenting desire to parade his professional prowess and personal wealth through artworks can also be seen at the Montmartre cemetery, where a large portrait bust of the surgeon is placed above the door to his tomb (Figure 32). Péan is portrayed with a straightforward gaze, his chin raised, and signature bushy sideburns covering his cheeks. As in *Avant l'opération*, he is wearing the red pin of the Légion d'honneur. Large letters spell out his name above

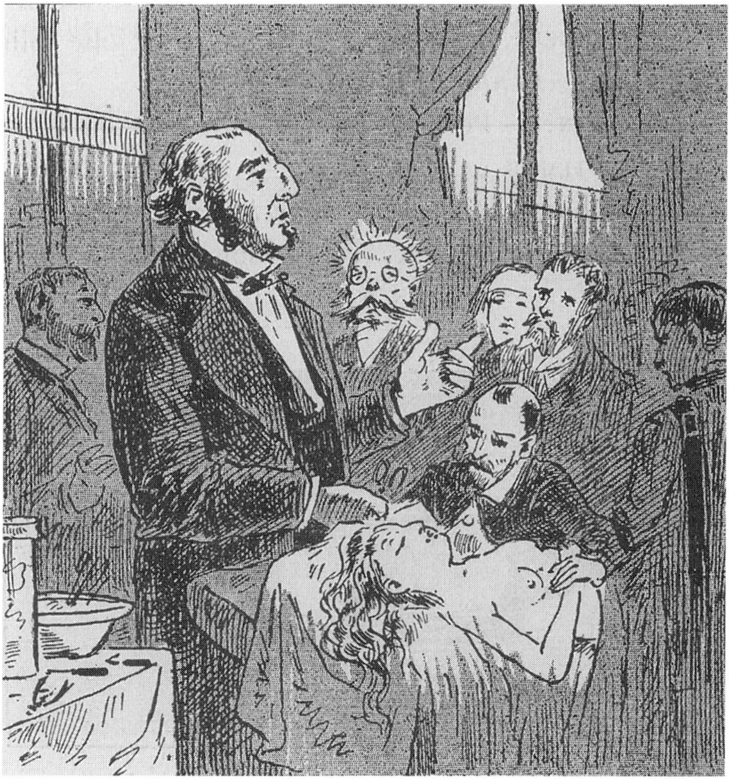

Engraving from 'Le Salon', from *L'Univers illustré*, 7 May 1887, p. 295. 31

the mausoleum's door; inside, Péan's numerous titles and professional affiliations are engraved in marble. Like many representations of Pasteur, particularly Gsell's 1887 portrait of the chemist, Péan's tomb highlights the importance of medical science and its practitioners not only in France, but also internationally, listing Péan as a member of the medical academies of Paris, Saint Petersburg, Constantinople, Madrid, Lisbon, Rio de Janeiro, and Mexico. Above the text-filled marble square is a large stained-glass window portraying Christ's resurrection. Here, modern surgical procedures are connected to god's work, and demonstrate the belief that Péan, like Pasteur, had god-like abilities to prevent impending death. 'Science is one. It is universal, like God', wrote Dr G. Rappin around 1895. 'Religion is aging, Science is growing. Science is the mother of all freedom. Poor Science! If people did for you just a little of what they do for religion. Where are your altars?'[27] Furthermore, light shines through the windows of Péan's tomb to illuminate the surgeon's professional feats just as light enters the surgical theatre to spotlight Péan's surgery in *Avant l'operation*, suggesting that the divine light of heaven and the rational enlightenment of modern science united to light his path.

Gervex utilised Péan's identity to produce his own. He inserted himself symbolically into the contemporary scene of Péan's surgical theatre as a documenter and witness to scientific medical progress through the great attention he gave depicted objects. As Gustave Ollendorf wrote:

> Here, since irony cannot be introduced into the scene, Monsieur Gervex has slipped it into the accessories. Our eye is irresistibly arrested, not by the main character, the person to be operated on nor by the secondary character, whose role is nonetheless important, the surgeon, but instead by a table on which are depicted the accessories for the operation – some scattered instruments – and a marvellous jar of sponges.[28]

These tools, signifiers of Péan's revolutionary role, become emblems of the artist's hand and evidence of his talent. They evoke Gervex's paintbrush and palette, and pictorially link the two men as modern skilled professionals. Gervex's blood-red signature beneath the empty stool implies his bodily presence and importance in the scene. This crimson signature interrupts the subtle colours of the painting's realist effect, thus connecting Gervex's name with the red labels of the jars, the spots of blood staining the white tablecloth, and the red Légion d'honneur pin attached to Péan's lapel. Blood, honour, and order stand not only as symbols of modern surgery, but also compositionally opens a space for both Gervex's and the viewer's body. This demarcation locates both Gervex and the implied viewer at the head of the operating table, providing visual priority and direct contact to both Péan and the operation; artist and spectator are invited to join the medical elite and momentarily perform medical manhood. The life-size figures depicted on the canvas and the open space offered to the viewer at the head of the table contributed to critics' understanding of the painting as a realist work since both artist and viewer become witnesses to, and participants in, cutting-edge surgical practice.

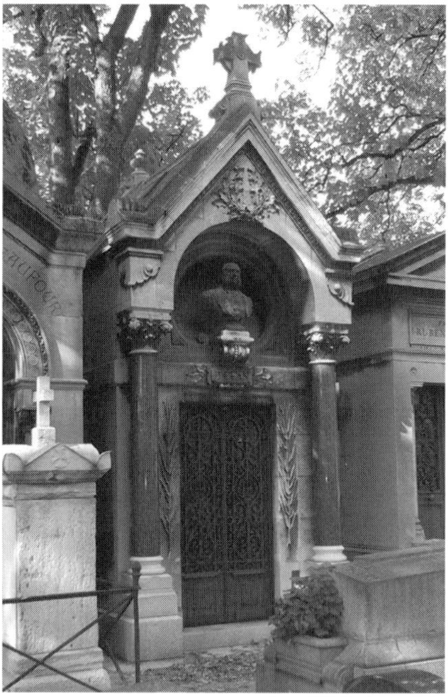

32 Péan's tomb, Montmartre cemetery, Paris.

Although *Avant l'opération* was described as a modern painting by Salon critics, they also noted that Gervex consciously engaged with earlier artistic conventions for painting

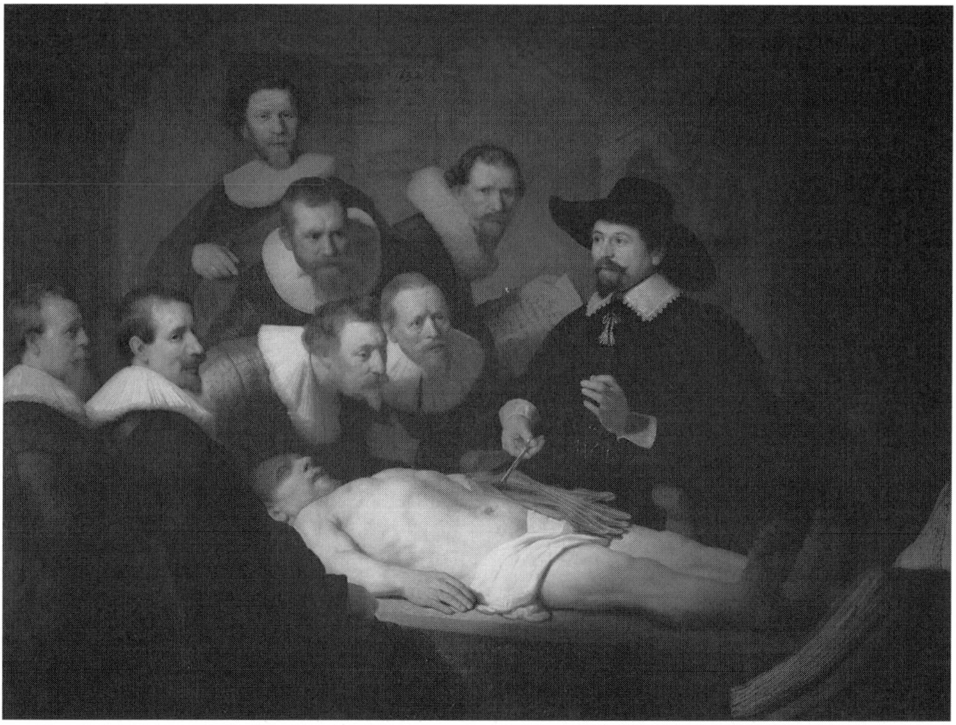

Rembrandt van Rijn, *The Anatomy Lesson of Doctor Nicolaes Tulp* (1632), oil on canvas, 170 x 217cm. 33

a medical theme. Looking to the past, Gervex rejected the single portrait format that he had used in his portrait of Dr Blanche from around 1880 and instead created a large-scale painting showing professional men in action. Paul Mantz referred to Gervex's work as 'more or less related to the anatomy lessons that seventeenth-century Holland so loved'.[29] Other contemporary observers commented that *Avant l'operation* was a modern rendition of Rembrandt's medical group portraits, especially his 1632 *Anatomy Lesson of Dr Tulp* (Figure 33). 'All in all, it is the subject of Rembrandt's *Anatomy Lesson*, attuned to modern reality, and we must be grateful to Monsieur Gervex for having been as sincere, as true to his times as the Dutch master must have been to his own', wrote Ballu.[30]

It is not at all surprising that the two paintings would invite comparison. *Avant l'opération* and *Anatomy Lesson of Dr Tulp* are both large oil paintings portraying known medical men at work. They are similar in narrative and composition: both show dark-suited men standing around a naked immobile body. The unconscious and unclothed figures are concurrently represented as the objects of art and science: their horizontal dominance in the canvases is evidence of the naked body's central role in the paintings' narratives and compositions, as well as its importance in medical and artistic study and the production of medical and artistic knowledge.

Although there were no painted Dutch group portraits in France in the nineteenth century, reproductions of these works were plentiful. French artists were familiar with Rembrandt's oeuvre and with other seventeenth-century Dutch group portraits. Improved modes of travel from France to the Netherlands made the study of Dutch art easier. Furthermore, at least 150 prints after Rembrandt were available in France between 1830 and the 1890s; from the mid-1880s, these prints dominated the Salon.[31] Léopold Flameng's engraving of Rembrandt's *Anatomy Lesson of Dr Tulp*, published by Cadart and first shown at the 1876 Salon, was one of the most exhibited and distributed prints.[32] Significantly, the engraving presents a mirror image of the Dutch master's painting and therefore is compositionally similar to Gervex's. The rise in value of Rembrandt's work, along with an increase in the number of his paintings and prints sold, attests to the popularity of his art in France.[33] Most critics who praised nineteenth-century French art with realist tendencies also praised seventeenth-century Dutch painting and Rembrandt in particular. They believed that Dutch artists were equally concerned with producing sincere representations of the visible world. Paul Lenoir, in his 1889 book, *Histoire du réalisme et du naturalisme dans la poésie et dans l'art depuis l'antiquité jusqu'à nos jours*, described Rembrandt as a 'realist genius'.[34] Louis Viardot, in 1860, similarly argued that Rembrandt 'clearly shows the highest extreme of pure "naturalism"'.[35]

The connections drawn between nineteenth-century French painting and seventeenth-century Dutch painting went beyond superficial formal strategies. Many nineteenth-century French art critics, art historians, and theorists, including Charles Blanc, Théophile Thoré, and Léon Bonnat, believed that ideological and political thought was articulated through visual means. The similarities between French and Dutch group portraiture were understood as transhistorical alliances and worldviews. By considering Gervex's painting in relation to Alois Riegl's 1902 work on group portraiture, *Das holländische Gruppenporträt,* it is clear that many nineteenth-century scholars turned to the art historical past for a visual language to explain their present.

Although Riegl's study was printed in German fifteen years after the 1887 Salon, his approach to the visual arts shares similar concerns with nineteenth-century French artists and critics regarding portraiture, realism, and politics. Riegl, like many nineteenth-century French critics, was interested in the relationship between aesthetics and historical periods. In 1863, Baudelaire addressed this relationship when he wrote:

> Every painter of the past has had his own modernity. Most of the fine portraits that remain to us from earlier times are dressed in costumes of their period. They are perfectly harmonious, because the costume, the hairstyles and even the gestures, the gaze and the smile (each period has its bearing, its gaze and its smile) form a whole of complete vitality.[36]

Alison McQueen argues that most French art critics believed that seventeenth-century Dutch art was a mirror of Dutch society, morals, politics, and values.[37] 'A gallery of Dutch paintings is a complete history of Holland during its Golden Age, a history that is simultaneously moral, political and natural', the art critic Charles Blanc claimed in his 1883 book *L'École hollandaise*.[38] Riegl's approach to art history was informed by his positivist education at the University of Vienna, which, like many French artists and critics, followed the belief that scientific methodologies could provide a solution to humanistic and social concerns.[39]

Riegl conceived of art and art history through the concept of *Kunstwollen*, often translated as 'the will of art'. The *Kunstwollen*, evident in historical periods, genres, traditions, and artists, was understood as an independent force that paralleled the ideas and views of a particular historical period and its people.[40] As Frauke Laarman states, '*Kunstwollen* in the visual arts regulates the relationship between human beings and the appearance of things as perceived by the senses: it generates the means of expression, how that individual wishes to see those things shaped or coloured'.[41] Riegl focused on Dutch group portraiture from the early sixteenth to the mid-seventeenth century in *Das holländische Gruppenporträt*, to argue that group portraiture was the most comprehensive expression of the Dutch *Kunstwollen*. He claimed that certain pictorial elements in Dutch art, such as the depiction of gestures, the placement of figures, and the compositional integration of the spectator into the portrait, were representative of social, historical, and political changes within Dutch society, particularly the shift towards a more secular, individualist, and mercantile society.

For Riegl, the coherence of seventeenth-century Dutch portraits lay not only in the objects, but also in the consciousness of the spectator who completes the scene. In many Dutch group portraits, including *Anatomy Lesson of Dr Tulp*, the figures interact with one another, and actively bring the viewer into their time and space through hand gestures and eye contact.[42] Both Gervex's and Rembrandt's portraits offer viewers unrestricted access to the painting's action. To achieve this, Rembrandt framed his foreground with two men to the left and a large book to the right. Gervex did the same with the still life on the left and the medic on the right. Both paintings position the majority of the people behind the naked body so that the spectator can occupy the frontal viewing position. Neither Tulp nor Péan makes eye contact with any individual in the canvas, nor do they look directly out at the viewer – both men gaze out at audiences not portrayed within the portraits. Rather than isolating viewers through their lack of direct engagement, the surgeons' gazing outside of the represented space constructs a three-dimensional world for the spectator. Instead of being the observer of a two-dimensional picture, the viewer is 'sandwiched' between the men depicted in the canvas and the audience implied by the doctors' active looks.

Although neither Péan nor Tulp occupy a much greater space than the other clothed bodies in the paintings, both men are portrayed as leaders through the rendering of their hands, which gesture to the crowd and hold medical tools. Benjamin Binstock argues that the hand motif in *The Anatomy Lesson of Doctor Tulp* symbolises the priority of sight over speech as a vehicle for human understanding.[43] The same can be said in relation to *Avant l'opération*, where observing and touching bodies is paramount. Sight was essential for learning surgical procedures and acquiring medical knowledge, yet of greater significance was the synchronisation of sight and touch. Surgeons, like artists, required acute hand-eye coordination to successfully fulfil their roles. Riegl claimed that hands were important in Dutch group portraiture because they denoted mental expressions and allowed the figures within the canvas to communicate to one another and to the portrait's beholder. Although Rembrandt's painting, unlike Gervex's, does not provide a detailed portrayal of the surrounding surgical space, the active involvement demanded of the viewer in both paintings contributed to the portraits' claims to truth and reality.

Riegl reasoned that the active participation of spectators in everyday scenes was a manifestation of republican values in Dutch society. As Margaret Iversen claims, the writing of Théophile Thoré, a French republican who wrote art criticism under the pseudonym William Bürger after exile from France in 1848, influenced Riegl. Thoré was interested in the role of the implied viewer, and expressed his belief that Dutch art embodied the principles of political and religious freedom – ideals that were valued and essential for a republican France.[44] Émile Leclercq expressed a similar sentiment when he wrote in 1882 that 'All Dutch art is fundamentally popular and democratic'.[45] The historic and artistic parallels between the secularisation of late nineteenth-century France and seventeenth-century Holland are also evident in Emile Michel's 1893 book *Rembrandt – sa vie, son œuvre et son temps*:

> After the definitive triumph of the Reformation in the Netherlands, religious painting – at least that whose object was the decoration of churches – no longer existed. As the Catholic clergy disappeared, the courts ceased their sponsorship of artists; but the corporations, assuming the place that had been thus vacated, were to open new paths for the activity of Dutch painters. As might have been expected, the heads of these associations had themselves painted wearing the insignia of their rank, and their portraits, hung in assembly halls, served, for the members, as so many exhortations to continue the examples of piety,

> patriotism and charity provided to them by these forebears whose images now hung before their eyes.[46]

Although Michel's work is primarily concerned with Holland, the shift from church patronage to government commissions that he described was also occurring during the French Third Republic. Republican governments sponsored artists, including Gervex, to paint secular themes for public buildings, and bourgeois professionals, including doctors, commissioned artists to paint their portraits – in both instances, visual representations secured this group's newfound status and evidenced the desire for a shared republican identity and iconography.[47]

Gervex's use of the group portrait, understood by Salon critics as intimately tied to seventeenth-century Dutch group portraits, points to the anti-clerical and republican values that he shared with Péan.[48] Republicanism was promoted by its followers for being rational and logical, particularly in contrast to the mysticism and faith associated with Catholicism. As Petra ten-Doesschate Chu argues, after 1848, the French linked seventeenth-century Dutch art with the Reformation, revolution, and republican government.[49] In 1883, Blanc argued that Holland's political independence allowed its art to progress towards a pure imitation of reality: 'The republican form, once recognised, liberated them from the purely decorative art commissioned by the courts and princes'.[50] Thoré was perhaps the critic who most ardently tied seventeenth-century Dutch republicanism with that of nineteenth-century France, claiming that France must follow Holland's lead by ridding itself of Catholicism and the monarchy to form a democratic republic.[51] The reformation of the hospital system was part of secular restructuring.[52] Unlike earlier forms of medical care that depended on nuns and priests, new scientific medicine was executed by physicians according to republican policies. 'It is quite true that the medical profession is fundamentally liberal and republican, that it shapes the mind to hate prejudice and love progress', wrote Jules Guérin, the editor of *La Gazette médicale de Paris*.[53] Gervex referred to the lingering religious presence in the medical sphere by including a nun.[54] Segregated in a back corner, her identity is signified by her black habit, a uniform associated with the spiritual past, which stands in opposition to the men's contemporary black suits.

In the painting, Péan's portrayal as a surgeon, rather than an anatomist, further inscribes republican ideals. Unlike anatomy, which was associated with intellectual capabilities, surgery was considered as a more physical act because of its historical ties to barbarism. In François Nicolas Augustin Feyen-Perrin's 1864 portrait, *La Leçon d'anatomie de Docteur Velpeau*, Velpeau is shown as an anatomist even though he was also a practising surgeon and physician (Figure 34).[55] Unlike *Avant l'opération*, Feyen-Perrin's painting does not depict or stress cutting-edge medical practice, nor is Velpeau presented as a modern

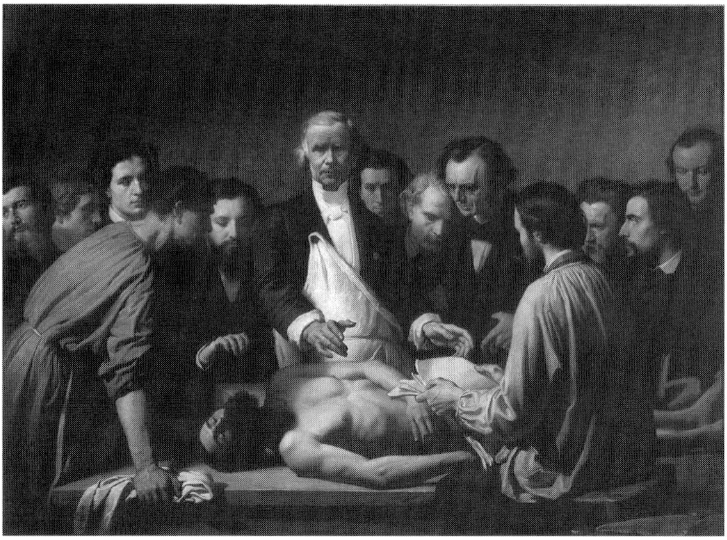

34 François Nicolas Augustin Feyen-Perrin, *La Leçon d'anatomie de Docteur Velpeau* (1864), oil on canvas, 170 x 233cm.

surgeon: the setting is non-specific and timeless, and there are no modern tools or technologies on display. Although some of these omissions can be partially explained by the painting's creation at a time before certain medical procedures, such as anaesthetic, were commonly used, it is clear that Feyen-Perin was more interested in using art historical precedents to identify his sitter as a leading medical man.

Péan, however, was portrayed as a modern surgeon. He wanted his class, social status, and modernity on view. Péan was very proud of his past and, in turn, his success. Numerous publications documented the story of how he moved from rural France to become one of the richest medical men in Paris.[56] Still, Gervex did not depict the doctor in the midst of surgery: there are only a few drops of blood, the white surgical aprons are unstained, and the patient's body is unscarred. Here, surgery is as an act of control, cleanliness, and restraint rather than brute physicality, and Péan is a skilled surgeon, calm and rational in the face of impending bloodshed.

Avant l'opération, like Gsell's 1887 painting of Pasteur and Brouillet's painting of Charcot, occupies a precarious position in relation to its status as history painting and/or group portrait. On the one hand, the men in the painting were named in some Salon reviews: young Dr Zacharian checks the patient's pulse, white-haired Dr Collin stares at Péan, the bearded Mathieu peeks out from behind the surgeon's shoulder and Dr Arbeau holds a shiny white bowl.

Yet, unlike most group portraits, in which all of the people depicted in the canvas were known and formed a collective identity, many in Gervex's work remained nameless.[57] For example, it is evident that Gervex re-used the model for the orderly from *Autopsie à l'Hôtel-Dieu* in the later painting: the moustachioed man at the head of the dissection table has his back to the viewer in *Avant l'opération*. This anonymous worker helps stage a medical scene in both paintings, serving as a modern type rather than an actual person. As an uneducated working-class man, he acts as a foil to accomplished physicians.

The patient and nurses in *Avant l'opération* are also props rather than known individuals. Like the surgical tools and sponges in the foreground, they are objects that construct medical personae. In this respect, *Avant l'opération* differs from Riegl's conceptualisation of seventeenth-century Dutch group portraiture as democratic and equal. It does not consist solely of individual portraits of people who have volunteered to be portrayed to achieve a common goal or display a collective identity. Rather, it contains known and unknown people who were depicted together to form Péan's desired identity.

The portraits of Péan, Charcot, and Pasteur that were on view in 1887 all displayed the identities of their protagonists through the representation of named and nameless people, but the anonymous in many respects paid a far more central role to the paintings' narratives than the portraits of specific individuals. Despite the detailed rendering of the leading men, the patients painted by Gervex, Brouillet, and Gsell are all types – hysteric, foreigner, nurse, child, and mother – rather than identifiable individuals. In these paintings, Pasteur's vaccines, Péan's clamps, and Charcot's hypnosis, are used on the bodies of the unknown. The patients' objectification is essential to the performance of medical and scientific male identities and subjectivities. Not only are Péan, Charcot, and Pasteur's roles as leaders indicated by these unnamed bodies, but as objects of medical study and experimentation, the female and foreign patients symbolise the discoveries of these men. The spectacle of medical innovation was produced by the curative potential of men's work yet guaranteed by exhibiting these bodies.

Libidinal looking: the artist/doctor/client and his model/patient/prostitute

The spectacle of modern medicine fascinated both men and women. They read about medical feats in newspapers and magazines, viewed the photographs, paintings, and sculptures of medical men on display in Paris, and integrated hygiene and other medical practices into their daily routines.[58] Although women were admitted to medical school in France from the late 1860s onwards, they were predominantly in the hospital environment as nurses, nuns, or patients; the active roles of diagnosis and analysis were considered male pursuits.[59] In *Avant l'opération*, women are shown as passive: the anaesthetised woman lies with her eyes closed; the nurse's face is turned away from the operation, looking at neither doctor nor patient. Although one could argue that the nun is facing the operation, her roughly rendered eyes are unfocused, and Dr Aubeau's standing body restricts her access to the patient. In contrast, the canvas shows looking as a privileged male activity. The men are all engaged in the act of looking: Mathieu, Dr Larrivé, and the medical attendant all twist and tilt their heads to get a better look, Dr Collin focuses directly on Péan, and Dr Zacharian fixes his gaze upon the patient's face. Although Dr Brochin, the chief editor of the *Gazette des hôpitaux*, is barely visible, hidden from view by Péan's imposing body and Mathieu's leaning form, Gervex nonetheless provided him with an eyeglass. Gervex also offered the painting's viewers the ability to see. They stand amongst these men, empowered with an active and privileged gaze. The life-size figures contribute to the sense of an all-encompassing reality and, in turn, this demarcated space places them in a position of authority from which to gain knowledge through the acute observation of the female body.[60]

Looking at naked bodies was understood, for the most part, as an educational pursuit for medical professionals and artists. Émile Zola drew upon the social respectability given to artists and doctors in order to justify his detailed and intricate account of Parisian sex lives in his 1867 novel, *Thérèse Raquin*.[61] In response to critics who saw his highly detailed descriptions of bodies and sexualities as pornographic, Zola wrote, in the 1868 preface to the second edition, that he was simply applying 'to two living bodies the analytical method that surgeons apply to corpses'.[62] He continued:

> While I was busy writing *Thérèse Raquin* I forgot the world and devoted myself to copying life exactly and meticulously, giving myself up entirely to precise analysis of the mechanism of the human being, and I assure you that the ferocious sexual relationship of Thérèse and Laurent meant nothing immoral to me, nothing calculated to provoke indulgence in evil passions. The human side of the models ceased to exist, just as it ceases to exist for the eye of the artist who has a naked woman sprawled in front of him but who is solely concerned with getting on to his canvas a true representation of her shape and colouration … Amid the concert of voices bawling: 'The author of *Thérèse Raquin* is a hysterical wretch who revels in displays of pornography', I waited in vain for one voice to reply: 'No, the writer is simply an analyst who may have become engrossed in human corruption, but who has done so as a surgeon might in an operating theatre'.[63]

The attacks against Zola's writing, which was described by critics as realist and naturalist, demonstrate how realism, despite its association with science, was considered a style of scandal, gratuitous detail, and pornography. Although Zola used the figures of the surgeon and artist to rid his work of its pornographic

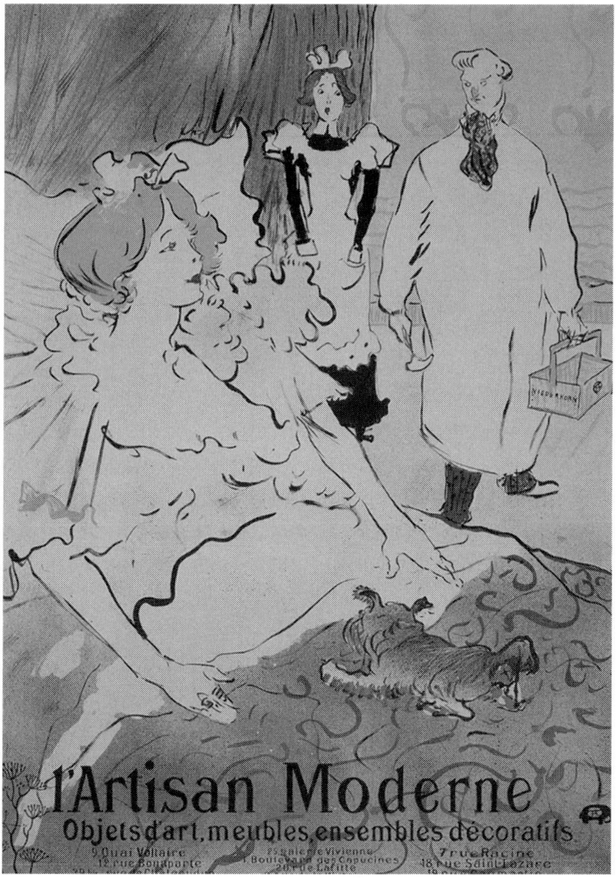

Henri de Toulouse-Lautrec, *L'Artisan moderne* (1896), 35
lithograph, 92 x 65cm.

categorisation, neither artist nor doctor were free of public criticism regarding their professional access to naked bodies, particularly female ones.

The relationship between male artist and female model, like that between male physician and female patient, was sexually fraught. Heather Dawkins, Susan Waller, and Marie Lathers, as well as numerous other scholars of the nineteenth century, have discussed the sexual potential of the relationship between artists and their models at length.[64] As they have pointed out, women posing naked in front of men as a form of employment was socially frowned upon because many models were in need of more money than modelling could provide. Financial strain led some into prostitution, thus modelling was often equated with harlotry. Although the study of the female body was institutionally justified by the Academie des Beaux-Arts, the relationship between a naked model and an artist within the artist's private studio was unregulated, which contributed to the questionability of modelling as a proper occupation. Like the relationship between artist and model, that between doctor and patient was loaded with fear and fascination. The looking at and touching of female bodies required by the medical profession wove threads of desire, immorality, and distrust through public conceptions of modern medicine and its practitioners. Many nineteenth-century cartoons parodied this relationship: an illustration from *L'Assiette au beurre* from around 1905, for example, shows a husband exclaiming, 'I hope he's not going to charge me for this operation!' while he watches a physician embrace his wife (Figure 8).[65] The access that medical men had to bourgeois wives, mothers, and daughters was fraught with anxiety because it threatened faithful bourgeois relationships. Furthermore, female patients were often considered highly sexed beings with deviant sexualities, as is most obvious in the case of hysteria (see Chapter 3). It was even suggested that women seduced doctors in order to take pleasure in medical inspections; some believed that the use of the speculum awakened a woman's sexual desire.[66] Henri de Toulouse-Lautrec parodied the sexual relationship between female patients and male doctors in his 1894 advertisement for an interior decorating store, *L'Artisan moderne*, which shows a young woman in bed awaiting the arrival of a fashionable decorator (Figure 35). The man's smock, tool kit, and predatory stance visually linked him to caricatures of lecherous medical men who, armed with occupational apparatus, probed and penetrated the bodies of the bourgeoisie. The salacious nature of the impending 'inspection' is symbolised by the woman's well-coiffed blonde hair, the shocked expression on the maid's face and the small fluffy dog on the woman's lap, a well-known symbol of eroticism.

The highly publicised connection between doctors and prostitutes that arose from discussions of the regulatory medical inspections of prostitutes contributed to the potentially scandalous nature of this relationship.[67] These mandatory examinations were established in France in 1810 as a means to stop the spread of venereal diseases, particularly syphilis.[68] Prostitutes were required to register with the *police des moeurs*. Those who lived in *maisons closes* were inspected once every week or two at the brothel while those who worked at *maisons de tolérance* or on the street went to a neighbourhood dispensary.[69] The inspection consisted of a gynaecological examination with the use of a speculum, as well as an examination of the woman's hands, face, back, mouth, urethra, and anus.[70] A doctor and police officer were always present, and, if in a *maison close*, the madam of the house. Although some women tried to avoid registration through police records because it posed a threat to their reputation and forced them to submit to an unpleasant examination, most sex workers held a card on which their health was recorded. A prostitute who did not show up for the mandatory inspection or who did not have her card was arrested

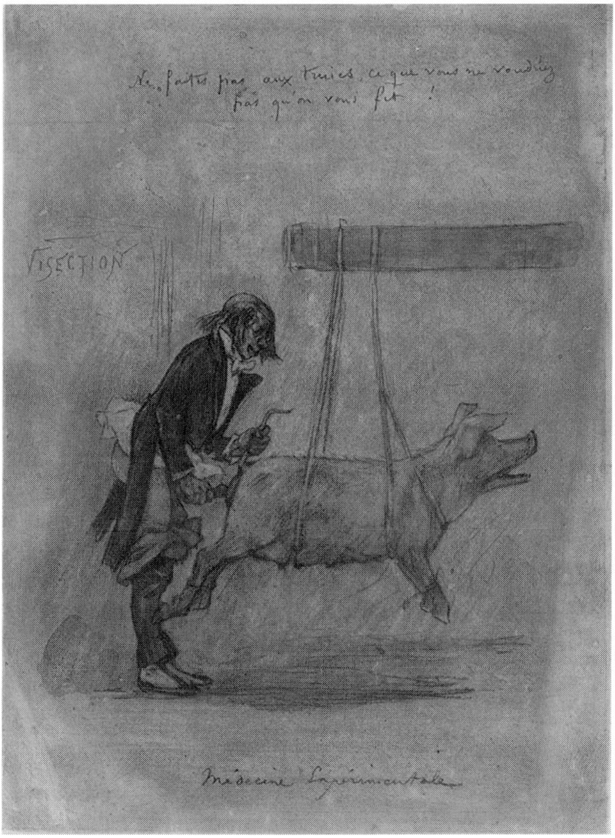

Félicien Rops, *Médecine expérimentale* (c.1880), heliogravure, 25.5 x 17.7cm. 36

and forced to submit to a gynaecological examination. Brothel customers were exempt from genital exams.

Although the medical inspection of prostitutes was understood as a matter of public health because syphilis was blamed for weakening national strength, poisoning families, and decreasing the population, the relationship between doctors and prostitutes was often questioned. Félicien Rops parodied this troubled relationship in his humourous print *Médecine Expérimentale* c.1880, which shows a doctor having sex with a suspended pig (Figure 36). Not only does this image picture the sexuality of medical men as deviant and perverse, but the pig – a symbol of prostitution – also suggests that a physician's contact with prostitutes was sexual. Rops's image implies that physicians' close contact with prostitutes' bodies combined the libidinal delights of looking and touching naked women with the authoritative power and social legitimacy of medicine:

under the guise of medical experimentation, doctors could satisfy their every desire.

The focused medical examination of bodies – including those of syphilitic women – is evidenced by the series of hand-coloured photo negatives reproduced in Alfred Louis Philippe Hardy's and A. de Montméja's 1868 book, *Clinique photographique de l'hôpital Saint-Louis*. Montméja, a physican who trained as a photographer, was particularly qualified for a project that merged the diagnositic with the aesthetic. The photographs taken at the hospital required interactions between photographers and doctors: doctors advised on what colours and details were required to produce lifelike representations, 'touching up' the photographs to make them appear more real. Montméja and Hardy emphasised the connection between the photograph and the patient's living body to attest to the truth claims of photography. In addition to the text on the bottom of each photograph that stated that the photograph and colouring were created directly from nature, they wrote 'We can say that these plates represent nature caught in the act'.[71]

Some of the photographs in this book show syphilitic women at Saint-Louis as ageing and deformed while others draw on popular stereotypes that associated specific diseases with particular populations; prostitution and syphilis were commonly linked. The photograph of a patient with vesicular syphilis, for example, shows a young naked woman, posing coyly with her arms behind her back (Figure 37). Small red dots, added to the black-and-white photograph, decorate the curves of her body, running from her shoulder, down her breasts, and around her abdomen until they disperse around her fuzzy pubis. The woman's sexual allure is symbolised by her accessible and naked body, and the fashionable black ribbon – a popular accessory for young working girls – around her neck. This photograph evinces how medicine borrowed from the popular visual culture of prostitution to make its representations legible for diagnostic – or perhaps even licentious – purposes, fashioning certain diseases and bodies as sexually alluring despite their sick status.

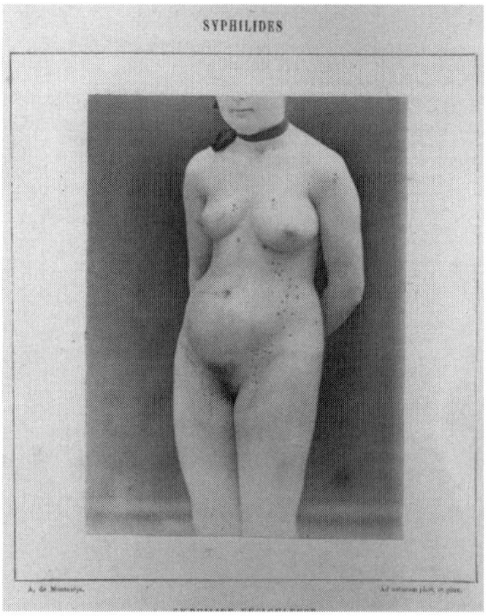

37 A. de Montmeja, 'Syphilide Vésiculeuse – II', from *Clinique photographique de l'hôpital Saint-Louis*, 1868, p. 120.

Péan's spectacular theatre: competing constructions of reality

Dissection and operating theatres were sites of modern entertainment that staged procedures and practices for the medical community and public.[72] Dr Péan, like other medical men in Paris (most famously Charcot), held weekly events in which he performed surgery on as many as six bodies over the course of a few hours in front of a large crowd.[73]According to one contemporary, Péan welcomed the audience's participation in the performance, often yelling out, 'Move aside, gentlemen, so that everyone can see!'[74] Operating theatres encouraged viewers' looking and invited them to partake in the spectacle of modern medicine. The ability to take part in the pleasure of looking differentiated the spectators from the patients whose bodies were on display. The operating theatre, as a site where the healthy were distinguished from the sick by the former's ability to see and act and the latter's imposed blindness through anaesthetics and forced immobility through surgical restraint, was one of many places where the public's fascination with the classification and categorisation of bodies was staged.

Gervex's depiction of Péan's surgery differs significantly from the accounts of his contemporaries who offered competing constructions of reality. Horace Bianchon, doctor and medical biographer, described his experience of Péan's surgery as follows:

> I was amazed. I had never imagined such dexterity, such speed, such impeccable sureness of hand, such consummate skill. It was more astonishing than horrible, this useful and beneficial butchery, this parade of unconscious patients being operated on and carried off in the blink of an eye, coming one after another on the bloody table in the gleam of bristling blades and clamps, instruments invented by him.[75]

For Bianchon, the atmosphere was one of urgency, speed, blood, and clanking metal. The operating theatre was a site where looking at bodies being dissected and dismembered is encouraged and expected. Although Ollendorf, in his book on the 1887 Salon, praised Gervex's realistic representation of Péan at work, he also criticised its ability to mislead both contemporary and future viewers:

> The figures in the background are not part of the scene, and since Monsieur Gervex sought the truth, he should have omitted them. When a professor is teaching in our hospital rooms, the students are gathered attentively around him; the ward nurses who have brought in the patient withdraw, and the leather straps of the harnesses are not left lying around on the bed. Finally, since this was a work that was meant to be preserved, and that, to use the expression that is currently fashionable, was supposed to serve as documentation, we would have liked the patient to keep on her hospital cap. Her tousled hair, spread against the white sheet, so effectively setting off the healthy glow of the patient's

> flesh, would, at the Salpêtrière, be explicable as the aftermath of some sort of attack, some nervous convulsion that would have caused a hysteric to suddenly become dishevelled. Here, at the Hôpital Saint-Louis, at an operation whose every detail will be pedantically and learnedly explained, this is misleading to the viewer.[76]

Ollendorf's comments – if they are to be trusted – demonstrate the instances in which Gervex departed from the realist quest of objective documentation in order to create an image that fulfilled his own desires as an artist, as well as those of Péan, as a paying customer. Ollendorf recognised that Gervex used the iconography of hysteria to render a female body that could retain its sexual allure despite its diseased identity. The pale and sickly, yet young and attractive patient fits easily within images of fashionable female illness. As discussed in Chapter 3, visual representations of hysterical women in the popular press and some Salpêtrière publications often showed eroticised female bodies seductively out of control. Although female illnesses, including hysteria, were often linked to prostitution, women's sickly surfaces were also considered fashionable by the bourgeoisie. The desire for pallor manifested itself commercially in women's cosmetics, particularly the aptly titled white facial powder, *Poudre Ophélie*. Undressed, unconscious, and horizontal, the woman in *Avant l'opération*, like Charcot's star hysteric, Blanche Wittman in Brouillet's *Une leçon clinique*, provided a pathological body for viewing pleasure.

Henri de Toulouse-Lautrec's numerous paintings and sketches of Péan provide other accounts of operating procedures at Saint-Louis. The artist frequented Péan's surgeries during the early 1890s, often accompanying his cousin, Dr Tapié de Celeyran, who was one of Péan's interns. Unlike Gervex, who painted a perfectly groomed Péan with an erect posture, the majority of Lautrec's images show him as a large and chunky man whose tiny head and feet destablise his rotund body. The artist's numerous sketches of Péan's face provide various takes on the surgeon's character: elegant profiles portray him as a grand orator while rough caricatures that exaggerate his hooked nose, heavy brow, and bushy facial hair show a barbarous thug. Despite their major differences in terms of style, medium, and exhibition history, Lautrec's images of Péan and Gervex's painting are both historical documents that record the details of Péan's body and depict his innovative procedures. Lautrec's multiple sketches, which show the surgeon washing before surgery, addressing the audience, and operating on a body, serve as a flipbook, symbolically bringing Péan and his procedure to life through the quick turning of pages. Although these images lack the detail, intricacy, and polish of Gervex's painted work, they nonetheless make claims to truth: the number of images, the multiple vantage points, and their status as sketches imply that they were created in the presence of Péan. Like Gervex, who referred to sketching in his memoirs to indicate his direct

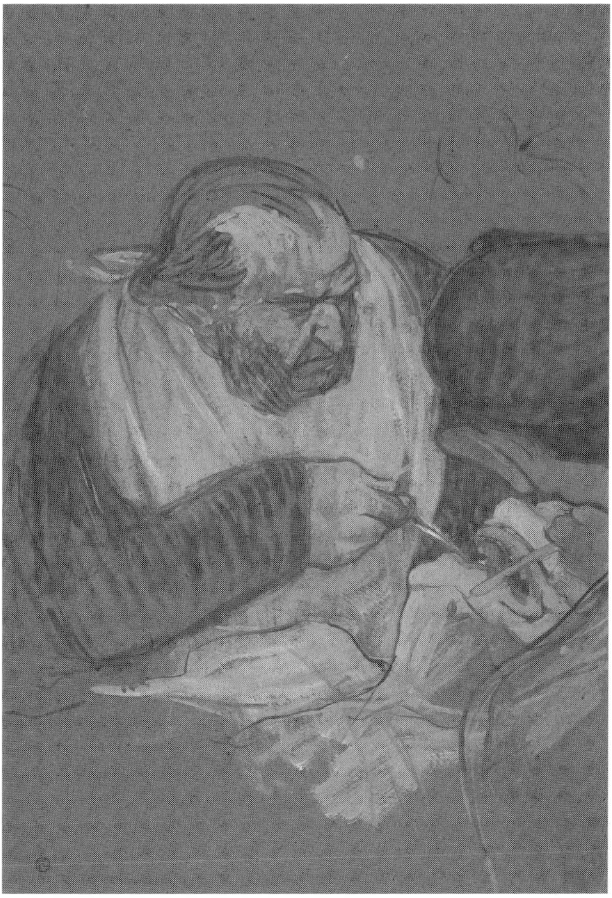

Henri de Toulouse-Lautrec, *Dr Péan Operating* (c.1891–92), oil on laminate cardboard, 73.9 x 49.9cm. 38

experience of an event, Lautrec's sketches also mark the artist as witness. Despite the differences between the two artists' work, the swiftness of Lautrec's studies produces a competing sense of reality that rivals the highly finished painted façade of Gervex's canvas.

Lautrec made only two paintings of Péan: *An Operation by Doctor Péan at the Hôpital International* and *Doctor Péan Operating* are both oil sketches on board made in 1891 (Figure 38). Like *Avant l'opération*, *An Operation by Doctor Péan at the Hôpital International* shows Péan standing at the head of an operating table surrounded by recognisable doctors.[77] Although both artists depicted daylight illuminating the operation through large open windows, Lautrec portrayed Péan with his back to the viewer, in the midst of surgery. The theatre is rendered as a busy and chaotic space where bodies crowd around the operating table to get a closer look, and patients wait to be cured. Lautrec's loose brushwork and dynamic composition contribute to this sense of movement. In this respect, the painting is more aligned with Bianchon's description of Péan's operating theatre than Gervex's ordered portrait.

In *Avant l'operation*, the spectacle of Péan's theatre is primarily created by the young, bare-breasted woman who dominates the canvas and its narrative. In contrast, the focus of *An Operation by Doctor Péan at the Hôpital International* is on the clothed bodies that are involved in the operation and its related procedures: the men seated on chairs watching the event, the medic crouched on the floor next to a patient, the nurse standing at the ready, and Péan and his interns performing the surgery. The seated medic shields the patient's body on the stretcher, and Péan's standing form, arms raised in action, disallows the spectator the viewing access to the patient that is granted by Gervex. Lautrec limits the viewer's access to the body being operated upon to foreground medical practice; the performance of medicine is the drama.

Lautrec's other painting, *Doctor Péan Operating*, provides an up-close look at Péan in action. With a white napkin around his neck and a silver tool in hand, he is shown delving into the mouth of an unconscious patient like a hungry man cutting into food. Unlike *Avant l'opération*, which portrays him gesturing elegantly, Lautrec's Péan is hunched over and is concentrating on the tracheotomy he is performing. The viewer is given full access to the patient and the operation through the composition's open foreground, and by Tapié de Celeyran whose tilted head and fleshy ear frame the viewer's position. In contrast to Gervex, Lautrec did not draw attention to his painting through the detailed rendering of naked female flesh. Rather, the unconscious patient's sex is unspecified – dressed simply in a white shirt the patient's features are hidden by the chloroform-soaked cloth that covers the eyes and nose. The patient's crude features, drooping jaw, and thick neck rid the painting of sexual allure.

Gervex's nudes

Contemporary critics located the sexual appeal of *Avant l'opération* in Gervex's painterly touch and in the painting's similarity to the artist's other salacious works, including *Rolla* – his notorious representation of an unclothed 'fallen' woman, Marion, that was rejected from the 1878 Salon because of its ostensible obscenity (Figure 39) – and *Femme au masque*, which was exhibited at the 1886 Salon to great fanfare since viewers tried to identify the nude masked woman.[78] Hippolyte Devillers wrote in his 1887 Salon review:

> No one plays with whites like Monsieur Gervex, but as he mixes in some kind of aphrodisiac substance that is not to be disdained, let him re-paint *Marion* – the horror of the jury – for us, or the *Femme au masque*. It is a good thing to

borrow one's subject from one's words. Monsieur Gervex has saucy remarks on his palette; let him use them![79]

Deviller's comments are typical of the sexual metaphors used by nineteenth-century artists and critics. In relation to *Avant l'opération*, Olivier Merson claimed, 'One could not better paint … the torso of the young patient, an accomplished piece, caressed by a self-assured brush'.[80] The seductiveness of Gervex's painting practice was also noted by A.M. de Bélina in 1883: 'Gervex is not only a talented painter, but also a charmer; much like his master Cabanel, he possesses the distinction and the seductive language that attract us'.[81] Mantz also focused on Gervex's rendering of naked female flesh when he wrote in his 1887 review that the Salon crowd was drawn to the canvas by 'both the interest of its subject matter and certain details of its beautifully developed execution, notably the woman's flesh, luminous and delicate against the whiteness of the sheets'.[82] The aphrodisiacal lure of the patient's pale skin was enhanced as Gervex's touches of white paint and naked female flesh became one. This sense of eroticised touch is emphasised by young Dr Zacharian, whose pink hand wraps around the patient's pale wrist and whose heavy arm lies across her pelvis.

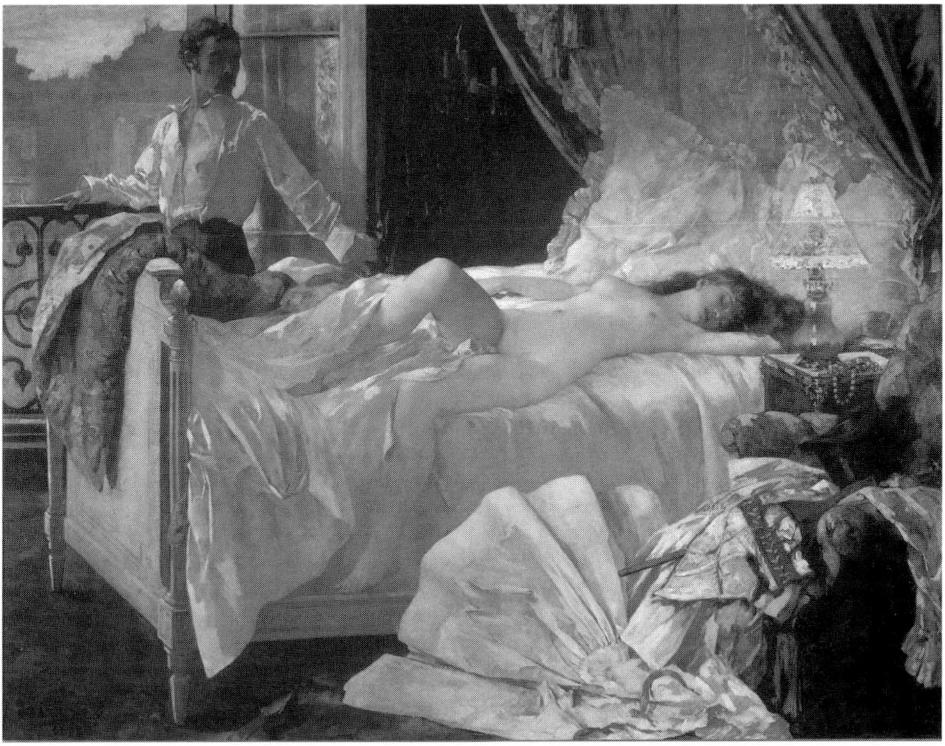

Henri Gervex, *Rolla* (1878), oil on canvas, 175 x 220cm. **39**

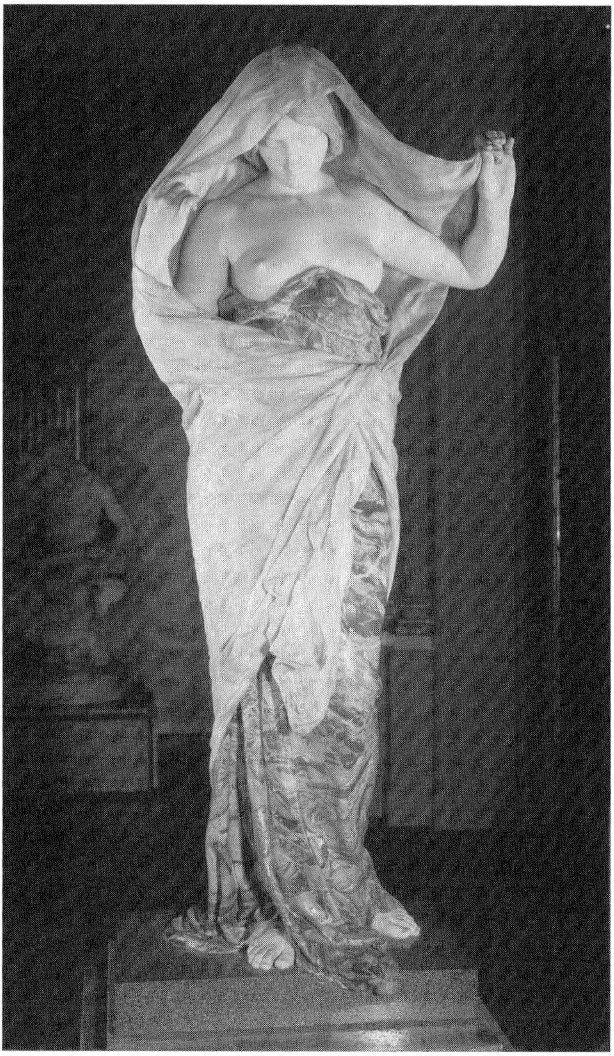

40 Louis Ernest Barrias, *Nature unveiling herself before Science* (1899), marble and polychrome onyx.

The neutrality of the clinic is potentially shattered in this moment of touch, where slipping sheets, gifted fingers, pink nipples, and young flesh converge. The doctor's touch, like Gervex's stroke, invokes a bodily desire that belies the assumed objectivity of rational documentation. Yet, Gervex symbolically contained this sensuality by invoking symbols of constraint, such as knotted curtains, a leather restraining belt slung around the orderly's shoulder, and the claustrophobic crowd of standing bodies. Furthermore, he pictured the patient according to many nineteenth-century academic conventions for painting the female nude: milky skin and closed eyes, a white cloth draping the lower body, light falling on young breasts, and dark hair cascading across crumpled sheets.[83] These elements reined in the possibility of passion and chaos (albeit fleetingly), returning the scene to one of clinical calmness and control.

Academic nudes, such as those painted by Gervex's teacher, Cabanel, spawned little criticism from the Salon jury: Cabanel's *Nymphe enlevée par un faune* (1860) and *La Naissance de Vénus* (1863), for example, were both popular, celebrated Salon nudes. As idealised bodies in timeless settings created by smooth academic brushstrokes, these images were not considered pornographic or obscene.[84] They did not show actual women's bodies, replete with pubic hair, fuzzy armpits, ageing skin, or genitals. Rather, these pristine nudes were used to symbolise nations, mythological figures, virtues, and professions. Medical and scientific spheres often relied upon artistic conventions when decorating their buildings. Numerous sculptures of female nudes, symbolising Truth, Medicine, and Nature, were scattered around the Académie de Médecine amongst the marble portrait busts of clothed medical leaders. A bas-relief of classical male and female nudes sits above the entrance to the main building, nude female figures symbolising Science and Truth flank the funerary sculpture of Dr Brouardel in one of the courtyards, and a version of Louis-Ernest Barrias's sculpture *Nature unveiling herself before Science* of 1889 is positioned to the left of the grand staircase leading to the medical library (Figure 40).[85]

Shown bare-breasted with long flowing hair, the young patient in *Avant l'opération* also recalls images of heroic female nudes – or semi-nudes – that personified France, such as Marianne, Liberté, and La République.[86] Although the patient's immobility contrasts with highly active portrayals of Liberté, as in Delacroix's 1830 *La Liberté guidant le peuple*, she can nonetheless be read as a sick Marianne. Marianne regularly appeared weak and ill during the late nineteenth century as a way to refer to France's loss in the Franco-Prussian war. For example, an 1871 postcard shows a bare-breasted and bound Marianne being sent to a Prussian camp.[87] Perhaps Gervex staged the scene of Marianne's resuscitation, where she is transported from the battlefield to the operating table to be brought back to life by Péan's innovative tools and procedures.

Although Gervex attempted to veil the patient's nakedness by referring to other symbolic nudes and by drawing on academic conventions (her body is pale and smooth, complete and untainted, chaste and intact), it is apparent that this was intended to be read as a real, observed body, not an imagined one, as is evident from the patient's creased skin and rough hands. Realist representations of unclothed female bodies were often considered obscene: unlike conventional nudes, these bodies exposed, or hinted at, a femininity that defied society's moral and sexual norms.[88] As demonstrated by the removal of *Rolla* from the Salon and most famously by the reactions against Manet's *Olympia* at the 1865 Salon, nudes were considered indecent for any number of reasons, including when body hair was shown; when there was obvious evidence of undress; when the woman was recognisable as a prostitute; when the body was painted in a way that challenged the smooth, contained, and 'sexless' body of conventional nudes; or when the body was associated with a scandalous contemporary setting or narrative. Gervex's *Rolla*, which was based on Alfred de Musset's 1833 poem, shows an unclothed woman sleeping on a bed while a young bourgeois man looks on the streets of Paris and considers suicide after having spent all his money on gambling and sex. As Hollis Clayson has aptly argued, the painting alludes to the debauchery of modern Paris because the woman's discarded corset in the foreground symbolised prostitution to nineteenth-century audiences.[89] This scene, and the corset in particular, modernised Gervex's nude: no longer veiled by the idealisation and timelessness of academic nudes, the woman in *Rolla* became scandalous through her identification as a prostitute despite being painted according to academic norms. Clayson suggests that the critics' dismay at this picture reflected fears and anxieties surrounding female sexuality and the spread of sexually transmitted diseases. Although *Avant l'opération* also modernised the nude by its contemporary scene, its setting is one in which an unclothed female body is controlled and made healthy through the medical intervention of male hands. In contrast, the woman in *Rolla* stretches out on the bed, carefree and unselfconscious. It is Rolla himself, not the naked woman, who is being punished for his sins.

Significantly, Gervex's professional identity was based upon *Rolla*. The young prostitute, Marion, stripped naked on a bed, brought the young Gervex fame and artistic credibility within the circle of artists praised by Zola as naturalists and exemplified by artists such as Manet and Degas. In 1881, Zola praised Gervex and named him as one of the younger generation of artists who would follow in their footsteps: 'of all the rebels at the École des Beaux-Arts, Gervex, Bastien-Lepage, Butin, Duez, have gone over to the camp of the moderns and seem to want to place themselves at the head of the movement'.[90] The painting's rejection from the Salon helped position Gervex as the new *enfant terrible*. Yet his rendering of undressed women in the 1880s, exemplified by *Avant l'opération* and *Femme au masque*, hovers between acceptability and scandal. Henry Houssaye's 1886 Salon review demonstrates that by the mid-1880s, Gervex's undressed women were considered pleasant rather than notorious, and his 'naturalism' was alluring and pleasurable: 'if Henri Gervex's *Femme au masque* is a work of naturalism, it is certainly a naturalism that is entirely lovable, full of seduction'.[91] This shift in Gervex's practice, and critics' responses to his work, demonstrate the flexibility and un-fixedness of the terms realism and naturalism, and also show the changing attitudes towards modern nudes.

By the late 1880s, the modern nude was not as contested a category as it had been during the time of *Olympia* and *Rolla*. This historical shift is exemplified by Zola's noting in 1881 that mythological and historical nudes at the Salon were being replaced by scenes of contemporary life, and most obviously by the 1889 campaign to buy *Olympia* for the national museum.[92] Although nudes in contemporary settings were becoming more commonplace by 1887, representations of unclothed female bodies nonetheless produced both pleasure and anxiety in Salon critics and audiences, particularly since women were simultaneously pictured as innocent, sickly, and seductive. The perceived duality of women remained because of the uncertainty and unknowability of female sex and sexuality. Despite intrusive medical examinations, the 'secrets' of the female body could never be solved. As demonstrated by the frequent personification of Nature and Truth as female forms, women's bodies were commonly conceived of as objects from which knowledge could be gained, and therefore direct observation and constant study were deemed necessary and socially justified. Barrias' *Nature unveiling herself before Science* illustrates this point and exemplifies the sexualisation of scientific inquiry. As Jordanova argues, the sculpture implies that science is a masculine viewer who can achieve full knowledge of nature through the examination of a female body.[93] She points out that what is significant about Barrias's work is that the female body is not a naked body, exposing all, but is rather one that needs to be unveiled. To disrobe this body would provide pleasure through the act of revealing, but it would also indicate that there is something to conceal.

In *Avant l'opération*, the female body is never completely unveiled nor is it ever fully stripped of academic conventions. The gap in the creased sheet which covers her lower half exposes pink flesh and forms a delicate opening that is clean and penetrable. The sheet's literal ability to hide the body is simultaneously used to mask and draw attention to the female genitals. As Peter Brooks argues in his psychoanalytic account of realist novels and paintings, the unveiling of the female body is impossible because narratives that involve this unveiling 'sooner or later reach the problem of unveiling the female sex, which they find to be itself a veil – perhaps from the anxiety that its final unveiling would reveal that there is nothing to unveil or, rather, that apparent nothing is indeed something'.[94] To 'de-nude' the patient in *Avant l'opération* would ultimately lead toward the unveiling of the female sex, considered in psychoanalytic theory to be the locus of male anxiety and female power. Although Brooks claims that this reflects the realist artist's inability to leave the conventional nude behind, it also points to the female body as a site of realism's irrationality and subjectivity. It is worth noting that an unidealised naked patient in a contemporary context would have been refused by Salon judges.

Gervex's reliance on artistic conventions allowed him to create a scene in which the sexual gratification of viewing the unclothed female body was untainted by medical constructions of women as diseased, fertile, and fragile.[95] Yet, the aestheticisation of the patient belies the illness that the medical theme suggests and ultimately exposes the trouble with realist claims to objective documentation. Unlike the nudes in Gervex's earlier paintings, such as *Satyre jouant avec une bacchante* (1874) and *Baigneuse endormie* (1873), this naked body cannot be unproblematically consumed as a playful young nymph in the woods or a sleeping nude in an idealised landscape. Rather, this is a modern woman, a medicalised *parisienne*, a clinical Ophelia. Removed from a mythological setting and placed in a medical sphere, the body is transformed into an object of medical inquiry. Unlike the contained vessels of academic femininity, where the robust health of female figures is indicated through their intimate connection with nature, the medical setting in *Avant l'opération* transforms the female body into an object to be read and monitored. Gervex's rendering of the patient's smooth, young body disavows the signs of illness that her position on the operating table purports. Furthermore, the body's idealisation contrasts with the attempted realism of the patient's face, whose large nose and furrowed brow indicate that this is a modern woman rather than a classical beauty. The representation of Woman in *Avant l'opération* fluctuates between sickness and health, purity and contamination, idealism and realism, thus exposing the fragility and impossibility of a perfect and static femininity.

Another example of Gervex's adherence to the conventions of painting a nude is displayed in his attempt to mask the patient's identity. Although the painting's title and Péan's presence indicate that this woman is a patient at Saint-Louis, nowhere is this illness indicated on her body. Unlike the patients photographed at the hospital, who were often covered in rashes and open sores, her body is smooth and white, contained and solid. Relatively devoid of nature's flaws and the signs of living, Gervex's patient resembles an anatomical wax model, a medical Venus. Medical Venuses, such as those displayed in the Spitzner collection, stood in stark contrast to the realities of lived female bodies – bodies that bled and hosted disease, bodies that were contagious, bodies that died and rotted.

Realism beyond reason: sleeping beauties in wax

Wax models and anatomical Venuses were used as teaching aids because wax, more than any other medium, was believed to best resemble human flesh. Reporting on the production of wax figures for the Musée Grévin, Alber wrote in *La Nature* in 1894 that 'The only malleable material capable of perfectly rendering the effect of flesh, with [its] velvety transparency, is wax'.[96] Wax was associated with feminity because of its soft, malleable, and subtle materiality. It was also linked to socially acceptable femininity since bourgeois women made wax models of flowers and fruit – symbols of femininity due to their associations with nature, fertility, fragility, and decoration – as a pastime. The pliability of wax and desired malleability of women were united in the fantasy of a medical Venus. The life-size models – adorned with pearl necklaces, closing glass eyes, and long flowing hair (human or animal) – often contained removable parts that allowed the models to be taken apart and put back together, giving the viewer access to inner organs, including the uterus, which was often accessorised with a fetus (Figure 41). Unlike wax models of male bodies that were customarily shown standing in active poses, displaying exterior musculature and bones, medical Venuses lay horizontally with half-shut eyes, suggesting sleep.

Clemente Susini and Gaetano Giulio Zumbo created the most famous of these wax models for La Specola in Florence in the eighteenth century (Figure 42), though models and Venuses were made in France until the late nineteenth century.[97] Gaston Le Breton describes their popularity in his 1891 'Essai historique sur la sculpture en cire', in which he provides a history from early Egyptian wax figures to nineteenth-century medical *moulages* (moulds).[98] The public fascination with wax models was sustained by Spitzner's display of pathological and celebrity wax bodies in his Grand Musée d'Anatomie, which opened to the Parisian public in 1856. Spitzner further propagated the idea of medicine as spectacle by hiring doctors and nurses to lead visitors through the exhibitions.[99] The popular demand for such entertainment provoked the opening of similar displays in Paris in the second half of the century, including the Musée Grévin, which opened in 1882.[100] The public's fascination with waxes was linked to the nineteenth-century obsession with

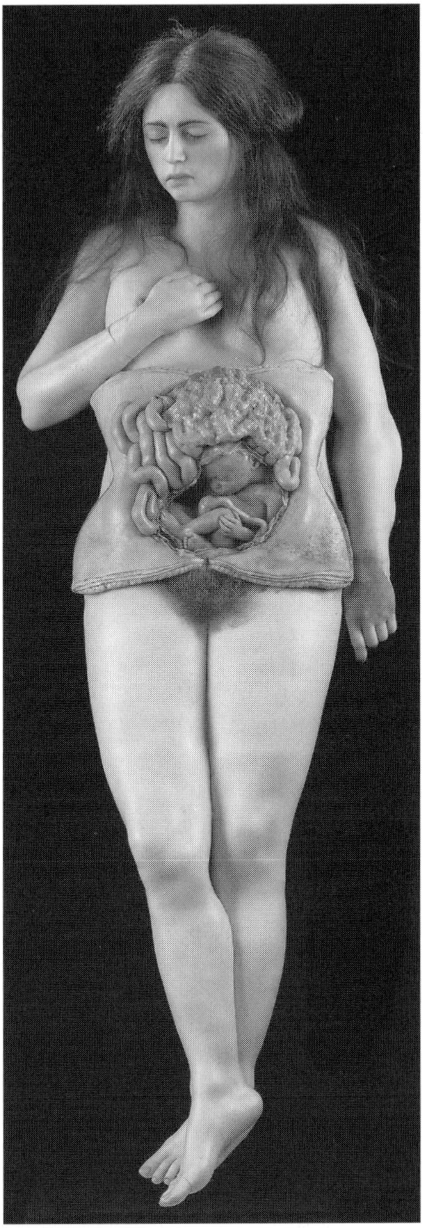

41 Anatomical model of a pregnant woman (nineteenth century), wax and hair.

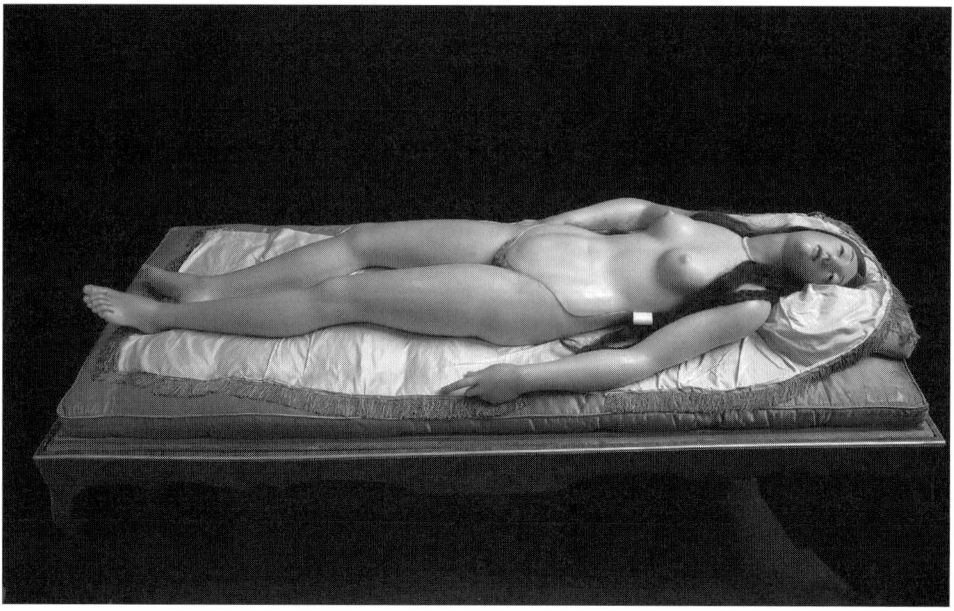

42 Anatomical Venus (eighteenth century), wax, hair, pearls.

representations of real bodies, as Vanessa Schwartz argues. The pleasure and entertainment arose from wax's striking verisimilitude to 'real' life. As reported in the *Moniteur Universel*, 'at the Musée Grévin resemblance is perfect, striking, extraordinary. You begin to ask yourself whether you are in the presence of a real person'.[101]

The female body in *Avant l'opération*, like a medical Venus, is an idealised yet pathological body ready to be dismantled and observed by the skilled eyes and hands of medical professionals. In contrast to Péan, whose masculinity is symbolised by his erect posture, gesturing hands, formal attire, facial hair, and prominent position, the patient's femininity is symbolised by nudity, pallor, and passivity. The woman's comatose state becomes representative of a femininity that allows for the total empowerment of the male gaze and touch; she is a foil against which male agency can be asserted. The female body has no agency: she is pure body, pure material, ready to be manipulated, prodded, and penetrated. Be it by Péan's scalpel or Gervex's brush, the body becomes both the object of male performance and its source of knowledge. Like a medical Venus, this female body contains the promise of revealing all. It is a potential body in pieces that could be taken apart and reassembled by Péan's skilled hands. The fragmentation of the human body was necessary for the acquisition of medical knowledge since, as Jonathan Sawday argues, the violent reduction of the complete body into pieces forms a new 'body' of medical understanding.[102] In medical Venuses, the female body is an object that improves medical knowledge and whose purpose is the advancement of medical learning. These wax figures embodied the pluralistic and often contradictory understandings of femininity and female sexuality in medical discourse because they were conceived of as bodies in need of medical attention, as well as decorative fertile vessels. Wax, unlike human flesh, is a material that can be easily cut into without encountering bones or organs. It can be melted and moulded to hide any signs of trauma. By drawing on artistic conventions, as is evident in the clear complexions, the loose flowing hair, and the figures' states of rest, these waxes provided a palatable femininity that passively revealed all.

In her scandalous novel *Monsieur Vénus,* published in 1884, Rachilde made the connection between wax and a submissive and pathological femininity. In this text, Raoule de Vénérande, an aristocratic woman, cunningly seduces a beautiful and young working-class painter, Jacques Silvert, through a series of actions that reverse conventional nineteenth-century gender roles. Raoule is an active seductress: she dresses as a man, financially supports Jacques, and controls his actions. Throughout the novel, Jacques becomes increasingly feminised by Raoule: he obeys her commands, he wears luxurious clothing that she gives him and, in the bedroom, he takes on the traditional female role of passive receiver. Diana Holmes argues that by having Raoule subject Jacques to the objectification, violence, and humiliation usually inflicted upon women, Rachilde reversed and parodied nineteenth-century conceptions of gender, and therefore reconfigured gender identity as fluid.[103] The ultimate objectification and feminisation of Jacques occurs at the end of the novel when Raoule crafts a wax model out of Jacques's dead body. By adding his blond eyelashes, white teeth, and fingernails to the model, thus making it as lifelike as possible, Raoule creates her own Monsieur Vénus. Transforming Jacques from a living man into a pliable model rid him of the active and domineering characteristics understood to belong to the male sex. Jacques's transformation into wax transgressed conventional gender roles because medical Venuses were primarily representations of female bodies made for male viewers and wax was associated with femininity's malleability not masculinity's stiffness. Significantly, Raoule's Monsieur Vénus is not only an effigy of her lover, but is also an instrument of sexual pleasure. Once again subverting gender roles, the novel ends with Raoule, here conceived as both a young woman in mourning and a young man in evening dress, visiting the wax model:

> They come to kneel beside the bed, and after contemplating at length the marvellous lines of the wax statue, they embrace it, kiss it on the lips. A spring hidden inside the flanks connects with the mouth and animates it at the same time that it spreads apart the thighs.[104]

Along with being 'feminised' by the new material of his body, Jacques's sexual actions are mechanically made female as his legs are made to separate upon sexual arousal. Death, sex, and femininity are intricately bound in the figure of the wax Venus, who remains sexually available despite her (or in this case, his) lifeless, lifelike body.

Anaesthetised states

Representations of sleeping, anaesthetised, hypnotised, and dead women were prominent in nineteenth-century visual culture: Bram Dijkstra argues that they were popular because they symbolised a femininity that appeared untouched by the emerging feminist movement,[105] while Elisabeth Bronfen, in her psychoanalytic examination of the aestheticisation of death in Gabriel von Max's 1869 painting *Der Anatom*, argues that the female body could materialise into an immaculate aesthetic form because it was a dead body, transformed into Art. She argues that such figures expose how death functions in the aesthetic construction of beauty since beauty becomes contingent on the transformation of an animate body into an inanimate one; while depictions of unconscious female bodies may signify beauty, completeness, and perfection, they also anticipate the dissolution of such attributes.[106] In relation to *Der Anatom*, Bronfen suggests that the fear of death is masked by the idealisation of a female corpse. Following similar conventions, Gervex hid the pain and suffering of Péan's patient by painting a semi-idealised nude body. In both works, the aestheticisation of the inanimate female body stands in for the unstable and ultimately unachievable representation of unknowable states.

In *Avant l'opération*, Gervex was confronted with the problem of how to depict a body under anaesthesia realistically. Anaesthetics were first used in 1846, yet how they worked was still debated.[107] Although they were praised for allowing longer operations and for removing pain during surgery, some contemporary critics believe that the process was brutal and violent, and therefore propagated the use of hypnotism during surgery instead.[108] At the Salpêtrière, anaesthesia was a common form of punishment and control used on hysterical women.[109] In *Avant l'opération*, Gervex portrayed the controversial act of making the subject unconscious by presenting the viewer with a relatively passive and peaceful female body. The only harmful signs of anaesthesia are the traces of blood on the white cloth, the patient's slightly furrowed brow and the display of her unruly hair. The woman is depicted in a constant state of being put to sleep; her consciousness is controlled by the young doctor holding the chloroformed cloth. Although anaesthetics were celebrated by the medical community because surgeons could perform operations more swiftly without the interference of a struggling patient, the public feared surgeons' full power over anaesthetised bodies. Martin S. Pernick argues that the link between anaesthetics and power was often understood in terms of sexual dominance: in Victorian humour magazines, where images showing women being tamed by anaesthetics became popular, anaesthesia exemplified male power and female passivity.[110] The ties between sexual desire and the application of anaesthetics remain at play pictorially in *Avant l'opération* through the hands of the young doctor: one lingers near a nipple while the other is positioned to cover her mouth.

Most contemporary critics recognised the patient as anaesthetised or chloroformed.[111] In many ways, she was visually similar to the wax model of an anaesthetised woman at the Musée Orfila, which opened in Paris in 1847. Both bodies were depicted with long flowing hair, pale skin, and smooth surfaces. Notably, Gervex painted the patient's lips slightly parted to indicate that this was a living and breathing body despite its inanimate status. Both bodies evidenced the nineteenth-century fascination with a body living on the cusp of life and death – at the Orfila, the wax Venus's mechanical lungs simulated the act of breathing. The electricity that coursed through the wax at the Orfila and the modern chemical substance that surged through Gervex's anaesthetised patient imbued both nudes with the blood of modernity. The timelessness of myth and the contemporaneity of technology unite in representations of sleeping female bodies, Nina Auerbach argues; their slumbering surfaces contain the epoch's power.[112]

The state of anaesthesia, a state between life and death, the animate and the inanimate, found its ideal medium in wax. In 1919, Freud used E. Jentsch's example of waxwork figures as the source that most keenly aroused the distinct sense of the uncanny. He described it as arising out of the feeling of 'doubt as to whether an apparently animate object really is alive and conversely, whether a lifeless object might not perhaps be animate'.[113] The sense of the uncanny was produced by the hyperrealism of wax models. Freud was familiar with wax figures through the widespread popularity of wax museums as forms of entertainment throughout Europe in the late nineteenth century. Furthermore, since he attended many of Charcot's lectures at the Salpêtrière between 1885 and 1886, it is likely that he was familiar with the wax models at Parisian hospitals and in public venues.

Although wax provided the verisimilitude that science demanded and benefited from the rhetoric of objectivity when displayed in a medical context, it nonetheless provoked feelings of fear because of its historical connections with cruelty. The inability to distinguish reality from fiction when viewing waxworks provided entertainment as much as it provoked anxiety, as is evident from de Bury's tale in *Les Bonhommes de cire* that began this chapter. For de Bury, the realism associated with wax models was connected to hysteria, fear, and repulsion rather than reason or delight. Wax often stood in when the human body fragmented or died, as is evident in wax death masks, religious votives, and the wax heads of those killed under the guillotine on show at Madame

Tussaud's and the Musée Grévin. Norman Bryson suggests that waxworks are most real in their excessive detailing, but that they are never real enough: the displeasure of viewing wax models is caused by its inability, as a medium, to maintain the desired stability of idealisation and bodily wholeness despite the realism of its surface. Wax melts, crumbles, and deforms; it presages a body in pain, mutilation, and potential termination.[114] Like medical Venuses, the anaesthetised state lingers between the interplay of idealisation and abjection, the wholeness of the body's exterior veiling the instability and unknowability of its interior.

In *Avant l'opération*, Gervex attempted to create an image in which the promise of female flesh remained safely contained through the use of artistic conventions and the depiction of anaesthetics. He staged a voyeuristic scene in which the gaze could enjoy the spectacle of modern medicine, specifically its object of enquiry – the female body – without having to turn away from the brutality promised by the scene's ultimate narrative: that of an operation in which a patient will be cut open. Rather than paint the violent event, he depicted the moment before the operation, the moment of cleanliness, hygiene, and control, the moment before the surgeon's clean hands and white shirt would be stained with the woman's blood, the moment before the erect bodies of suited medical men would be transformed into hunched-over butchers. The tiny drops of blood are an intimation of what is to come. They also work pictorially to bring out the artist's blood-red signature. The crimson paint used to form Gervex's name foreshadows Péan's impending cut to connect the specialised manual skills of both artist and surgeon. This painting epitomises what Bronfen calls the 'crucial moment of hesitation' where the aesthetically pleasing unity of the female body appears to draw 'added power from the fact that implicitly we know it is about to be cut into'.[115] Péan was a man who cut and cured bodies. In *Avant l'opération*, he is presented, tool in hand, ready to puncture the immaculate vessel as the female body becomes the site of his performance. The perfect contours of flesh are ready to be destroyed. The female body as it is now represented will never be the same again but will be scarred and marked by the surgeon's cut. Unlike other paintings of surgical theatres, like Thomas Eakins's *The Gross Clinic*, that show bodies mid-surgery – bloodied and fragmented – the unpunctured body on the operating table in *Avant l'opération* does not repel the viewer because it is not yet disfigured.[116]

Péan, as a surgeon, fragmented and fixed bodies. His profession demanded the repetitive act of cutting and sealing. Péan's invention was used to seal arteries, yet the mark of his knife left his seal in human flesh. Such bloody displays were not suitable for a Salon audience, nor could such a portrayal present Péan as a perfect icon of rational republican masculinity. The painting required an idealised depiction of a pure and contained femininity even though the painting's narrative, sitter, and scene demanded a body cut open. Despite the safety of artistic conventions and the assumed reason of realism, the painting remains haunted by the inevitability of incision. Restricted by societal constraints, Péan's occupational necessity to cut up bodies could not be fully realised within the confines of painted portraiture. It is not surprising, therefore, that Péan turned to another form of realism that, through its association with the production of medical knowledge, was also cloaked in social respectability.

Péan's collection of wax body parts

During the last decades of the century, Péan commissioned roughly 615 *moulages* of diseased body parts. These waxes were displayed in the large lecture theatre and museum at Saint-Louis hospital, which was built in 1889 to host the first international conference of dermatology and to celebrate the progress of French medicine during the Exposition Universelle of that year (Figure 43).[117] During the nineteenth century, *moulages* became a primary form of recording diseases affecting the surface of the body because they could provide more realistic representations than living bodies: sealed in jars, human flesh discoloured and disintegrated while wax maintained its applied form and pigments. Wax modelling, like photography, was introduced into the Parisian hospital system as a means of recording the intricacies of diseases and diseased bodies.[118] A *moulage* was created by a plaster cast that, moulded on the human body, provided a negative into which wax could be poured.[119] Following the moulding process, the *mouleur* (mould maker) and doctor would work together to craft an object that was understood to be an exact replica of the human body. Hair and coloured pigments were often added to aid the viewer in determining who the patient was and what illness was present. *Moulages*, as imprints of the body's surface, provided the easiest visual access to illness and allowed doctors and medical students to test their own knowledge of diseases and their symptoms without the presence of the patient. The examination of the *moulage*, unlike the examination of a living human body, particularly the body of a woman, was not regulated by the confines of bourgeois comportment and spectatorship. Rather, these wax bodies, contained within the privileged and regulated medical sphere, allowed, stimulated, and encouraged the visual scrutiny of naked bodies and body parts.

Péan's waxes show in detail how diseases attack particular body parts: wax *moulages* of genitalia, tongues, arms, faces, and torsos are covered with signs of illness, including pus and multicoloured rashes (Figure 44). The detailed imitation of fleshy skin tones, the redness of infection, minute hair follicles, and goose bumps produced images of sick bodies that were considered as lifelike as possible. These wax body fragments were mounted on black painted wood and framed by white plaster-soaked cloth. They were accompanied by a printed label that indicated the name of the doctor who commissioned the piece and

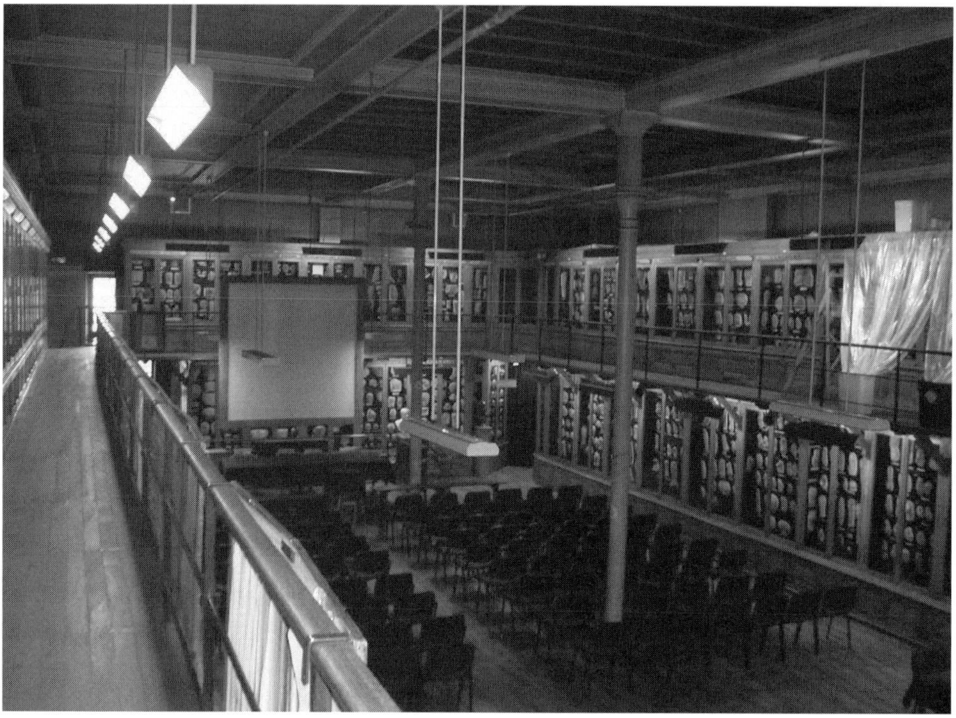

43 Musée des moulages at Hôpital Saint-Louis, Paris.

the name of the disease; another label provided the wax's catalogue number. Each one was signed in white paint by the *mouleur*.

From the outset, these works were intended to be collected and displayed within the medical sphere. They were used for documenting disease and teaching. However, by drawing on such artistic conventions as the practice of signing an artwork, the *moulages* were also aligned with the seemingly more subjective art world. The personally marked works and aestheticised presentation undermined the waxes' status as impartial models made for scientific study and situated them as part of a privileged and personal collection. Although collecting and exhibiting objects were integral to the production of medical knowledge, they also reflected the subjective fantasies of the collector. In this respect, the Saint-Louis waxes were tied to Péan and to the 'reality' he wished them to represent. Like Péan, the *mouleur* at Saint-Louis had an invested role in the production of the waxes – his signature was inscribed near the doctor's name. Although this united the model-maker with the physician, symbolically imbuing him with a medical professional's claim to accuracy and objectivity, it was the doctor's experience and orders – his expert eye – that were needed to construct the 'reality' of a disease.

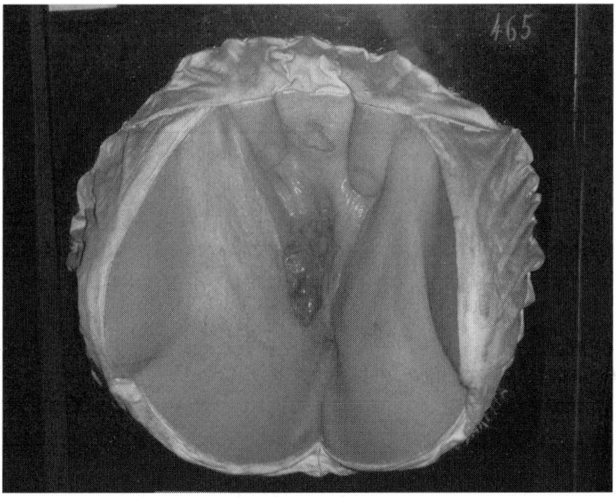

Moulage from Dr Péan's collection, Hôpital Saint-Louis, Paris. 44

Jules Baretta, who made the majority of waxes at Saint-Louis during the nineteenth century, began his process by making a plaster cast of the diseased body part. Casting was a process used in medical and artistic millieux to produce indexical objects. It was a method of image production that promised accurate replicas, yet it was often socially linked to sexual desire, particularly in artistic spheres. The fantasy of making casts from naked bodies is staged in Édouard Joseph Dantan's painting *Un moulage sur nature* (shown at the 1887 Salon) (Figure 45) and Felicien Rops's *La Naissance de Vénus* of 1878. In Dantan's work, men are peeling dried plaster off a woman's naked body, while in Rops's, a sculptor pours liquid plaster onto a woman's bare stomach and genital region. Both images show healthy female bodies as the objects of casting; the casts produced would later be used as models of female bodies from which artists could work. Despite the professional setting, the close contact between naked female bodies and clothed men in these works elicits a sense of desire despite the veneer of professional obligation. This tension, and the wish to keep touch reined in as a specialist's task, is evident in Mantz's 1887 Salon review of Dantan's painting:

> The two artists who are carrying out this work bring to it a sort of priest-like gravity; they do not allow themselves to be distracted by the nearby spectacle; if such rites were entrusted to pure laymen, we might see their hands shake as they touched the amorous flesh; but there are states of grace for mould makers, and they are interested only in the success of their delicate operation.[120]

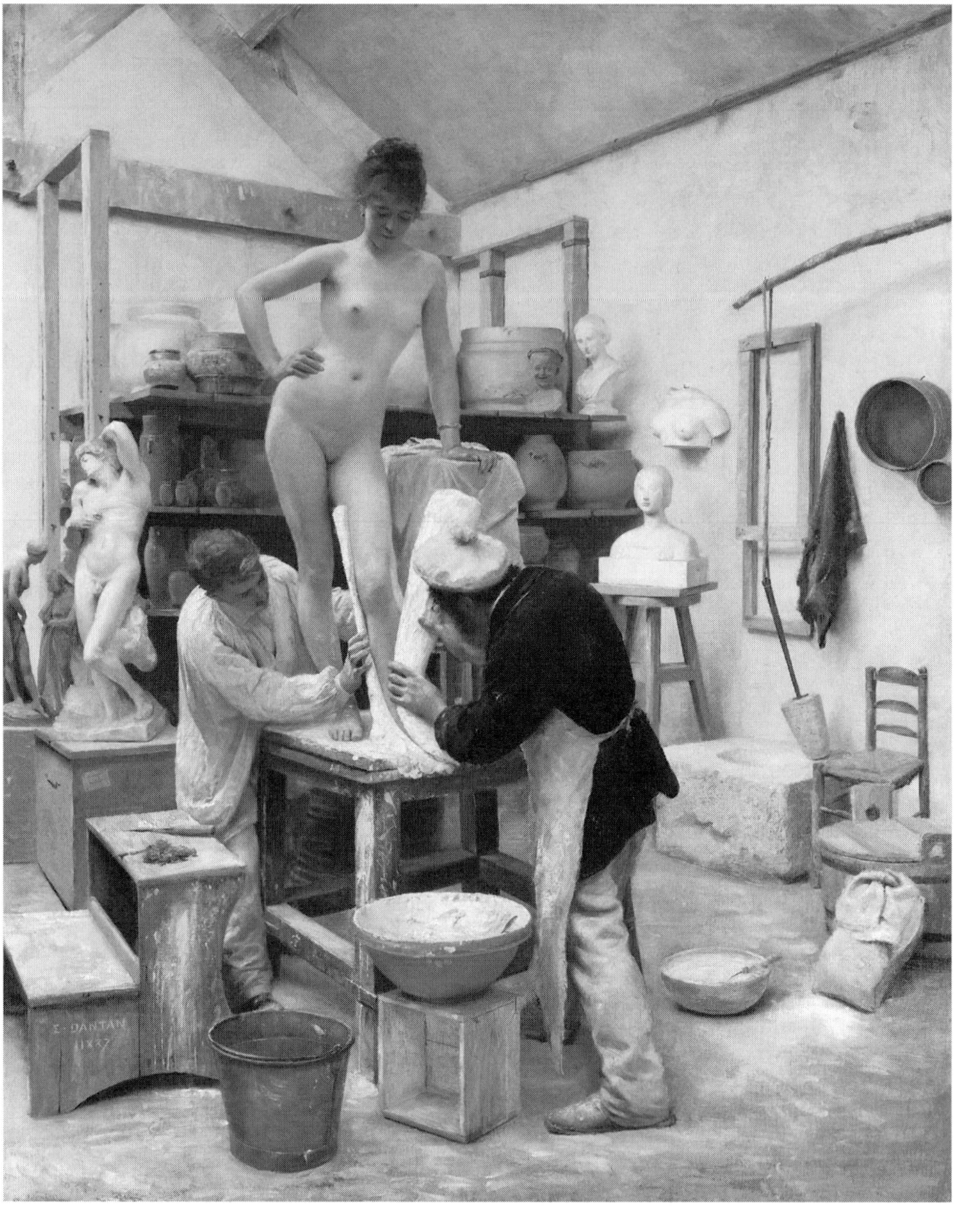

45 Édouard Joseph Dantan, *Un moulage sur nature* (1887), oil on canvas, 165 x 131.5cm.

Despite Mantz's purported belief that the *mouleurs* were indifferent to bare female skin, the painting's narrative used the occupational guise of casting as a socially justifiable means to display the contact between female flesh and male hands. Although Dantan created a modern nude by showing the model in a contemporary setting, with a Parisian coiffure, a brassy gold bracelet, and tanned face and hands, this image nonetheless adheres to many academic conventions of painting an idealised female nude: her body is white, her pubic mound is hairless, and her nipples are pink and erect. By drawing on these tropes, Dantan, like Gervex, pictured female sexuality as pure, accessible, and unthreatening for its display at the Salon. By surrounding the model with men in their specialised workplace, he portrayed artists' practice (including his own) as professional and detached, while the act of looking and touching naked bodies is shown as a valid requisite for the creation of female nudes.

The casting process in the medical sphere required the same intimate and lengthy contact with bodies as it did in the art world. As M. Sully Prudhomme wrote in 1891, the intimate process of making a medical cast at Saint-Louis required patience and kindness:

> Monsieur Baretta is an invaluable scientific collaborator. Without roughness, with a mother's gentleness and unfailing patience, he applies the plaster apparatus and as the material sets, he chats with the patient, takes an interest in his illness, gets him to talk about its progress, and, without seeking to, wins his trust, so greatly does he inspire sympathy. If the patient prefers not to speak – since it takes some time for the plaster to harden, and since the sight of a cast in progress is by no means pleasant – Monsieur Baretta shows him his paintings … then he sits down at his piano and soon is lulling his client with some old melody.[121]

Although Sully Prudhomme's account describes Baretta as compassionate and caring, the wax tongues and genitalia displayed at the hospital leave no doubt that casting was an invasive and uncomfortable process that required wet plaster on open sores, rashy skin, and the body's most sensitive openings. The exhaustive touching is showcased in Péan's collection of *moulages* of diseased genitalia. In a few of these waxes, fingers pry open vaginal lips and pull down foreskin to reveal interior illness (Figure 44). The thickness, length, and position of the fingers, cast from life along with the genitalia lead us to ask 'to whom do the fingers belong?' Although they may allude to masturbatory pleasure, itself conceived of as a sign of sexual deviance and illness in nineteenth-century medical discourse, by being cut off from the body, the fingers also act as a medical tool, much like the speculum, holding open cavities for medical male eyes. The function of the fingers and their fragmentation from an identifiable body helped rid the wax models of the salaciousness invoked by their close iconographic ties with pornographic images, which showed probing fingers as a means of pleasure and exposing further flesh.[122] The wax casts also stood as proof of medical touch itself, as they held in wax the intimate moment of bodily contact between doctor, *mouleur*, and patient. Significantly, the scrutiny and handling of diseased genitalia pointed to a pleasure that was not necessarily libidinally charged. The gratification of studying the intricate detailing of diseases, and the pleasure taken in cataloguing and collecting *moulages* of diseased body parts, are evidence of a curiosity and delight with representations of reality that exceeds medical and taxonomic requirements. Yet, displayed in a medical setting and labelled *ad nauseam* with the names of doctors, diseases, and catalogue numbers, the fingering of genitalia was exhibited as a legitimate professional pursuit.

Created primarily as objects of study and medical training, dermatological waxes were examined by medical students and doctors as a way to practise diagnostic skills and see rare diseases. Patients had limited access to the waxes and could not always see what was happening, and was going to happen, to their bodies. As learning tools and models of illness, the realism of the waxes was of utmost importance. Life-size, three-dimensional, and in colour, these hyper-real objects were believed to provide more lifelike models than those made by other media used in medical instruction, such as photography, painting, drawing, and print.[123] An article in *Annales de dermatologie et de syphiligraphie* described the waxes in 1889 as pure reproductions, captured from nature itself.[124] However, *moulages* were expensive to commission, time-consuming to create, delicate to handle, and only allowed fragments of bodies to be rendered (fragmentation focused the viewer's eye on the symptom, but could not give a sense of bodily wholeness). For these and other reasons, photography was increasingly integrated into the hospital system as the primary means of recording diseases. Photography was first used at Saint-Louis by Dr Montméja in the late 1860s, and the production of photographs increased during the 1890s when a photography studio was installed at the hospital.

An atlas of skin diseases produced by the Saint-Louis doctors and edited by J.J. Pringle in 1895 contains coloured photo-lithographs of wax models and black-and-white photographs of living patients.[125] These photographs show how wax models of bodies, photographs of patients, and actual human beings were used interchangeably in the teaching of medicine. At times, wax and photography were more desirable because through the intervention of artists and the input of doctors, the colours, size, and shapes of symptoms could be made more obvious. Although photographs could fray at the edges and wax models could melt, neither decomposed nor rotted, as did the human body. The signs and symptoms of diseases could be frozen in time in both print and wax, unlike the human body and its illnesses, which were organic, ever-changing, and contagious. Such instances expose moments in which real bodies failed to fulfil the realist demands of modern medicine. They also expose how reproductions were more desirable than the real thing, especially at a time when physicians and scientists, like Pasteur, Lister, and Koch, were studying the dangers of contagion.

Medical waxes also served as trophies of medical conquests. As new illnesses were 'discovered', medical men and scientists named diseases, tools, and processes after themselves to propagate their status as leading men. Péan's forceps and hemostatic clamps, like his waxes, helped display his professional rank. Péan's name was printed in large letters above his collection at Saint-Louis and was also exhibited next to each wax along with his diagnosis. The expense of creating *moulages* exhibited the economic status of medical men and their nations. By the mid-century, the State provided funding for, and encouraged donations to, French hospitals and scientific institutions like the Pasteur Institute. Hospitals and individual physicians began their own collections of medical objects, tools, sculptures, and paintings as a means to compete against other countries, particularly Prussia and England, whose medical collections were well known.[126] The French medical academy publicly displayed a long list of benefactors near their main library in Paris to demonstrate the important role of medical men in the funding of new medical museums, chairs, and specialities. Medical museums not only strengthened medical knowledge, but also exhibited the superiority of a country's medical progress internationally, thus serving to attract foreign doctors and students. Parisian doctors further promoted France as a leading medical force by hosting the first international congress of dermatology at Saint-Louis in the large lecture theatre that was filled with *moulages*; this event coincided with the Exposition Universelle and the centenary of the French Revolution. Through the exhibition of these waxes in a newly completed building, French medicine was displayed as modern, rich, and progressive to an international crowd. Significantly, Péan's collection, the largest in the hospital, was visible to the visitor who stood in the main lecture theatre while other doctors' collections were displayed behind walls, thus affirming Péan's key role in the documentation and discovery of diseases.

In order to secure the waxes' use as educational tools, medical *moulages*, such as Péan's, were displayed as scientifically as possible. In 1883, Dr Doyon wrote that without a proper scientific museum for the display of anatomical models, they would be objects of curiosity rather than instruction.[127] In comparison to the lavish velvets and decorative cabinets housing curiosities in the eighteenth century, or the spectacular wax exhibition venues like the Musée Grévin and the Spitzner in the late nineteenth century, the simple wood cabinets with black backdrops at Saint-Louis constructed the waxes as rational objects of medical study rather than spectacular items displayed to satisfy bizarre curiosities.[128] Displayed in a room made specifically for the exhibition of medical models, every *moulage* at the hospital was labelled, catalogued, and displayed behind glass in an attempt to rid them of voyeuristic delight.

Although Péan performed numerous surgeries, he was best known as a doctor who specialised in operations on female reproductive organs.[129] Hirschler's contemporary account of Péan in *Nos Docteurs* claims that, 'It was at the Hôpital Saint-Louis that he became known above all for the admirable ovariotomy operations that placed him in the uppermost ranks of the great surgeons … Today Dr Péan is surely the most famous surgeon known.'[130] Péan was the first to perform a vaginal hysterectomy in France. He also designed medical tools specifically for operations on women's bodies and publicised his charitable operations on female, not male, patients.[131] *Moulages* of diseased and distorted female genitalia comprise a portion of his collection. Rows of wax representations of diseased genitalia were, and still are, hung behind glass under a sign that lets the visitor know that these wax body parts belonged to the famous surgeon. Like Courbet's *L'Origine du monde*, these *moulages* of female genitalia were commissioned by, and produced for, a specific and privileged male gaze.[132] Although it was claimed that they were made directly from nature, indicating that they were cast directly from a human body and finished with the utmost realism in the presence of that body, the waxes' details reveal nonetheless the phantasmatic and subjective side of realist fantasies. For instance, Dr Fournier's wax female genitalia, exhibited across the room from Péan's, were covered in fluffs of pubic hair and coloured with bright tangerine-pink pigment, while Péan's collection remained relatively hairless and flesh-toned (Figure 46). Significantly, the process of detailing the wax model was one that united the *mouleur* with the medical professional, as the medical man directed the *mouleur* on how much colour was needed, how much intricate detailing was required and how much hair to insert. This moment allowed the physician to become both surgeon and sculptor, and perhaps even pornographer. Despite the objects' uses and display within the seemingly objective medical sphere, the personal and subjective tastes of collectors remained on show.

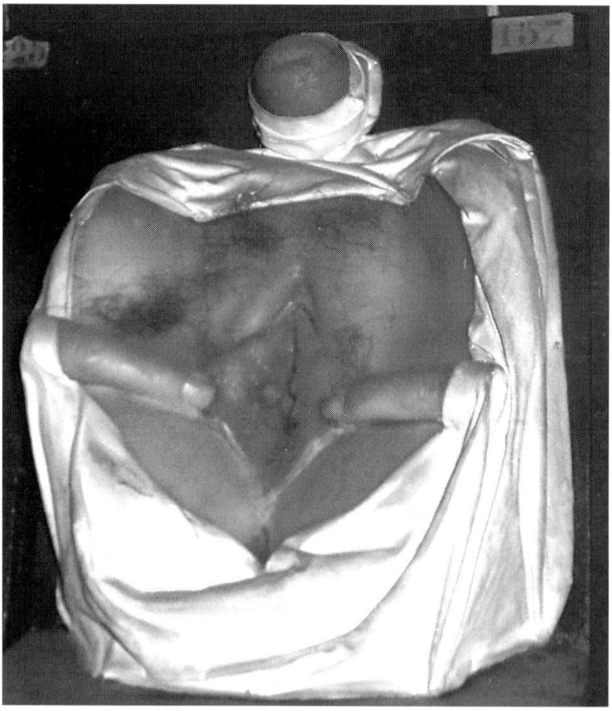
46 *Moulage* from Doctor Fournier's collection, Hôpital Saint-Louis.

Conclusion: 'éffroyable réalisme'

Péan's professional identity as a rational man of modern scientific medicine imbued him with the social qualifications to both produce and authenticate reality. His commission, *Avant l'opération*, required the image of an idealised femininity for its display at the Salon, but his commissioned pieces for the walls of Saint-Louis demanded that female sexuality be depicted as degenerate, diseased, and dismembered. Péan's wax genitalia demonstrate an erosion of the perfect femininity that Gervex attempted to create. Péan's identity as a reasonable republican in *Avant l'opération* stood in opposition to the identity invoked by the wax body parts. As Roger-Milès wrote in his 1890 book *La Cité de misère*, these medical waxes represented

> the entire army of dermatoses, in their exact representation, in their extraordinary crudeness, in their dreadful realism; the ugly, the monstrous, the painful … these representational human fragments, collected right at the hospital, are like souvenirs in which treacherous infections come back to life.[133]

The frightening and horrifying realism of Péan's waxes contrasts with Gervex's work, which was considered a rational painting that provided pleasure through the artful portrayal of a bare-breasted young woman. Unlike Gervex's rendering of a relatively flawless female body, the waxworks expose Péan's intimate contact with disease, contagion, and female genitalia. The number of waxes commissioned and the intricate detailing of every fleshy fold, deformity, and pustule point to a fascination with the female body, female sexuality, and diseases that goes beyond the demands of professional scientific duty and into the realm of fantasy and desire. Unlike *Avant l'opération*, in which the unharmed surface of the female nude helped portray Péan as a controlled and rational man, the diseased wax fragments construct a collector and collecting practice that bordered on obsession.

Wax, in the nineteenth century, was considered a medium of realism and reason, yet was also regarded as the material of fantasy and spectacle as is evident by the popularity of exhibition venues like the Musée Grévin and the Spitzner anatomical museum. Its smooth surface could best represent the body's exterior as solid and complete while its mimetic properties produced an indexical mould of every physical imperfection, thus seeming to reproduce a body without the mediation of materials like paint which displayed an artist's touch. Yet casting was a process that required bodily contact and, in turn, became the product and evidence of this intimate encounter. Furthermore, the lifelike quality of the waxes provoked feelings of horror, fear, and fascination rather than simply rationality and reason.

Avant l'opération was understood as a form of realist documentation. The painting was the end-product of the interactions between a paying customer and a portrait painter, a surgeon and an artist who was recognised – and who self-identified – as a realist. Gervex's use of realist techniques helped portray both himself and Péan as modern, rational men. Yet Gervex's realism failed to mask the irrational desire that was signalled by a naked female body on display. Similarly, the personally invested and highly charged waxes could not remain hidden behind the detached façade of modern scientific medicine. Neither Péan's representation of female bodies in wax, nor Gervex's in paint could guarantee a purely objective, accurate, and stable recording of reality or femininity. Surely such a desire itself reveals a madness because of its obvious impossibility. Péan's collection of sick female figures in paint and in wax demonstrate the vulnerability, instability, and unfeasibility of the claims to truth and the real made by realistic representations. The creating and collecting of images and objects that portrayed female bodies always threatened to erode the rational façade of modern scientific medicine and professional duty, as fantasy and pleasure were never far from the surface. Both *Avant l'opération* and the wax genitalia reveal a desire, obsession, and fascination with the female body, particularly for Monsieur le Docteur Jules Émile Péan: creator and collector of realistic representations of bodies and body parts.

Notes

1 Henri Blaze de Bury, *Les Bonhommes de cire* (Paris: Michel Lévy, 1864), p. 38. 'Vous connaissez l'étrange et mystérieuse impression qui vous saisit, en compagnie de ces bizarres figures, d'une réalité si vivante et auxquelles un certain sentiment d'effroi vous empêche d'adresser la parole, car vous n'êtes pas bien sûr que ces lèvres ne vous répondraient pas … On recule et on se rapproche; c'est comme une curiosité malsaine, hystérique, une sorte d'attrait répulsif.'

2 M. Desjardin, 'À travers le Salon', *La République française* (30 April 1887), 1–2: 'une œuvre à sensation'.

3 Charles Darcours, 'Beaux-arts et Théâtre', *Le Journal illustré* (8 May 1887), 146. 'M. Gervex accapare presque tout le bruit de la salle 13 avec son tableau.'

4 Georges Lafenestre, '1887 Salon', *Revue des deux Mondes*, 81 (1 June 1887), 586: 'de n'intervenir personnellement en aucune façon ni dans l'éclairage de la salle, ni dans la disposition des figures, ni dans le groupement des accessoires, c'est de rester, en un mot, le pur et simple copiste de la réalité …'

5 M. Hamel, 'Le Salon de 1887', *Gazette des beaux-arts* (June 1887), 479: 'aucune intention tragique ou larmoyante'; 'l'éloquence de la vérité'; 'Nul mystère, rien qui vise l'émotion: tout est dit simplement avec la certitude de la science quand elle affirme'.

6 Louis de Fourcaud, 'Le Salon de 1887', *La Revue illustré*, I (1887), 314: 'la sincérité dans l'observation, et, dans l'exécution, la logique'.

7 De Fourcaud, 'Le Salon de 1887', p. 323: 'sentiment juste de la situation, attitude naturelle, harmonie sobre, effet franc, nullement mélodramatique'.

8 Josh Ellenbogen, *Reasoned and Unreasoned Images: the Photography of Bertillon, Galton, and Marey* (University Park: Pennsylvania State University Press, 2012), pp. 4–5.

9 Louis de Fourcaud, 'L'Art contemporain – École Française', in *Revue de l'Exposition universelle 1889* (Paris: Librairie d'art, 1889), p. 5: 'des personnages vrais en des actions variées, dans des milieux vrais, éclairés de la même lumière qui nous enveloppe, respirant le même air que nous respirons. Donnez-nous la vérité …'

10 Ballu, 'Salon de 1887', n.p. 'Il est impossible de donner mieux l'impression d'un jour intérieur, de cette atmosphère impalpable, éclairée par la fenêtre aux rideaux blancs relevés, modelant de reflets froids les visages, et circulant sur les murs nus de la salle de l'hôpital. Ce qu'il y a d'air dans cette perspective restreinte, en somme, est inimaginable. On y pénètre, on y est, on y respire.'

11 Michael Fried, *Realism, Writing, Disfiguration in Thomas Eakins and Stephen Crane* (Chicago: University of Chicago Press, 1987), p. 63.

12 Gervex, *Souvenirs recueillis par Jules Bertaut*, p. 252. 'C'était l'époque où la découverte de la pince hémostatique révolutionnait les anciennes méthodes. Le docteur Péan, debout devant le corps endormi d'une jeune femme qu'il allait opérer, parlait, tenant entre ses doigts la fameuse pince. En un clin d'oeil j'aperçus le tableau à faire; je pris quelques croquis et j'abandonnais définitivement le banal profil du portrait classique.'

13 Charles Baudelaire, 'Salon of 1846', in *The Mirror of Art, Critical Studies by Charles Baudelaire*, ed. and trans. Jonathan Mayne (London: Phaidon Press, 1955), p. 129.

14 Darcours, 'Beaux-Arts et théâtre', p. 146. 'C'est une peinture intéressante et dont le thème réaliste est préférable aux sujets galants trops souvent traités par un artiste de grand talent.'

15 For a history of antiseptic surgery and Lister's use of antisepsis, see Michael Worboys, *Spreading Germs: Disease Theories and Medical Practice in Britain, 1865–1900* (Cambridge: Cambridge University Press, 2000); and Bynum, *Science and the Practice of Medicine in the Nineteenth Century*, pp. 112–114, 132–137.

16 This painting went missing during the Second World War, but a study can be found at the National Gallery in Washington, DC.

17 Larousse, *Grand Dictionnaire universel du XIXe siècle [deuxième supplément]*, p. 1314. 'M. Gervex aborda, en 1876, avec *L'autopsie à l'Hôtel-Dieu*, les sujets modernes qui devaient établir sa réputation et le placer au rang des artistes les plus en vue de la jeune école.'

18 Larousse, *Grand Dictionnaire universel du XIXe siècle [deuxième supplément]*, p. 1314: 'on doit lui savoir gré de la franchise de son exécution et de la sincérité qui règne dans son œuvre. La lumière frise les objets et elle pénètre les corps, ses attitudes sont justes, son dessin est honnête et ses moyens sont francs.'

19 Gervex wrote, 'Ce sujet réaliste entre tous n'avait pas été choisi par moi, il m'avait été fourni par le hasard. J'avais découvert, au cours de mes flâneries, la salle d'autopsie du vieil Hôtel-Dieu comme les Parisiens découvrent les coins pittoresques ou peu connus de leur ville. Et j'avais été bouleversé de ma trouvaille.' (This realist subject among all others was not chosen by me; it was provided to me by chance. I had

discovered, in the course of one of my *flâneries*, the autopsy room of the old Hôtel-Dieu, much like Parisians discover the picturesque or less known corners of their city. And I was bowled over by my discovery.) Gervex, *Souvenirs recueillis par Jules Bertaut*, p. 26. For a discussion of Gervex's approach to painting, see Petra ten-Doesschate Chu, 'Into the Modern Era: The Evolution of Realist and Naturalist Drawing', in Weisberg (ed.), *The Realist Tradition: French Painting and Drawing 1830–1900*, p. 292.

20 Gervex, *Souvenirs recueillis par Jules Bertaut*, p. 26: 'le plus complètement ma théorie de l'art moderne'.

21 A.M. de Bélina, *Nos Peintres dessinés par eux-mêmes – notes humoristiques et esquisses biographiques* (Paris: E. Bernard et cie, 1883), p. 53.

22 Victorien Maubry, 'Le Salon', *Le Témoin* (16 May 1887), 41–42: 'une source de gloire et de profit'.

23 'Le Salon', *L'Univers illustré* (7 May 1887), 295.

24 '*Avant l'Opération:* Tableau de M. Gervex (Salon de 1887)', *Paris illustré* (28 May 1887), 76: 'conserver le souvenir de l'invention de la célèbre méthode chirurgicale de M. le Dr Péan.'

25 For nineteenth-century accounts of the invention of hemostatic clamps, see '*Avant l'Opération:* Tableau de M. Gervex (Salon de 1887)', p. 76, and A.C., 'Le Docteur Péan', *La Chronique médicale – Revue bi-mensuelle de médecine, historique, littéraire et anecdotique* (15 February 1898), p. 8. For discussions of surgical instruments, see Knut Haeger, *The Illustrated History of Surgery* (London: Harold Starke, 1989); and John Kirkup, *The Evolution of Surgical Instruments. An Illustrated History from Ancient Times to the Twentieth Century* (Novato: Norman Publishers, 2003).

26 For a discussion of *Avant l'opération* at the Exposition Universelle of 1889, see Walton, *Chefs-d'œuvre de l'exposition universelle de Paris, 1889*, pp. 87–88.

27 Doctor Gustave Rappin, 'Pensées' (c. 1895), as cited in Jacques Léonard, *La France médicale: médecins et maladies au XIX*[e] *siècle* (Paris: Gallimard/Julliard, 1978), p. 240. 'La Science est une; elle est comme Dieu universelle. La Religion vieillit, la Science grandit. La Science est la mère de toute liberté. Pauvre Science! Si l'on faisait pour toi un peu seulement de ce que l'on fait pour la religion! Où sont tes autels?'

28 Gustave Ollendorf, *Salon de 1887* (Paris: L. Baschet, 1887), p. 51. 'Ici l'ironie ne pouvant pas se mettre dans la scène, M. Gervex l'a glissée dans les accessoires. Notre oeil s'est trouvé invinciblement arrêté par lui, non pas sur le personnage principal, celui qu'il s'agit d'opérer, non pas sur le personnage secondaire, mais dont le rôle est encore important, l'opérateur; mais sur une table où figure les accessoires de l'opération, quelques instruments épars – et un merveilleux bocal d'éponges.'

29 Paul Mantz, 'Le Salon – I', Supplement to *Le Temps*, 8 May, 1887, n.p.: 'plus ou moins parents de ces *Leçons d'anatomie* que la Hollande du dix-septième siècle a tant aimées et dont Rembrandt a fourni deux modèles inégalement fameux'. Mantz referred to Rembrandt's *Anatomy lesson of Dr Tulp* and *Anatomy lesson of Dr Joan Deyman*.

30 Ballu, 'Salon de 1887', n.p. 'C'est en somme le sujet de *La Leçon d'anatomie* de Rembrandt mis au point de la vérité moderne, et il faut savoir gré à M. Gervex d'avoir été aussi sincère, aussi exact à son époque que le maître hollandais a dû être à la sienne.'
31 Alison McQueen, *The Rise of the Cult of Rembrandt: Reinventing an Old Master in Nineteenth-Century France* (Amsterdam: Amsterdam University Press, 2003), pp. 15, 264.
32 McQueen, *The Rise of the Cult of Rembrandt*, p. 266.
33 Petra Ten Doesschate Chu, like McQueen, offers a detailed account of the influence of seventeenth-century Dutch art on nineteenth-century French artistic practice. See Chu, *French Realism and the Dutch Masters: The Influence of Dutch Seventeenth-Century Painting on the Development of French Painting between 1830 and 1870* (Utrecht: Haentjens, Dekker & Gumbert, 1974).
34 Lenoir, *Histoire du Réalisme et du Naturalisme dans la poésie et dans l'art depuis l'antiquité jusqu'à nos jours*, p. 563. 'Le sujet, d'ailleurs fort connu, n'exigeant d'autre invention que celle de l'ordonnance, et nul idéal, convenait merveilleusement au génie réaliste du peintre de *Gueux*.'
35 Louis Viardot, *Les Musées de France* (Paris: Hachette et Co., 1860), p. 148: 'marque bien l'extrême hauteur du pur "naturalisme"'.
36 Charles Baudelaire, 'Le Peintre de la vie moderne – IV. La modernité', *Le Figaro*, 26 November 1863. 'Il y a eu une modernité pour chaque peintre ancien; la plupart des beaux portraits qui nous restent des temps antérieurs sont revêtus des costumes de leur époque. Ils sont parfaitement harmonieux, parce que le costume, la coiffure et même le geste, le regard et le sourire (chaque époque a son port, son regard et son sourire) forment un tout d'une complète vitalité.'
37 McQueen, *The Rise of the Cult of Rembrandt*, pp. 39–41.
38 Charles Blanc, *L'École hollandaise* (Paris: Librairie Renouard, 1883), p. 12: 'une galerie de peintures hollandaises est une histoire complète de la Hollande du beau siècle, une histoire à la fois morale, politique, naturelle'.
39 For an account of Riegl's education and relationship to positivism and realism, see Margaret Olin, *Forms of Representation in Alois Riegl's Theory of Art* (University Park: Pennsylvania State University Press, 1992), pp. 3–16.
40 For discussions of Riegl's concept of *Kunstwollen*, see Margaret Iversen, *Alois Riegl: Art History and Theory* (Cambridge, MA: MIT Press, 1993) and Richard Woodfield (ed.), *Framing Formalism: Riegl's Work* (Amsterdam: G+B Arts International, 2001), particularly Frauke Laarman, 'Riegl and the Family Portrait', pp. 195–218 and Benjamin Binstock, 'I've got you under my skin: Rembrandt, Riegl, and the Will of Art History', pp. 219–264.
41 Laarman, 'Riegl and the Family Portrait', p. 199.
42 For an in-depth discussion of Riegl's concept of 'attention' and the role of the spectator, see Iversen, *Alois Riegl*, pp. 101–147.
43 Binstock, 'I've got you under my skin: Rembrandt, Riegl, and the Will of Art History', p. 226. For a further discussion of Dr Tulp's hand gesture, see William Schupbach's *The Paradox of Rembrandt's 'Anatomy of Dr Tulp'* (London: Wellcome

Institute for the History of Medicine, 1982), which claims that Tulp's raised left hand demonstrates the operation of the corpse's exposed tendons.

44 See Théophile Thoré's account in his *Musées de la Hollande: I Amsterdam et la Haye-Études sur l'école hollandaise, II Musée van der Hoop à Amsterdam, et Musée de Rotterdam* (Paris: Vve J. Renouard, 1858 and 1860) and his article 'Nouvelles tendances de l'art', in *Salon de Théophile Thoré 1844, 1845, 1847, 1848* (Paris: Librairie internationale, 1868).

45 Émile Leclercq, *Caractères de l'école française moderne de peinture* (Brussels: Librairie Renouard, 1881), p. 151: 'tout l'art hollandais est d'essence populaire et démocratique.'

46 Émile Michel, *Rembrandt: Sa vie, son œuvre, et son temps* (Paris: Hachette, 1893), p. 122. 'Après le triomphe définitif de la Réforme dans les Pays-Bas, la peinture religieuse, celle du moins qui avait pour objet la décoration des églises, n'existait plus. En même temps que le clergé catholique disparaissait, la cour cessait de patronner les artistes; mais les corporations, en prenant la place ainsi laissée vacante, allaient ouvrir des voies nouvelles à l'activité des peintres hollandais. Comme il était naturel de le penser, les chefs de ces associations se firent représenter revêtus des insignes de leur dignité, et leurs portraits placés dans les salles de réunion étaient pour les affiliés autant d'exhortations à continuer les exemples de dévouement, de patriotisme ou de charité que leur avaient donnés ces devanciers dont ils avaient sous les yeux les images.'

47 For an examination of Gervex's republican state commissions, see Jean-Christophe Gouvennec, 'La République triomphante: les années 90', pp. 164–189 and Roselyne Hurel, 'Le Panorama de l'*Histoire du siècle 1789–1889* par Henri Gervex et Alfred Stevens', in Jean-François de Canchy (ed.), *Henri Gervex, 1852–1929* (Paris: Paris-Musées, 1992), pp. 190–205.

48 For a discussion of Péan's republicanism, see Dr Aubeau, 'La Psychologie de Péan', *La Chronique médicale – Revue bi-mensuelle de médecine, historique, littéraire et anecdotique* (15 February 1898), pp. 106–108.

49 Chu, *French Realism and the Dutch Masters*, p. 14. Although Chu bases her assumptions primarily on historian Edgar Quinet's texts from the mid-nineteenth century, it is evident that these associations, particularly the association between Dutch art and republicanism, were carried into the last decades of the nineteenth century.

50 Blanc, *L'École hollandaise,* p. 19. 'La forme républicaine, une fois reconnue, les a délivrés de l'art purement décoratif que commandent les cours et les princes …'

51 See McQueen, *The Rise of the Cult of Rembrandt* for a discussion of Thoré's republican views, pp. 37–38, 109–121.

52 For accounts of the secularisation of medicine in France, see Jan Goldstein, *Console and Classify: the French Psychiatric Profession in the Nineteenth Century* (Cambridge: Cambridge University Press, 1987); Ruth Harris, *Murders and Madness: Medicine, Law and Society in the Fin de Siècle* (Oxford: Clarendon Press, 1989); and Ellis, *The Physician-Legislators of France.*

53 Jules Guérin, *La Gazette médicale de Paris* (4 March 1848), as cited in Léonard, *La France médicale au XIXe siècle*, p. 255. 'Il est bien vrai que la profession médicale

est d'essence libérale et républicaine, qu'elle façonne l'esprit à la haine du prejugé et à l'amour du progrès.'

54 For an account of the institutional changes that affected nursing, see Katrin Schultheiss, *Bodies and Souls: Politics and the Professionalization of Nursing in France, 1880–1922* (Cambridge, MA: Harvard University Press, 2001).

55 For a discussion of the specialisation of medicine, see George Weisz, *Divide and Conquer: A Comparative History of Medical Specialization* (New York: Oxford University Press, 2004).

56 Aubeau, 'La Psychologie de Péan', p. 107; and Bianchon, *Nos grands médecins d'aujourd'hui,* pp. 317–318

57 Alsdorf, *Fellow Men: Fantin-Latour and the Problem of the Group in Nineteenth-Century French Painting.*

58 For a discussion of the relationship between women and popular medical culture, see Mary Lynn Stewart, *For Health and Beauty: Physical Culture for French Women 1880s–1930s* (Baltimore: Johns Hopkins University Press, 2000).

59 The American woman, Mary Corinna Putman Jacobi, was the first woman admitted as a student to the Faculté de Médecine in Paris in 1867. Three other women, including the well-known English physician, Elizabeth Garrett Anderson, were admitted in 1868. For an account of the integration of women into the Parisian medical system, see Joy Harvey, 'La Visite: Mary Putnam Jacobi and the Paris Medical Clinics', in La Berge and Feingold (eds), *French Medical Culture in the Nineteenth Century*, pp. 350–371; G. Despierres, 'Histoire de l'accession de la femme aux études médicales et plus particulièrement à Lyon', *Conférence d'histoire de la médecine à Lyon*, pp. 51–70 (Lyon: Fondation Marcel Mérieux, 1984); Pierre Darmon, *Le médecin parisien en 1900: la vie quotidienne* (Paris: Hachette, littératures, 2003), pp. 25–29, 211; and G. Nicole-Genty, M. Chapuis, J. Chapuis *et al.*, *Les Premières femmes médecins en France*, exhibition catalogue, Bibliothèque de l'Académie nationale de médecine (Paris: Académie national médecin, 1975).

60 Both men and women viewed the canvas at the Salon. There is no doubt that women were interested in medicine and also viewed nudes at the Salons. Nonetheless, the touching and looking at women's naked bodies within the medical sphere was understood as a more male than female pursuit. For a discussion of male viewing within operating theatres see Marcia Pointon's discussion of Eakin's *Gross Clinic* and *The Agnew Clinic* in *Naked Authority: The Body in Western Painting 1830–1908* (Cambridge: Cambridge University Press, 1990), pp. 16–58; and Callen, 'Doubles and Desire: Anatomies of Masculinity in the Later Nineteenth-century', 669–699. For a pioneering work on the notion of a gendered gaze, see Laura Mulvey, 'Visual Pleasure and Narrative Cinema', *Screen*, 16:3 (1975), 6–18.

61 Zola's story was first published in serial form in *L'Artiste* between August and October 1867 under the title *Un mariage d'amour*. The title was changed to *Thérèse Raquin* when the story came out in book form.

62 Zola, 'Introduction', in Leonard Tancock (trans.), *Thérèse Raquin* (2nd edn, London, [1868] 1962), p. 23.

63 Zola, *Thérèse Raquin,* p. 23.

64 For feminist discussions of models' relationships with artists, see Heather Dawkins, *The Nude in French Art and Culture, 1870–1910* (Cambridge: Cambridge University Press, 2002), pp. 86–133; and Marie Lathers, *Bodies of Art: French Literary Realism and the Artist's Model* (Lincoln: University of Nebraska Press, 2001). For a social history of models, see Susan Waller, *Invention of the Model: Artists and Models in Paris, 1830–1870* (Aldershot: Ashgate, 2005).
65 'J'espère qu'il ne va pas me faire payer cette opération-là!'
66 Carole Groneman, 'Nymphomania: The Historical Construction of Female Sexuality', in Jennifer Terry and Jacqueline Urla (eds), *Deviant Bodies: Critical Perspectives on Difference in Science and Popular Culture* (Bloomington: Indiana University Press, 1995), p. 233.
67 For discussions of the medical inspection of prostitutes, see Jill Harsin, *Policing Prostitution in Nineteenth-Century Paris* (Princeton: Princeton University Press, 1985); Charles Bernheimer, *Figures of Ill Repute: Representing Prostitution in Nineteenth-Century France* (Cambridge, MA: Harvard University Press, 1989), pp. 8–33; and Alain Corbin, *Women for Hire: Prostitution and Sexuality in France after 1850*, trans. Anne Sheridan (Cambridge, MA: Harvard University Press, 1990).
68 Mary Spongberg, *Feminizing Venereal Disease: The Body of the Prostitute in Nineteenth-Century Medical Discourse* (Basingstoke: Macmillan, 1997), p. 36.
69 Corbin, *Women for Hire*, p. 87.
70 Harsin, *Policing Prostitution*, p. 16.
71 Alfred Louis Philippe Hardy and A. de Montméja, *Clinique Photographique de l'hôpital Saint-Louis* (Paris: Chamerot et Lauwereyns, 1868), p. III: 'nous pouvons dire que ces planches représentent la nature prise sur le fait'.
72 Kemp and Wallace, *Spectacular Bodies*, p. 23.
73 Bianchon, *Nos grands médecins d'aujourd'hui*, pp. 316–317, and L. Marc, 'Le Docteur Péan', *L'Illustration* (31 December 1887), 480.
74 Bianchon, *Nos grands médecins d'aujourd'hui*, p. 316. 'Écartez-vous, messieurs, que tout le monde puisse voir!'
75 Bianchon, *Nos grands médecins d'aujourd'hui*, pp. 316–317. 'Je fus émerveillé. Je n'avais pas idée d'une pareille dextérité, d'une telle rapidité, d'une sûreté de main si impeccable, d'une habileté si consommée. C'était plus étonnant qu'horrible, cette utile et bienfaisante boucherie, ce défilé de malades endormis, opérés, emportés en un clin d'oeil, se succédant sur la table sanglante parmi tout un hérissement clair de lames et de pinces, d'instruments inventés par lui'.
76 Ollendorf, *Salon de 1887*, pp. 51–52. 'Les personnages du fond ne font pas partie de la scène, et puisque M. Gervex a cherché la vérité, il aurait dû les supprimer. Quand un professeur enseigne dans nos salles d'hôpital, les élèves, attentifs, l'entourent, les infirmiers de service qui ont apporté la malade se retirent et l'on ne voit pas traîner sur le lit les courroies de leurs atteles. Enfin, puisqu'il s'agissait d'une œuvre qui sera conservée, qui devra, suivant l'expression à la mode aujourd'hui, servir de document, nous aurions voulu que la patiente ait gardé le bonnet d'hôpital. Les cheveux en désordre, qui s'étalent sur le drap blanc, et qui mettent d'ailleurs si bien en valeur la chair lumineuse et saine de la malade, s'expliqueraient à la Salpêtrière

à la suite de quelque attaque, de quelque convulsion nerveuse qui aurait échevelé tout d'un coup un sujet hystérique. Ici, à l'hôpital Saint-Louis, en présence d'une opération dont tous les détails vont être doctoralement et sagement expliqués, ils font faire fausse route au spectateur.'

77 Drs Delaunay and Baumgarten are among those portrayed. Gerstle Mack, *Toulouse-Lautrec* (New York: Knopf, 1953), pp. 258, 234–235.

78 For a discussion of *Rolla*'s removal from the Salon, see Hollis Clayson, *Painted Love: Prostitution in French Art of the Impressionist Era* (Los Angeles: Getty Publications, 2003), pp. 79–93.

79 Hippolyte Devillers, 'Salon de Paris', *La Jeune Belgique*, VI (5 July 1887), p. 236. 'Nul ne joue des blancs comme M. Gervex, mais comme il y mêle je ne saurais dire quelle substance aphrodisiaque qu'il n'est pas à dédaigner, qu'il nous réédite *Marion*, l'épouvante du jury, ou la *Femme au masque*. Il est bon d'approprier son sujet à son mot. M. Gervex a de la polissonnerie sur sa palette, qu'il s'en serve'.

80 Olivier Merson, 'Salon de 1887 – II', *Le Monde illustré* (14 Mai 1887), 315: 'on ne pourrait mieux peindre … le torse de la jeune malade, morceau acompli, caressé d'un pinceau sûr de lui …'

81 De Bélina, *Nos peintres dessinés par eux-mêmes*, p. 52. 'Gervex n'est pas seulement un peintre de talent, mais c'est aussi un charmeur; comme son maître Cabanel, il possède cette distinction et ce langage sédusisant qui attire'.

82 Mantz, 'Le Salon – I', n.p.: 'aussi bien par l'intérêt du motif que par certains détails d'exécution d'une très bonne venue, notamment les chairs de la femme, lumineuse et délicates sur les blancheurs du linge'.

83 For influential feminist analyses of the female nude, see Lynda Nead, *The Female Nude: Art, Obscenity and Sexuality* (London: Routledge, 1992); Linda Nochlin, *Women, Art and Power: and Other Essays* (New York: Harper & Row, 1988); and Susan R. Suleiman (ed.), *The Female Body in Western Culture: Contemporary Perspectives* (Cambridge, MA: Harvard University Press, 1986).

84 For censorship of the nude during the late nineteenth century, see Dawkins, *The Nude in French Art and Culture*, pp. 7–85; and Jennifer L. Shaw, 'The Figure of Venus: Rhetoric of the Ideal and the Salon of 1863', *Art History*, 14:4 (1991), 540–570.

85 For a brief history of the acquisitions of the Paris Medical Faculty, see Louis Landouzy and Noe Legrand (eds), *Les Collections artistiques de la faculté de médecine* (Paris: Faculté de médecine, 1911).

86 I am grateful to Sander Gilman for pointing out the prevalence of healthy and sick Marianne figures in nineteenth-century French art and literature.

87 For a detailed examination of the signification of Marianne, see Maurice Agulhon, *Marianne into Battle: Republican Imagery and Symbolism in France, 1789–1880* (London: Cambridge University Press, 1981).

88 For a discussion of how realism was often equated with dirt and ill morals, see Alan Krell, 'Dirt and Desire: Troubled Waters in Realist Practice', in Richard Hobbs (ed.), *Impressions of French Modernity* (Manchester: Manchester University Press, 1998), pp. 135–147.

89 Clayson, *Painted Love*, p. 83.

90 Émile Zola, 'Après une promenade au Salon', *Le Figaro*, 23 May 1881. Zola also praised Gervex's naturalism in *La Naturalism au Salon 1880* and *Lettres de Paris: Nouvelles artistique et littéraire – Le Salon de 1879*: 'des révoltés de l'École des beaux-arts, Gervex, Bastien-Lepage, Butin, Duez, sont passés dans le camp des modernes et semblent vouloir se mettre à la tête du mouvement'.

91 Henry Houssaye, *Le Salon de 1886* (Paris, 1886), p. 6: 'si la *Femme au masque* de M. Henri Gervex est du naturalisme, c'est assurément du naturalisme tout à fait aimable et plein de séduction'.

92 Zola, 'Après une promenade au Salon'.

93 Ludmilla Jordanova, *Sexual Visions: Images of Gender in Science and Medicine between the Eighteenth and Twentieth Centuries* (Madison: University of Wisconsin Press, 1989), p. 87.

94 Peter Brooks, *Body Work: Objects of Desire in Modern Narrative* (Cambridge, MA: Harvard University Press, 1993), p. 159.

95 The strength of female bodies was noted in medical discourse, as doctors were studying why women lived longer than men. For a critique of how feminist accounts may over-emphasise the nineteenth-century construction of women as being weak and closer to nature, see Ludmilla Jordanova, 'Linda Nochlin's "Women, Art and Power"', in Norman Bryson, Michael Ann Holly and Keith Moxey (eds), *Visual Theory: Painting and Interpretation* (Cambridge: Polity in association with Blackwell, 1991), pp. 54–60.

96 Alber, 'Les Personnages en Cire', *La Nature*, 21:1 (1894), 325. 'La seule matière plastique capable de rendre absolument l'effet des chairs, leur velouté et leur transparence, est la cire'.

97 For accounts of La Specola and other collections of medical waxes, see Roberta Panzanelli and Julius Ritter von Schlosser (eds), *Ephemeral Bodies: Wax Sculpture and the Human Figure* (Los Angeles: Getty Research Institute, 2008); and Anna Maerker, 'Anatomy and Public Enlightenment: the Florentine Museo "La Specola"', in J.M.M. Alberti and Elizabeth Hallam (eds), *Medical Museums: Past, Present, Future*, pp. 88–101.

98 Gaston Le Breton, 'Essai historique sur la sculpture en cire', in *Précis analytique des travaux de l'Académie des Sciences, Belles-Lettres et Arts de Rouen pendant l'année 1891–1892* (Rouen: Impr. de P. Periaux, 1893), pp. 250–303.

99 Pamela Pilbeam, *Madame Tussaud and the History of Waxworks* (London: Hambledon and London, 2002), p. 136.

100 Anne Pingeot (ed.), *Le Corps en morceaux* (Paris: Ministère de la culture, de la communication, des grands travaux et du bicentaire; Réunion des musées nationaux, 1990), pp. 53–54 and Pilbeam, *Madame Tussaud and the History of Waxworks*, p. 149.

101 *Moniteur Universel* (6 June 1882) as cited in Vanessa R. Schwartz, *Spectacular Realities: Early Mass Culture in Fin-de-Siècle Paris* (Berkeley: University of California Press, 1998), p. 119. Schwartz points out that wax museums added many elements of the real to contribute to the verisimilitude of wax figures such as accessories, ornaments, and framing effects. The sense of reality was heightened by scenes from recent history or realist novels, thus drawing connections between

the truth of journalism and the aesthetics of wax. See pp. 89–148 for her discussion of waxworks.

102 Jonathan Sawday, *The Body Emblazoned: Dissection and the Human Body in Renaissance Culture* (London: Routledge, 1995), p. 2.

103 Diana Holmes, *Rachilde: Decadence, Gender and the Woman Writer* (Oxford: Berg, 2001), p. 120.

104 Rachilde, *Monsieur Vénus*, trans. Melanie Hawthorne (New York: Modern Language Association of America, 2004), p. 210.

105 Bram Dijkstra, *Idols of Perversity: Fantasies of Feminine Evil in Fin-de-Siècle Culture* (Oxford: Oxford University Press, 1986), p. 35.

106 Elisabeth Bronfen, *Over Her Dead Body: Death, Femininity and the Aesthetic* (Manchester: Manchester University Press, 1992), p. 5.

107 For overviews of the rise of anaesthetics, see Stephanie J. Snow, *Blessed Days of Anaesthesia: How Anaesthetics Changed the World* (Oxford: Oxford University Press, 2008); and Bynum, *Science and the Practice of Medicine in the Nineteenth Century*, pp. 121–123.

108 Dr Azam, *Hypnotisme double conscience, et altération de la personnalité* (Paris: J.B. Ballière et fils, 1887), pp. 31–33.

109 Bronfen, *The Knotted Subject: Hysteria and its Discontents*, p. 196.

110 Martin S. Pernick, *A Calculus of Suffering: Pain, Professionalism and Anesthesia in Nineteenth-Century America* (New York: Columbia University Press, 1985), p. 86.

111 Mantz, 'Le Salon – I', n.p; Meurville, 'Le Salon – La nature au Salon', *Gazette de France* (27 May 1887), XII.

112 Nina Auerbach, *Woman and the Demon: The Life of a Victorian Myth* (Cambridge, MA: Harvard University Press, 1982), pp. 41–42.

113 Sigmund Freud, *The Uncanny*, trans. David McLintock (London: Penguin Books, 2003), p. 135. This description is the one that Freud borrowed from E. Jentsch.

114 My discussion on waxworks draws on Norman Bryson, 'Everything we look at is a kind of Troy', in Tracey Bashkoff and Nancy Spector (eds), *Sugimoto: Portraits*, exhibition catalogue (New York: Guggenheim Museum, 2000), p. 61. It is informed by Naomi Schor's discussion of wax models in 'Duane Hanson: Truth in Sculpture', in Schor, *Reading in Detail: Aesthetics and the Feminine* (New York: Methuen, 1987), pp. 131–140.

115 Bronfen, *Over Her Dead Body*, p. 5.

116 Fried claims that the wounded figure in *The Gross Clinic* invokes pleasure and pain. He argues that the violence of surgery is morally justified in the image because it emphasises curing and the anaesthetised state suggests that the patient is not in pain. See Fried, *Realism, Writing, Disfiguration*, p. 61.

117 Gérard Tilles and Daniel Wallach, *Le Musée des moulages de l'hôpital Saint-Louis* (Paris: Doin-AP-HP, 1996), p. 14.

118 For an examination of medical wax models in France, see Thomas Schnalke, *Diseases in Wax: The History of the Medical Moulage,* trans. Kathy Spatschek (Chicago: Quintessence Publishers, 1995), pp. 83–92; and Hélène Pinet, 'Cire anatomique', in Pingeot (ed.), *Le Corps en morceau*, pp. 51–56.

119 For a description of making *moulages*, see Schnalke, *Diseases in Wax*, p. 9, Gérard Tilles, 'Histoire des bibliothèques médicales et des musées des hôpitaux de l'Assistance publique. L'exemple de l'hôpital Saint-Louis', PhD dissertation, Université de Paris XII, 1995; and Édouard Papet, 'Technique: "saisir la nature sur le fait"', in Edouard Papet (ed.), *À fleur de peau: le moulage sur nature au XIXe siècle*, exhibition catalogue (Paris: Réunion des musées nationaux, 2001), pp. 74–77.

120 Mantz, 'Le Salon – I', n.p. 'Les deux artistes qui se livrent à cette besogne y apportent une sorte de gravité sacerdotale; ils ne se laissent point distraire par le spectacle voisin; si l'on confiait de pareils aveux à de purs laïques, on verrait peut-être leurs mains s'agiter au contact de la chair amoureuse; mais il y a pour les mouleurs des grâces d'état, et ils ne s'intéressent qu'au succès de leur opération délicate'.

121 M. Sully Prudhomme, 'Préface', in L. Roger-Milès, *La Cité de misère* (Paris: Marpon & Flammarion, 1891), pp. 160–165. 'M. Baretta est un précieux collaborateur de la science. Sans brutalité, avec des douceurs de mère et une patience qui ne se dément pas, il applique ses appareils et pendant que la matière prend, il cause avec le malade, s'intéresse à son affection, se fait raconter ses évolutions, gagne, sans le chercher, sa confiance tant il inspire de sympathie. Le malade aime-t-il mieux se taire, comme il faut un certain temps pour que l'appareil durcisse et que la vue d'une pièce en préparation n'a rien de réjouissant, M. Baretta lui montre ses tableaux … puis il se met au piano et le voilà qui berce son client avec quelque vieille mélodie'; Thomas Schnalke, 'Casting Skin: Meanings for Doctors, Artists, and Patients', in Soraya de Chadarevian and Nick Hopwood (eds), *Models: The Third Dimension in Science* (Stanford: Stanford University Press, 2004), pp. 207–241.

122 For a discussion of medical imagery and pornography, see Roberta McGrath, *Seeing Her Sex: Medical Archives and the Female Body* (Manchester: Manchester University Press, 2002).

123 Multiple visual sources were used for study and teaching at Saint-Louis. For a discussion of teaching models at Saint-Louis and other at Parisian hospitals, see Tilles, 'Histoire des bibliothèques médicales et des musées des hôpitaux de l'Assistance publique'.

124 P.G. Unna, 'Lettres de Paris par P.G Unna', *Annales de dermatologie et de syphiligraphie*, IX (Paris, 1889), p. 59: 'ces modèles sont de pures reproductions, la nature prise sur le fait'.

125 E. Bessnier, A. Fournier, Tenneson *et al.*, *Pictorial Atlas of Skin Diseases and Syphilitic Affections, from Models in the Museum of the Saint Louis Hospital, Paris*, ed. J.J. Pringle (London: Rebman Publishing Co., 1895).

126 For a discussion of the emergence of medical museums in France, see Tilles, 'Histoire des bibliothèques médicales et des musées des hôpitaux de l'Assistance publique', pp. 216–225.

127 A. Doyon, 'Du mode d'enseignement de la dermato-vénéréologie contemporaine. Vienne, Paris, Lyon', *Annales de dermatologie et de syphiligraphie* (1883), 4, pp. 189–196, 249–256, 309–311, as cited in Tilles, 'Histoire des

bibliothèques médicales et des musées des hôpitaux de l'Assistance publique', p. 106.

128 For an account of the history of waxes in France see Pilbeam, *Madame Tussaud and the History of Waxworks*, pp. 37–63; Schwartz, *Spectacular Realities*, p. 92; and Tilles, 'Histoire des bibliothèques médicales et des musées des hôpitaux de l'Assistance publique', pp. 217–219.

129 Ovariotomies became a common surgical procedure during the late nineteenth century. The removal of ovaries, like the removal of appendices, was considered a means by which surgeons could make money as it was not always a necessary medical procedure. See Léonard, *La France Médicale au XIXe Siècle*, p. 229.

130 J. Hirschler, *Nos docteurs* (Paris: J. Hirschler, 1896), p. 126. 'C'est à l'hôpital Saint-Louis qu'il s'est surtout fait connaître par d'admirables opérations d'ovariotomie qui l'ont placé tout à fait au premier rang des grands chirugiens … Le docteur Péan est certainement à l'heure qu'il est le plus célèbre opérateur connu'.

131 Dr Delaunay, 'Péan jugé par ses élèves', *La Chronique médicale* (15 February 1898), p. 104; and Aubeau, 'La Psychologie de Péan', p. 106.

132 Courbet's painting was commissioned in 1866 by Khalil Bey, an art collector and Turkish ambassador to St Petersburg for his collection of erotica. For a history of the painting, see Linda Nochlin, 'Courbet's "L'origine du monde": The Origin without an Original', *October*, 37 (1986), 76–86.

133 Roger-Milès, *La Cité de misère*, pp. 156–157: 'toute l'armée des dermatoses, dans leur représentation exacte, dans leur crudité exceptionnelle, dans leur effroyable réalisme; le laid, le monstrueux, le douloureux … ces débris humains figurés, collectionnés à l'hôpital même, sont comme des souvenirs où revivent de traîtresses infections'.

3 Hysterical realisms at the Salpêtrière: images, objects, and performances *chez* Dr Charcot

André Brouillet's painting *Une leçon clinique à la Salpêtrière* depicts a crowd of men from various disciplines – medicine, politics, art, and literature – watching the movements of a hypnotised female hysteric while listening to renowned neurologist, Dr Jean-Martin Charcot (Figure 4).[1] Declared 'the success of the Salon' by Hugues le Roux in *Le Temps*[2] and 'one of the most important artworks of the Salon' by *Le Journal des arts*,[3] *Une leçon clinique* was discussed and reproduced in multiple journals and Salon catalogues during the late nineteenth century. Louis de Fourcaud claimed it was Brouillet's most important painting to date,[4] Olivier Merson asserted that it was a masterpiece that characterised the times, prophesising that it 'could well be the most sensational painting of the Salon of 1887',[5] and both Meurville and Mantz mentioned the crowds that formed around the painting from the first day of its display.[6]

Brouillet and his painting's fashionable status is not surprising, considering that he combined themes that captured the popular imagination: hysteria, hypnosis, the illustrious Charcot, and the workings of the Salpêtrière and its female patients. The drastic rise in diagnosed cases of hysteria in the second half of the century, as well as the proliferation of pictures, plays, novels, and medical texts about hysteria, encouraged and sustained the public's fascination with this mystifying disease and the women it was believed to inhabit. Viewed by the Parisian public at the annual Salon, Brouillet's large canvas and life-size figures invited viewers into the modern medical world of Charcot's Salpêtrière, giving them a front-row seat to an otherwise sold-out show.[7]

Charcot became a physician at the Salpêtrière in 1862 after completing his medical training and worked at the hospital for the duration of his career. Although many of his patients were ageing women, alcoholics, and epileptics, he was best known for his work with hysteria, in particular his conception of *la grande attaque hystérique*, which was considered the most spectacular of hysterical conditions. Charcot and his supporters generally understood hysteria as a localised deformity in the cerebral cortex that, when exposed to a variety of factors – including heredity, sexuality, and psychic trauma – produced visible hysterical symptoms, including bodily seizures, paralyses, and social deviance.

Charcot's multi-volume *Œuvres complètes*, which contain many images of cross-sections of brains and spines, show how doctors sought, but could not find (despite emerging magnification tools), visible proof of disease in patients' bodies. Therefore, symptoms observable to the naked eye took on new potency as they became essential to diagnosis. By making hysteria perceptible on the body's exterior, it was transformed into a legible illness, thus securing it as an object of medical study.

Une leçon clinique is a product of hysteria's heyday, when the Salpêtrière was, in Charcot's words, a 'living museum of pathology', when its photographic studio and artistic atelier pumped out pictures and sculptures, when its doctors produced visual recordings, and its patients obediently performed.[8] Drawings, etchings, photographs, paintings, and wax and plaster casts of hysterical patients were created and consulted not only by the hospital's doctors, but also by those who frequented Charcot's public lectures: physicians, artists, politicians, actors, and writers huddled together to watch the celebrity doctor and his equally famous hysterics.

Brouillet's painting, widely reproduced in medical, artistic, and popular publications, embodies and illustrates the fertile and frenzied union of art and medicine in late nineteenth-century Paris, and highlights the significant role Charcot played in this merger.[9] This painting helped fabricate Charcot's scientific persona in the public imagination even though he did not commission the work or purchase it. Often discussed alongside Gervex's portrait of Dr Péan, *Une leçon clinique* was understood as a truthful historical document that accurately recorded Parisian medical culture. De Fourcaud claimed in *Revue illustrée* that 'it would be difficult to find a more honest painting by which to consecrate the memory of Dr Charcot's renowned experiments and of the exceptional crowds they have attracted to his lectures in recent years'.[10] Ollendorf emphasised the veracity of the work, writing that '[t]he composition conforms to the truth, is clear and coherent. It shows to advantage its principal subject – Dr Charcot – without aggrandizement or artifice'.[11] Although Roger Ballu criticised the painting's dull composition, he praised its sincerity when he wrote that on a second viewing, 'a certain reality seizes you'.[12] The painting's realist effect prompted Meurville to write in the *Gazette de France* that the painting did not demand lengthy viewing because everything was immediately visible: 'it takes only a minute to admire the truthfulness of the characters and the light. Beyond that, there is nothing more to discover'.[13] For these critics, Brouillet's realism was taken at face value; its truth claims were rarely questioned.

By focusing on Brouillet's *Une leçon clinique*, this chapter will explore the ways in which realist modes and media dealt with the challenge of representing hysteria. Since the 1980s, Brouillet's work has often accompanied chapters and articles dedicated to the study of hysteria, yet little attention has been given to the history of the painting, to the context in which it was produced, or to the contemporary criticism it generated. Salon criticism is of particular value, as it provides historical accounts not only of the painting, but also of how hysteria and hypnosis were understood. It reveals how medical knowledge permeated lay consciousness and demonstrates the connections between the worlds of art and medicine. Brouillet highlighted realism's essential role in depicting hysteria and, subsequently, in the construction of hysteria as a 'real' disease by including multiple modes of visualising the disease in *Une leçon clinique*. This chapter argues that the painting is both a realist rendering of hysteria and a realist portrayal of various realist forms of representing hysteria by demonstrating that paint, photography, wax, drawing, hypnosis, and electrotherapy were all forms of realism. Each section of this chapter focuses on a different mode of representing hysteria depicted or symbolised in *Une leçon clinique* by situating it within wider cultural contexts and debates.

Une leçon clinique foregrounds the central role that visualising hysteria played in formulating understandings of the disease and Charcot's identity. The imaging of hysteria contributed to Charcot's persona as a medical leader particularly since he encouraged the taxonomic project. However, the visualisation of hysteria at the Salpêtrière was excessive and extreme. Like Péan's medical collection at Hôpital Saint-Louis, there were occasions when it went beyond the demands of medical practice and was arguably as hysterical as the disease it purported to portray. As evinced by *Une leçon clinique* and other contemporary works on the subject, the hysterical female body, in representation and as a living body, was a site upon which realisms 'went mad'.[14]

Hysteria beyond construction and rebellion

Although critics of Charcot ridiculed his conception of hysteria, particularly Dr Hippolyte Bernheim from Nancy (who opposed Charcot's belief that hypnosis could diagnose hysteria), most physicians and the public accepted it as a genuine illness. Since the mid-twentieth century, however, the debate around hysteria has been more academic than medical. Most twenty- and twenty-first-century scholars have focused on hysteria as a socially constructed category invented out of sexual, professional, or institutional desire.[15] They have shown how its symptoms often aligned with characteristics that did not fit easily into nineteenth-century conceptions of proper femininity and masculinity. Homosexuals, childless women, effeminate men, amongst other types, were classified as hysterical.[16]

The scholarly fascination with hysteria resurfaced in the 1970s with the emergence of French psychoanalytic feminism and continued into the 1980s with Georges Didi-Huberman's seminal study of the iconography of hysteria at the Salpêtrière. He conceptualised the extraordinary quantity and character of the photographs of hysterical women as a 'paradox of spectacular evidence' by arguing that, despite the multiplicity of symptoms, hysteria arose out of nothing, as nineteenth-century physicians had not located hysteria's organic existence.[17] The 1990s saw a boom in interdisciplinary approaches to the topic, as the selected essays in *Hysteria Beyond Freud* attest.[18]

Since the late nineteenth century, hysteria has been a battleground for academic theories, as scholars search for the most 'real' and 'true' understanding of the disease. Freud famously rejected Charcot's emphasis on the visual and used language to create a concept of hysteria that fulfilled his aims.[19] In response to Freud, and Freudian theory, feminists such as Hélène Cixous, Catherine Clément, and Luce Irigaray employed psychoanalytic theory to produce new models of hysteria by questioning the exclusion of female subjectivity in patriarchal culture. Historians and philosophers, including Michel Foucault, explored the social, historical, and political forces that contributed to hysteria's discursive formation. More recent examinations of hysteria mimic nineteenth-century medical investigations of the hysterical body since many reveal more about the examiner than the examined.[20] To a certain extent, academic debates about hysteria remain grounded in feminist projects, as both Carol Armstrong's and Judith Surkis's reviews of the 2003 English translation of Didi-Huberman's book attest.[21] Although hysteria has been written out of current medicine, it still exists, Elaine Showalter claims, under different names and attached to different bodies; chronic fatigue syndrome and multiple personality disorder are 'new' hysterias.[22] For Showalter, hysteria is 'a mimetic disorder; it mimics culturally permissible expressions of distress'.[23] The images and objects that portray hysterical bodies emerging from the Salpêtrière, particularly those commissioned by Charcot, epitomise a historical moment when the visual legibility of diseases and their evidence on the body's surface was paramount.

During the nineteenth century, sick bodies were visually documented so that they could be studied. The hysterical body, however, posed problems because it could never be just one thing or hold just one pose. Definitions of hysteria were always shifting. The frenzied character of hysteria and the public's understanding are evident in Jules Claretie's 1881 novel, *Les Amours d'un interne*, when the character Pedro defines hysteria through contradictory and exaggerated characteristics:

> It is really the whole nervous system going haywire. It can be erotic – as in the vulgar understanding – it can be sombre, it can be mystical, it can be religious, it can be anything. The hysteric eats too much or eats nothing, sleeps too much or not enough, appears engrossed like an idiot or exalted like a madwoman; she loves noise, garish colours, romantic fantasies; wants people to take care of her, and only her; she stands outside the rules of both polite society and the demimonde; the theatre, the salons, all of Paris is filled with hysterics, text-book cases requiring treatment by Doctor Charcot … Hysteria! It could even

> be considered the great modern malady. Society is suffering from a gigantic neurosis or neuritis.[24]

As Pedro's description attests, the hysterical body had to be many things at once: it was eroticised for novels and public spectacles – including the Salon – but sick and disordered for medical study. It held the promise and threat of transformation. Like the mysteries of the unconscious mind and the anaesthetised body, the unknowability of hysteria was a part of its power; the body remained secret despite being subject to constant study, analysis, and dissection. Representational methods had to account for this malleability and transformation and, therefore, visual images of hysterical bodies were simultaneously products and producers of this representational insanity.

Medical texts from the Salpêtrière, as well as the Charcot Museum's models and anatomical specimens, merged artistic methods and media to produce images and objects that were considered as accurate and legible as possible. Charcot's *Œuvres complètes*, Bourneville and Regnard's 3-volume *Iconographie photographique de la Salpêtrière*, and the various volumes of the *Nouvelle iconographie de la Salpêtrière* are filled with lithographs, etchings, woodcuts, drawings, black-and-white photographs, and coloured graphs. Similarly, the medical museum that Charcot founded in 1878 had an assortment of images,

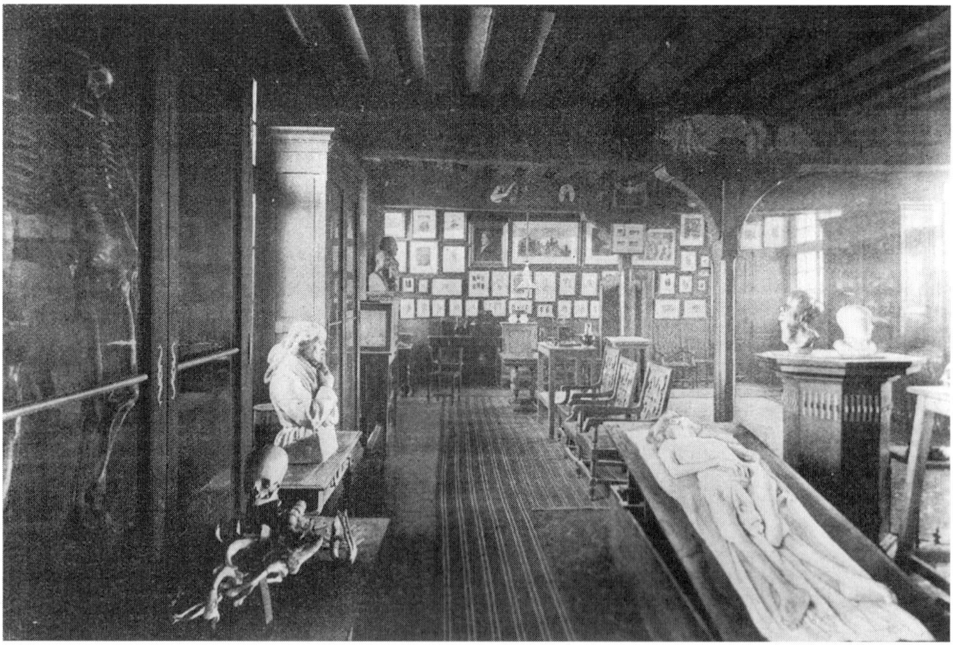

47 Photograph of Musée Charcot, c.1878.

objects, and sculptures on display.[25] A blurred nineteenth-century black-and-white photograph of the museum shows the diversity of the collection (Figure 47): a life-size wax model of a naked woman, twisted by ataxia, takes centre stage; a plaster sculpture by Richer portrays a clothed and aged woman holding a cloth to her mouth to catch drool; a glass cabinet to the left contains complete human skeletons, while other human bones are scattered around the room; on the back wall are an assortment of portraits and landscapes; plaster busts of idealised human heads are displayed on plinths and on top of cabinets. Different media were understood to have varying strengths, weaknesses, and uses: photography captured particularities, casting held poses, and drawing and painting showed drama, movement, and expression (all things that caused photographs to blur). Some methods, like photography, promised greater mechanical objectivity than others while drawings, at least on the surface, testified to witnessing events and lent images a sense of truthfulness through the participation of experts. Certainly, the graphs recording hysterical movements and tremors required an expert eye to comprehend zigzagging patterns. To make sense of the changes in scientific picture making, Daston and Galison explain that there was a chronological development to the relationship between scientific pictures and the concept of objectivity that moved from 'truth-to-nature' to 'mechanical objectivity' to 'trained judgement'. They argue that as scientists reimagined their scientific selves over the eighteenth to twentieth centuries, the 'truth' of pictures moved from a generalised universal image made by an illustrator's skilled hand to a specific case captured by a photographic apparatus to difficult data interpreted by an expert observer.[26] The Salpêtrière images and objects, however, provide an interesting historical example because they destabilise this linear history as multiple modes, methods, and procedures were used concurrently. The representations in these books and in the museum were intricately related to one another and to other iconographical precedents and artistic conventions outside the medical sphere. In many cases, they worked together to produce the effect of the real. Yet such depictions could not always provide the stable recordings required for medical study because they had to account for the vastness of hysteria's definition. Thus, the images and objects produced at the Salpêtrière demonstrate how medical men included and excluded elements of reality to produce a secure and readable iconography of hysteria.

Charcot's lessons and his audience

Newspapers and Salon reviews from 1887 focused on the audience depicted in Brouillet's canvas and printed a diagram with the sitters' names.[27] 'All of the faces are portraits, and the newspapers unfailingly named the people who posed for the young painter', wrote Mantz.[28] Ballu went so far as claiming that the painting 'will be successful, and not merely because of people's interest in trying to identify the individuals portrayed'.[29] Identifying the audience contributed to the fun of viewing the work and attested to the ostensible reality of the scene.

In *Une leçon clinique*, Charcot stands before an audience of recognisable men. Packed tightly into the amphitheatre of the Salpêtrière, suited male bodies dominate the canvas, forming a black block of uniformity. Eyes fixed forward, they watch Charcot discuss the hypnotic state of his patient, who lies in the arms of the young Dr Babinsky.[30] Two nurses stand at the ready, prepared to lower the unconscious woman onto a draped stretcher. Dr Paul Richer is positioned to Charcot's right, pen in hand, recording the movements of doctor and patient. His role as the Salpêtrière artist is emphasised by a depiction of one of his drawings of a hysterical woman in the midst of a *grande attaque* on the amphitheatre wall. Charcot first hired Richer, a physician and an artist, to illustrate and sculpt the bodily contortions of hysterical patients in 1878, claiming that 'one could base a diagnosis solely on these drawings!'[31] Richer was responsible for making an illustrated chart of Charcot's conception of the *grande attaque hystérique*. His individual drawings illustrate each phase of the attack, recording every movement of the hysterical body as it proceeded towards the climax of the arched-back *arc en cercle* (Figure 48). These drawings create a pattern of bodily movement that appears proto-cinematic and similar to flipbooks. The chart allowed doctors to diagnose the hysterical state of their patients by comparing actual bodies with those drawn by Richer. As photography could not clearly capture the body in motion until the 1890s, Richer's drawings provided the most accurate visual recording of the progress of a hysterical attack in the 1880s. Richer's desire to illustrate the bodily action that was central to hysterical fits is evident in both *L'Hystéro-épilepsie ou grande hystérie* (1881) and *Les Démoniaques dans l'art* (1887), where dotted lines form the pose of a figure in motion to symbolise movement (Figure 49).

Richer's respected position as both artist and physician exemplifies the nineteenth-century emphasis on the role of vision in medical diagnosis and study. His identity as a man who linked art and medicine was secured through his selection as professor of anatomy at the Académie des Beaux-Arts in July 1903.[32] As Raphaël Blanchard exclaimed in his address honouring Richer's appointment: 'Art and Science, long strangers to one another, now fraternise closely, and you are the principal author of this fertile union'.[33] Richer's work at the École des Beaux-Arts, particularly his encouragement of the use of photography, reinforced the intimate relationship between art and medicine, and stressed photography and the human body as sites of this union. Due to its association with mechanical objectivity, modernity, and science, photography eventually replaced drawing as the most accurate and detached medium for imaging the object world in a medical context.

Other audience members in Brouillet's painting include Dr Paul Berbez, head of the clinic of diseases of the nervous system (wearing a monocle) and

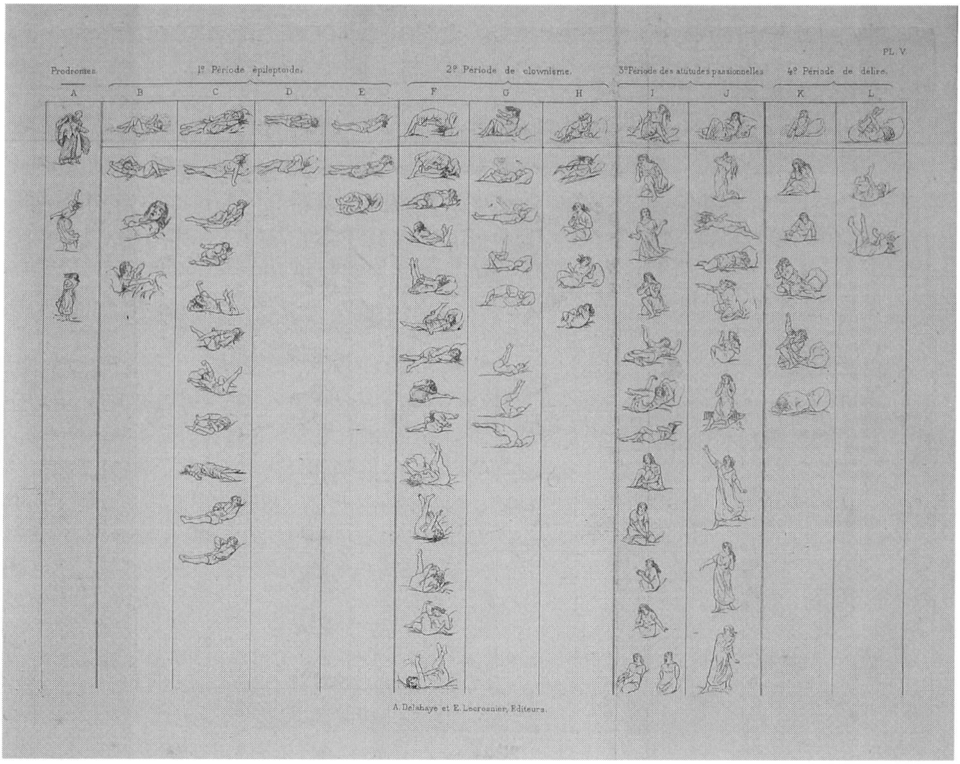

Paul Richer, Detail of 'Phases of hysterical attacks', drawings from P. Richer, *Études cliniques sur l'hystéro-épilepsie ou grande hystérie*, 1881 (Paris), p. v. **48**

Dr Bourneville, editor of the *Iconographie photographique de la Salpêtrière*, who leans his head against that of the politician Dr Alfred Joseph Naquet. The head photographer of the hospital, Albert Londe, sits in the far left foreground. Jules Claretie, who wrote the books *L'Obsession, moi et l'autre*, about a painter with a second personality, and *Les Amours d'un interne*, is positioned next to Naquet and in front of the novelist Paul Arène (who dedicated his 1889 novel *La Chèvre d'or* to Charcot). In the back row stand Philippe Burty, art critic, collector, and art adviser to Mme Charcot; Dr Maurice Debove, social crusader against syphilis; Dr Victor Cornil, a politician interested in medico-legal reform; and Mathias Duval, professor of anatomy at the École des Beaux-Arts as well as an expert on hypnosis.[34] Salon critics believed the hysterical woman was Blanche Wittman, one of Charcot's star hysterics who appeared in demonstrations.[35] The crowd depicted by Brouillet attests to the way in which hysteria required an 'interdisciplinary' representation: for these men, the hysterical body was an object of study, a seductive character for fashionable novels, a model to

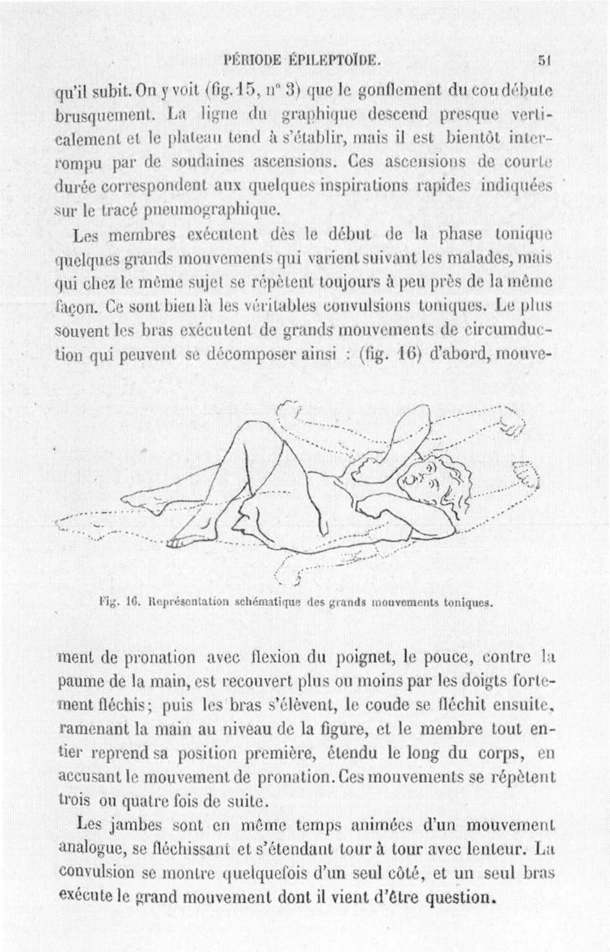

PÉRIODE ÉPILEPTOÏDE. 51

qu'il subit. On y voit (fig. 15, n° 3) que le gonflement du cou débute brusquement. La ligne du graphique descend presque verticalement et le plateau tend à s'établir, mais il est bientôt interrompu par de soudaines ascensions. Ces ascensions de courte durée correspondent aux quelques inspirations rapides indiquées sur le tracé pneumographique.

Les membres exécutent dès le début de la phase tonique quelques grands mouvements qui varient suivant les malades, mais qui chez le même sujet se répètent toujours à peu près de la même façon. Ce sont bien là les véritables convulsions toniques. Le plus souvent les bras exécutent de grands mouvements de circumduction qui peuvent se décomposer ainsi : (fig. 16) d'abord, mouve-

Fig. 16. Représentation schématique des grands mouvements toniques.

ment de pronation avec flexion du poignet, le pouce, contre la paume de la main, est recouvert plus ou moins par les doigts fortement fléchis; puis les bras s'élèvent, le coude se fléchit ensuite, ramenant la main au niveau de la figure, et le membre tout entier reprend sa position première, étendu le long du corps, en accusant le mouvement de pronation. Ces mouvements se répètent trois ou quatre fois de suite.

Les jambes sont en même temps animées d'un mouvement analogue, se fléchissant et s'étendant tour à tour avec lenteur. La convulsion se montre quelquefois d'un seul côté, et un seul bras exécute le grand mouvement dont il vient d'être question.

49 Paul Richer, 'Représentation schématique des grands mouvements toniques', from P. Richer, *Études cliniques sur l'hystéro-épilepsie ou grande hystérie*, 1887 (Paris), p. 48.

be illustrated, photographed, and sculpted, as well as a rebellious citizen in need of surveillance. Unconscious, diseased, and under the scrutiny of medical, political, literary, and artistic men, the hysterical female body in *Une leçon clinique* is shown as material and muse. Her identity was as dependent on Charcot, the audience, and Brouillet as their identities were on her.

Salon critics discussed the painting's narrative with ease and familiarity. They recognised Charcot, located the work at the Salpêtrière, and took pleasure in describing all the people portrayed. Charcot and his lectures were well known

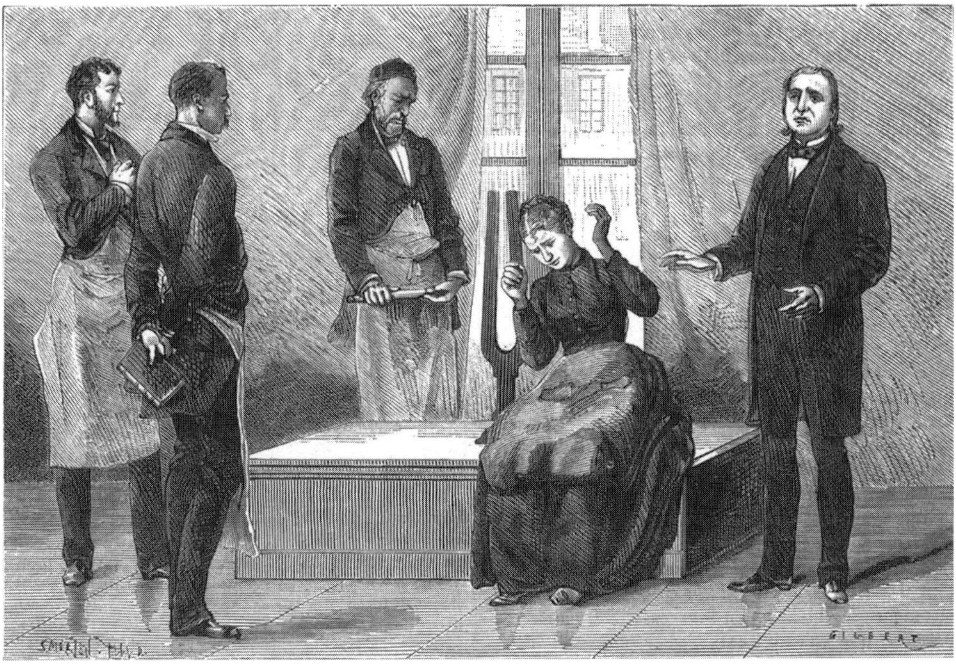

'Du Somnambulisme et du Magnétisme', from *La Nature*, 18 January 1879, p. 105, engraving after drawings done at the Salpêtrière. 50

in the last decades of the century – both before and after *Une leçon clinique*'s exhibition at the Salon – particularly his spectacular public Tuesday and Sunday lectures.[36] 'The podium was always decorated with pictures and anatomical schemata pertaining to the day's presentation', recalled Charcot's contemporary Henri Ellenberger.[37] The Salpêtrière lectures, that could barely contain the huge crowds that they drew, received ample attention in the press:[38] Gaston Tissandier noted that the lectures had 'considerable vogue'[39] while Félix Platel based Charcot's celebrity status on these events.[40]

Representations of Charcot's lectures were prevalent and contributed to his notoriety. In 1878, Dr A. Cartaz published black and white prints of Charcot performing medical procedures on hysterical women in his article in *La Nature*. In the first, the doctor projects light directly at a woman as a means of inducing her into a cataleptic trance. In the second, he is in the midst of a lecture; catalepsy is produced in a female patient through sound vibrations (Figure 50). His gesturing hands and outward look indicate that he is addressing a larger crowd that is not depicted. He is leading the lecture, whereas the hysterical patient is the object of scientific enquiry: on display and under study. Her pathological state is manifest in her sexual difference from medical men, whose health and intellect are signified by steady gazes, standing suited bodies, and the medical tools and books in their hands.

The prints' reproduction in *La Nature* imbued them with the truth claims of scientific journalism. The assumption that they were accurate was implied by their legibility, the correspondence between the article's descriptive text and the detailed images, and the words beneath the prints that claim they were 'drawn from life at the Salpêtrière'. Proclamations of authenticity were common in nineteenth-century medical atlases and textbooks; a close connection between image and its referent in the observable world was a noted sign of veracity. Charcot's *Œuvres complètes*, particularly the first volume, link visual representations with witnessed events; many images are labelled as 'Drawn by P. Richer, based on a sketch made as seen by Mr Charcot'.[41] Although Richer's drawings, in some cases, were not based on his own direct observation of a hysterical body, his images were imbued with a claim to truth by being based on Charcot's studies after nature. The distance of Richer's drawings from actual events did not decrease their validity as truthful, medically valid documents, but in fact quite the opposite. One could even suggest that Richer, one step removed, was perceived as being able to produce a more objective and legible rendering than Charcot's quick sketch. Richer's drawings were made to teach and therefore required mixing the authenticity of Charcot's witnessing – his expert eye – with Richer's aesthetic polish and his own diagnostic knowledge. He was, after all, artist and medical expert in one.

The second *La Nature* print is a typical example of nineteenth-century representations of Charcot lecturing at the Salpêtrière and shares many similarities with *Une leçon clinique*: the narrative is clear; men are knowledgeable professionals whose field of study is the female body; hysteria is a female disease; men are intellectually engaged while the female is unconscious or semi-conscious; the Salpêtrière is a spectacular site of medical innovation where Charcot and patients perform for a crowd. Prints in Salpêtrière-produced books, such as Bourneville and Regnard's various volumes of *Iconographie photographique de la Salpêtrière* and Regnard's *Les maladies épidémiques de l'esprit* (1887), contain similar images. Most imply that a crowd is present, since patients and physicians are shown facing out, but do not show spectators.

In contrast, the audience is central to Brouillet's painting. The men gathered here signify power and authority and, in turn, lend support to Charcot's theories. They build up his identity and enhance his celebrity status. It is likely that the men portrayed in *Une leçon clinique* attended Charcot's lectures at one point, but doubtful that they were present at the same event and that they all agreed with Charcot's beliefs. 'To my knowledge, Messieurs Jules Claretie, Alfred Naquet and Paul Arène do not regularly attend Monsieur Charcot's lessons', wrote Dr Dubray in his Salon review for *Union médicale*.[42] There were well-known conflicts between the men in the picture; it is unlikely that they gathered for the painting or were willing to sit next to each other. Although the canvas shows members of the audience taking notes, the interns who were responsible for recording Charcot's lectures, Drs Colin and Blin, are missing.[43] Therefore, it is certainly the case that *Une leçon clinique* is a fictional grouping whose purpose was to show Charcot's impact on various disciplines, to exhibit Charcot's and Brouillet's contact with the Parisian elite, and to build their reputations as leading men. The artifice of this gathering coincides with that of group portraiture: the rhetoric of realism and the genre of portraiture helped portray communities and identities as natural and cohesive (even when this was not the case).[44] Yet, *Une leçon clinique* does not fit easily into the genre of group portraiture because it contains unwilling participants and was not commissioned. The artificiality of the audience challenges the truth claims of Brouillet's realist strategies, which included the detailed renderings of recognisable Parisian figures. Paradoxically, however, it was this fictional grouping that contributed to Salon critics' praise for the painting's accuracy and ability to serve as a historical document.

Borrowing sources: Charcot's books and commissions

Visual representations were crucial to Charcot's identity as a prominent Parisian physician. The widely circulated depictions of hysteria commissioned by Charcot, and emerging from the hospital under his direction, contributed to the dominance of his theories and his medical persona. The non-medical public's access to images over texts contributed to Charcot's authority in the public imagination. Upon Charcot's death in 1893, Professor Joffroy argued that, 'As for hysteria, it can be said that Charcot created it almost from beginning to end'.[45] Charcot's students and colleagues, such as Dr Henry Meige, promoted the importance of visual observation and optical records for diagnoses as an innovation: observation extended and reinforced the empiricist faith in vision emerging from the Salpêtrière.[46] Most famously, Freud, who attended many of Charcot's lectures in the mid-1880s, emphasised Charcot's reliance on the visual when, on the occasion of Charcot's death in 1893, he recalled that Charcot called himself a '"visual", a man who sees … He used to look again and again at things he did not understand, to deepen his impression of them day by day, till suddenly an understanding of them dawned on him'.[47] Although, as discussed in Chapter 1, there was a tension between laboratory science – which proved that not everything was visible to the eye – and clinical study – which prioritised visual observation and haptic palpations – the anatomic-clinical method was nonetheless considered scientific, modern, and successful.[48]

Charcot wanted his patients to be undressed when he viewed them so that he could read their bodies for signs of illness. His former interns Souques and Meige described the examination as follows:

> He sits down near a bare table, and immediately has the patient to be studied brought in. The patient is then completely stripped. The intern reads the 'observation', while the Master listens attentively. Then there is a long silence during which he gazes; he gazes at the patient and drums his fingers on the table. The assistants are standing, crowded together, anxiously awaiting a word that will shed some light. Charcot remains silent. Then he instructs the patient to move in a certain way, makes her speak, asks for her reflexes to be measured, for her sensitivity to be examined. And again he falls silent, Charcot's mysterious silence. Finally he brings in a second patient, examines her like the first, calls for a third, and still without a word, compares them. This minute observation, primarily visual, is the source of all of Charcot's discoveries. The artist who, in this case, goes hand in hand with the doctor, is not extraneous to his discoveries.[49]

In order to make diagnoses and generate medical knowledge, bodies were categorised, symptoms listed, and illnesses named. Like his predecessors at the Salpêtrière, including Philippe Pinel, Charcot added to the iconography of hysteria to make it visible and participate in the republican project of strengthening French hospitals by assembling taxonomies of diseases. Classifying bodies and illnesses was essential to providing proof and improving professional skills. It was also crucial to the specialisation of medical fields taking place during the period. New taxonomies enriched and expanded the discipline, while naming diseases, procedures, and discoveries ensured one's historical legacy. The images, objects, and books commissioned by Charcot, like those produced at the Hôpital Saint-Louis, the Pasteur Institute, and the Académie de Médecine, contributed to the advancement of French medicine and its international reputation. Charcot, like Péan, was praised for his classifications and his modernisation of medicine. 'Charcot imposed order and precision on a multitude of medical questions that before him were nothing but disorder',[50] wrote Dr G. Daremberg, and Bianchon claimed that 'he is the reformer, the great initiator of the modern method. These scientific triumphs number in the hundreds, and the best of them, in Germany, were derived from Charcot or from our Pasteur'.[51]

Charcot's active role in making visual records encouraged his followers to see him as both a physician and an artist. The integration of art into medicine fulfilled a personal desire for Charcot, who, like Péan and Pasteur, was forced to choose between medical and artistic training.[52] Although Charcot drew his own images of hysteria, he was best known for those he commissioned. His role at the Salpêtrière was similar to Péan's at Saint-Louis and Pasteur's at the Pasteur Institute: he received government funding to produce images and objects that aided medical learning.

Charcot helped secure money for a photographic studio for the hospital in 1878. Drs Bourneville and Regnard thanked him for being the force behind this new room as well as the 3 volumes of the *Iconographie photographique de la Salpêtrière*.[53] The books are filled with descriptive medical text, line drawings, graphs, engravings, and photographs of women in different stages of hysterical attacks and in a range of states of undress and consciousness. Although they were made for the medical community, the images and ideas contained in the pages quickly influenced the popular press and lay consciousness.[54] Bourneville and Regnard's books fit into Charcot's taxonomic project: the layout and the emphasis on images helped doctors and medical students with diagnoses, ordered symptoms into cohesive sections, and provided a historical record of discoveries and experiments. To this day, many diseases remain known by the names of Salpêtrière doctors, such as Tourette's Syndrome and the Babinsky Reflex.

The *Iconographie photographique* series played a key role in visualising hysteria. It set a precedent for publishing books and periodicals dedicated to the depiction of the disease and encouraged the use of photography in medical books. Furthermore, the volumes showcased technological changes in photography and printing techniques: the first edition of volume 1 from 1875 contains 40 albumen prints mounted on card (each loosely inserted as issued) while in the later editions and volumes the callotype plates and engravings are reproduced directly onto the books' printed pages. Significantly, these books contain works from the history of art, such as a sketch by Rubens in the 1877 edition. This practice of mixing artistic and medical pictures continued in Salpêtrière publications well into the twentieth century. Charcot's museum fused these worlds too, as 'artistic' prints and portrait busts were hung next to skulls, skeletons, and a wax model of a hysterical patient.

The blurred boundaries between the medical and artistic spheres were promoted by Charcot throughout his life and work, and exemplified by the two books he wrote with Richer: *Les Démoniaques dans l'art* (1887) and *Les Difformes et les malades dans l'art* (1889). Intended for both a public and medical audience, they entertained and educated readers by merging contemporary medical thought, art history, and sensational tales of hysteria. Charcot and Richer rewrote the history of hysteria and the history of art by arguing that hysteria had a long past – was this not evident, they suggested, from the visual similarities between mad women in famous historical (and often religious) artworks and those in contemporary medical iconography? Charcot's success depended on the presence of hysteria in the nineteenth century and on its existence prior to his work at the Salpêtrière. In response to critics who accused him of inventing hysteria, Charcot 'proved' its actuality by ostensibly finding depictions of the disease in well-known paintings from the Renaissance and beyond. In turn, he argued that his commissioned medical photographs, drawings, and sculptures would be historical documents that would help future physicians. Albert Londe, head photographer at the hospital, also linked historical art with the images produced at the Salpêtrière:

> Let us admire in passing those scrupulous artists who were not afraid to reproduce nature itself in all its ugliness and deformities, thus leaving us with documents of the highest value. This role that they fulfilled belongs henceforth to doctors, who can now, thanks to photography, leave to future centuries iconographic documents of inestimable value.[55]

Londe's beliefs demonstrate how art no longer had a monopoly on 'deformed' bodies. Photographers, with the help of doctors, were the artists of the future.

Les Démoniaques dans l'art and *Les Difformes et les maladies dans l'art* also fulfilled a political role for Charcot. Jan Goldstein explains that the images within these books reflected Charcot's anticlerical stance: through a series of art historical examples, he argued that the past saints, particularly those in the throes of ecstasy or receiving heavenly visions, were hysterical. This critique undermined Catholic faith while promoting scientific medicine as a trusted leading force in modern society. The visual representations produced at the Salpêtrière, however, also drew on older religious precedents for historical credence.[56] For example, Richer utilised Rubens's drawings to illustrate a hysteric with a contorted body and exposed tongue in his drawing of a *Contorsion-attaque démoniaque*.[57] Although Richer's reliance on art historical models appears to undermine the truth claims made by Richer, Charcot, and others at the Salpêtrière, who insisted that their depictions of hysteria were objective recordings taken directly from nature, it also demonstrates the degree to which doctors trusted art historical models as accurate medical records.[58]

Une leçon clinique is like a patchwork quilt made of images collected and discussed by Charcot and Richer in *Les Démoniaques dans l'art*. Although Brouillet's canvas portrays a contemporary Parisian scene, its timely display at the Salon, shortly after the publication of *Les Démoniaques dans l'art*, linked his rendition of hysteria with the 67 images in this book, thus aligning the painting with the earlier religious sources discussed by Charcot and Richer. Paul Mantz referred to Charcot and Richer's book in his 1887 Salon review:

> [t]he volume *Les Démoniaques dans l'art*, a book that touched us deeply, as it taught us that even in the distant past, artists were familiar with diseases of the nervous system and the convulsions of the hysterical crisis, and that, if some of them left us with improved or romanticised representations, our friend Rubens was of the most exact in translating with a paintbrush the terrible spectacle of the phenomenon as it was honestly observed.[59]

Although we do not know the extent to which Brouillet was influenced by this book – nor do we know if he conceived the painting's composition before or after seeing *Les Démoniaques dans l'art* – he was very familiar with the Salpêtrière's

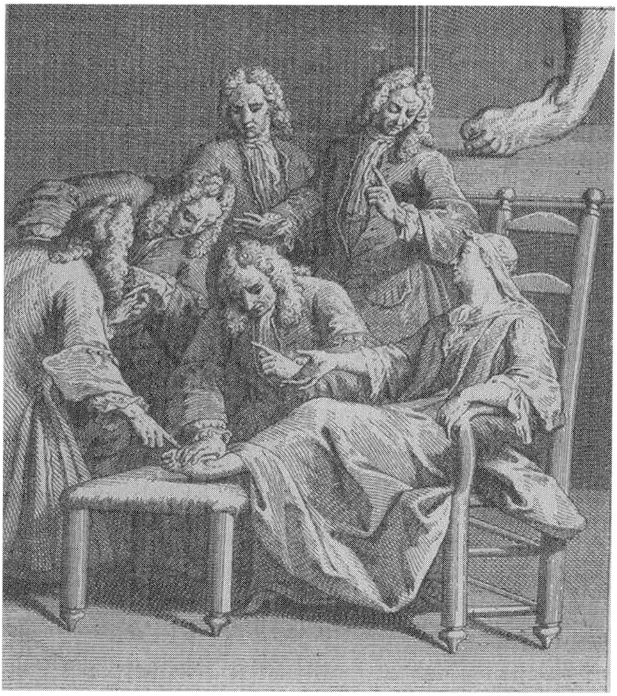

'Pied-Bot', from Louise Basile Carre de Montgeron, *La vérité des miracles* (1745–47), reproduced in J.M. Charcot and P. Richer, *Les Démoniaques dans l'art* (Paris, 1887), p. 81, engraving. 51

visual practices, and there are clear visual similarities between his painting and the works discussed. For example, the hysteric's pose in Brouillet's painting mimics the arched backs of the famous works reproduced in *Les Démoniaques dans l'art*, where possessed bodies fall into outstretched arms. The precedent of a sexualised semi-naked female figure is in an engraving after Adam van Noort's seventeenth-century work *Sainte Claire délivre une dame de Pise de cinq démons*. The depiction of a large crowd in an open space is similar to B. Picart's print *Grand secours* from 1808. Brouillet's decision to paint a copy of Richer's drawing to indicate the patient's illness appears to be based on the drawing of a pathological foot in Louis Basile Carré de Montgeron's *La vérité des miracles opérés par l'intercession de M. de Pâris et autres appellans démontrée contre M. l'archevêque de Sens* from 1745–47 (Figure 51). By painting a contemporary medical scene filled with doctors and a patient, rather than a religious one packed with priests and madmen, Brouillet transformed these pictures to align himself with the famed artists of the past; modern scientific medicine, rather than religion, was now a superior subject matter for significant French painting.

Brouillet pointed to the disintegrating role of religion in medical spheres by including two nurses. Unlike Gervex's painting, in which a nurse and a nun take part in the operation, *Une leçon clinique* depicts no religious figures, despite their presence in most French medical institutions. Similarly, nuns were not portrayed in photographs from the Salpêtrière.[60] Nursing was integral to a secular hospital system because nurses replaced nuns. Working as a nurse was well regarded as an essential role in the protection of French health, but was also problematic because it took women away from child rearing and put them in close contact with illness, disease, and potentially amorous doctors. It is significant that many employees at the Salpêtrière began as patients: Blanche Wittman, for example, worked in the photographic studio and radiology laboratory after her tenure as the hospital's star hysteric. Augustine, another hysterical *vedette*, was photographed as a patient in a nightgown and as a hospital worker in a nurse's costume in the 1879 volume of the *Iconographie photographique*, thus presaging the slippage between nurse and patient.

Brouillet alluded to the unstable position of nursing at this historical moment through the portrayal of the nurse, Mlle Écary, whose youth and uniform connect her to the hysterical patient, but whose occupational identity unites her with Mme Bottard, whose married status (indicated by her wedding ring) stages her social respectability as a caregiver.[61] This young nurse, like Augustine in the Salpêtrière photographs, occupies various positions. She is a symbol of anticlerical republican policies and one step away from hysteria. Nurses, like hysterical patients, were educated and managed by Salpêtrière doctors; they were marginalised figures, necessary in medical spaces, yet never a leading force. The young nurse in *Une leçon clinique* is barely present: only her face appears from behind the old nurse. In this work and in the many volumes of *Iconographie photographique*, nurses served iconographical and political roles; they exhibited the identities and political views of medical men by their uniforms, actions, and hospital presence rather than by their individual identities. Charcot used depictions of nurses to advance his anticlerical battles. His involvement in the creation of a new medical iconography reconfigured the relationship between medicine and religion into a political visual language linking medicine to a secular state.

Realism and light: 'It does not confuse fantasy with science'

Like Gervex, Edelfelt, and Gsell, Brouillet painted a fashionable, contemporary scene to get noticed by Salon reviewers, advertise his identity as a modern painter, and publicise his association with men of great import. Brouillet achieved success the previous year when his painting, *Le Paysan blessé*, was bought by the State after its display at the Salon.[62] Perhaps the success of Edelfelt's portrait of Pasteur at the 1886 Salon encouraged Brouillet to abandon a medical genre scene with unknown people for a painting that was considered more intriguing because of the specificity of its sitters and setting. Although a few critics denounced Brouillet's painterly ability, considering his work inferior to Gervex's, the painting's scene, figures, and style were unanimously regarded as modern.[63] Like laboratories and operating rooms, the Salpêtrière, with its electric lights, photographic studio, and electrotherapy units, was a pioneering scientific space *par excellence* and therefore an ideal venue for modern portraiture.

Brouillet exhibited his familiarity with cutting-edge medicine by painting a scene at the Salpêtrière; this made him a part of Charcot's privileged crowd. As Gervex, Edelfelt, Gsell, and Bonnat had done, Brouilllet displayed his connection with medical men through visual means, imbuing his painting and professional identity with the social qualifications to produce and document reality. Although Brouillet did not depict himself in the amphitheatre, the painting's detailed portraits and setting signified his presence and powers of observation; the painting purports to portray an actual event whether it happened or not. *Le Temps*, *Le Monde illustré*, and *L'Art français* remarked that Brouillet had first-hand experience of the scene. Javel wrote, '[H]e saw the poignant scene which he retraces with true emotion',[64] and Mantz claimed, 'Before painting, he educated himself. It was at the Salpêtrière, by watching the master's lessons, that he studied the arrangement of the scene, noted the details of the experiment and the patient's attitude'.[65] Brouillet's implied attendance and the use of realist strategies transformed him into a documenter of modern medicine and its elite. Like Nadar's photographic portraits of Pasteur – which were understood as exact images of a historical personality not only because of photography's assumed objectivity, but also because of the photographer's statements – Brouillet's painting was considered evidence of the artist's encounter with leading men.

Une leçon clinique's status as a realist work was enhanced by Brouillet's depiction of light. Although Mantz commented on its beauty ('Monsieur Brouillet remains what he has been from the beginning, a lover of light'),[66] it was also characterised as scientific. Mantz prefaced his discussion of both Brouillet's and Gervex's paintings with: 'As soon as science arrives, the house is flooded with true light',[67] and Ollendorf claimed that, 'Upon entering the home of the scientist, the light becomes calm, and politely cools. It takes on the tone of the house. It becomes austere and scientific. It does not confuse fantasy with science'.[68] In contrast to the artificial light of public theatres in Paris that heightened illusion and pleasure, the luminosity of the medical theatre in Brouillet's painting was discussed in terms of its scientific severity and objectivity. Georges Olmer noted the similarity between Brouillet's depiction of light in the clinic and the representation of laboratory light in Ferdinand Gueldry's painting *Au laboratoire municipal* (Figure 52). Olmer claimed that both were 'documentary paintings with meticulous exactitude and perfect

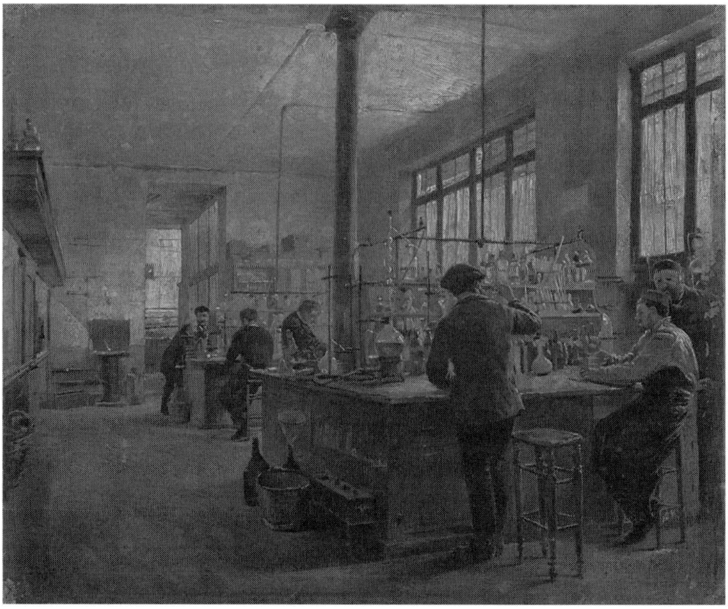

52 Ferdinand Joseph Gueldry, *Au laboratoire municipal* (1887), oil on canvas.

technique … It is but a short distance from the laboratory to the clinic, and the light we see in Monsieur Brouillet's painting is not perceptibly different from that which we have just admired in Monsieur Gueldry's painting.'[69] Merson praised his rendition of light for its clarity and ability to illuminate the faces and details of the picture.[70] Brouillet's light, though created by his brush, was considered real and austere rather than phantasmatic. Scientific narratives required bright and clear light; dark shadows and warm golden hues produced a sense of drama that was antithetical to the optics of modern scientific spaces.

Light was, after all, essential to sight and diagnosis. Brouillet included gaslights in the painting to show that hospitals were contemporary venues filled with new technologies, even though they are not lit. The room is illuminated by daylight that comes through the large windows, emphasising the actual over the artificial. Brouillet's work differs from Platel's account of Charcot's presentations:

> The long hall has been adapted into an auditorium. It is ten o'clock in the morning – and gaslight illuminates this theater, which has been carefully closed against the sunlight. The show begins without music, as at the Théâtre-Français. From the rear of the stage, stage right, enters the great Charcot. His patients follow him.[71]

Platel, who openly criticised Charcot's theatrics, described the rooms as devoid of sunlight, like theatres.[72] By rendering the clinic in daylight, Brouillet symbolically rid Charcot's lectures of their spectacular qualities. Here, medical practice is a day job that is prestigious and requires great skill, unlike evening labour such as performance or bar work, conducted under gas light by uneducated minds for common crowds.

Light was used metaphorically to describe the enlightenment of medical men, the discovery of truths, the unearthing of knowledge, and the illumination of ideas. Tissandier used these metaphors in Charcot's obituary: '[Charcot] sparkled with the greatest brightness', and he 'illuminated with a new light an entire realm of enquiry heretofore confined to the shadows'.[73] Meurville used light as a metaphor for knowledge in his 1887 Salon review when he advocated that medical knowledge be shared: 'several doctors contend that light is always beneficial'.[74] Light was also understood as a guiding force for modern medicine. André Sauger claimed medicine was 'the luminous discovery that will lead future generations toward absolute truth'.[75]

Light enabled vision and the pursuit of knowledge in scientific, medical, and artistic spheres. In the nineteenth century, it became charged with an ideological force as medical and artistic discourses merged in the gendering of light. Callen argues that as a metaphor and symbol of sight, light signified an authoritative masculine power, particularly when scientific optical theories, such as those by Helmholtz and Rood, located it within the overtly masculine space of science. Furthermore, art critics, including Félix Bracquemond and Charles Blanc, emphasised light's importance because it symbolised a male artist's mastery over colour (often personified as female), showed his ability to represent the world truthfully, and exhibited his observation skills.[76] Light was conceptualised as a sexualised masculine force that dominated female bodies. For example, Titian's *Danae and the Shower of Gold* exemplifies this sexual metaphor by showing Zeus's golden shower caressing – and ultimately impregnating – the young Danae's body.

The enlightenment of male minds was positioned in opposition to the dark mystery of the female body. Doctors and hysterical female patients epitomised this dichotomy. In Brouillet's work, the bright sunlight fosters the collective gaze of the male audience to focus on the female body, thus securing their roles as observers and her role as object. The hysteric's eyes, in contrast, are half-shut. Her vision is impaired, symbolically indicating that she has no access to knowledge, particularly medical knowledge that relied on visual observation. The inclusion of two nurses contributes to the power of vision staged here. Although they are looking at the hysterical woman, the old nurse's hands, which reach out to catch the falling body, prioritise touch and physical contact over sight; they are physical caregivers rather than intellectual onlookers.

Heroic men and sick women: precedents in paint and photography

The narrative of *Une leçon clinique* centres on the relationship between Charcot and Wittman: 'The doctor and his subject are what attracts and holds the spectator's gaze from the outset. That is where the drama lies', wrote Javel.[77] Charcot is represented as the guiding force: the men are listening to his words and taking down notes, thus showcasing Charcot's influence over the understanding of hysteria in various disciplines. In contrast, Wittman is Charcot's binary opposite: stripped, sexed, and semi-conscious. Brouillet's realistic rendering of bodies was praised. As Javel claimed, 'The listeners are depicted in realistic poses that attest to an absolutely remarkable sureness of vision on the part of Monsieur Brouillet.'[78] Scientific language helped critics decipher Brouillet's image and those shown in it. Merson credited the science of the composition for the likeness of the figures while others focused on the physiognomy of those portrayed.[79]

The diversity of the audience depicted by Brouillet in *Une leçon clinique* was one of its greatest attractions, yet it did not extend to sex and class. Javel described the audience as 'elite'[80] and surely, when Mantz wrote, 'In this learned audience, everyone will recognize someone he knows', he was intending to address his prestigious male peers and indicate his intimacy with them.[81] Darcours commended Brouillet for a painting that would allow Salon viewers to recognise 'all our doctors of repute' and show them how such men speak and gesticulate.[82] Since visible exteriors were understood to symbolise invisible interior qualities, the accurate portrayal of the body's surface was of great importance, particularly if moral and intellectual characteristics were to be easily read and emulated, as it was in the case of medical men. Dr Dubray praised Brouillet's depiction of Charcot:

> This likeness, one can say, is true from head to foot, since it is not only the well-known face of the professor that is of an irreproachable fidelity, but also his posture, the pose of his legs, and everything about his person, which is taken from life.[83]

Javel also focused on the doctor's physiognomy, claiming it 'exudes intelligence and goodness' and that 'it is very rare that genius is not complemented by goodness'.[84] The critic located Charcot's moral character and intellectual capabilities in Brouillet's rendition of the doctor's exterior.

Charcot's physical appearance had been under public scrutiny for years. In his biographical account of Charcot in *Les Hommes de mon temps* of 1878, Platel wrote a few paragraphs aligning Charcot's physical features with moral and scientific values:

> His hair – all of which he still has, almost in its original colour – bespeaks strength of will, which is also indicated by his nose. He needs his hair to

> resemble Bonaparte – and he does not want to lose his hair, just like the rest of us, even though we are far younger than he! There is something mystical in his gaze, astonishing in a materialist. His gaze is oblique – which is surprising in a mask of Bonaparte. The top of his cranium is narrower than the lower part of his face, which means that the man loves material pleasures. His mouth has a pinched quality, indicating that he is more inclined toward hatred than love. His nose is powerful and distinctive. All of Monsieur Charcot's strength is here. This Roman nose is solid and well defined. It is like the tip of the prow of a Roman galley, destined to cleave the waves, despite wind and tide.[85]

By emphasising Charcot's full head of hair, his greater aptitude for hate than love, his similarity to Bonaparte, his soldier-like character, and his materialism, Platel stressed the characteristics associated with medical masculinity in the late nineteenth century.[86] Like Brouillet, he portrayed Charcot as a republican leader: educated, rational, strong, and nationalistic. Yet, knowing that Platel was a critic of Charcot, it is evident that his description was tinged with cynicism and mockery: he was criticising Charcot's materialism and tenacity.

Although Salon critics discussed the healthy men in Brouillet's canvas, it was their sick counterpart, described in *Le Monde illustré* as 'the only variety introduced into this vast uniformity', who received the most attention.[87] Wittman is presented as Charcot's co-star in *Une leçon clinique*: light falls through the window onto her exposed chest while she swoons in the painted spotlight. Dr Jules Falret described hysterics as 'veritable actresses' in his 1890 medical text *Études cliniques sur les maladies mentales et nerveuses*.[88] It was commonly assumed that they were actresses, performing under Charcot's direction.[89] Yet it was also suspected that hiding behind these submissive surfaces were deceitful women. Dr Janet claimed that hysterical women were receptive to the desires of medical men, but always demanded something in return; they were simultaneously passive and demanding, diseased and desired, unconscious and conniving.[90] Hysterics' obedience to doctors' requests troubled the truthfulness of hysterical symptoms: were they signs of illness or a performance to please? Despite the seeming legibility of hysterical bodies in visual recordings, hysteria remained hard to read, the truth claims made by its representation constantly undermined by the instability of its definitions, causes, and existence, as well as by the threatening subjectivity and agency of hysterical patients.

Unlike the covered bodies of male professionals, whose high-buttoned black jackets, bearded faces, and white cuffs and collars only allowed for the exposure of pink hands and faces, Brouillet showed the swooning body of Blanche Wittman with a bare chest, smooth shoulders, and naked arms. Her dress is pulled down, her corset is loose, and her breasts are covered with the flimsy cotton of white undergarments. Brouillet portrayed hysteria as a sickness of undress by drawing on the lineage of the hysterical striptease staged in some of the photographs reproduced in the *Iconographie photographique* series and Tony Robert-Fleury's *Pinel freeing the insane* (1876), the largest painted representation of hysteria on show at the Salpêtrière in the late nineteenth century (Figure 53).[91]

Robert-Fleury's painting of Dr Philippe Pinel watching as a man unchains a motley crew of hysterical women at the Salpêtrière went against historical record by showing Pinel at the Salpêtrière rather than at the Bicêtre (the men's hospital where Pinel first unchained patients). Jane Kromm suggests that this historical inaccuracy was made in order for the artist to include women rather than men.[92] Female maladies were certainly more fashionable than male ones, as men's sickness provoked fear, particularly in light of the recent defeat in the Franco-Prussian war and the associated anxieties surrounding masculinity. Robert-Fleury's painting – especially his depictions of hysterics – iconographically corresponds to the medical books produced at the Salpêtrière in the mid-1870s that showed hysterical women with bulging eyes, open mouths, and fearful expressions. For example, the woman shown lying on the ground in Robert-Fleury's work is similar to the albumen print of a hysterical woman in the 1875 volume (Figure 54). In both works, a hysterical woman is lying in the

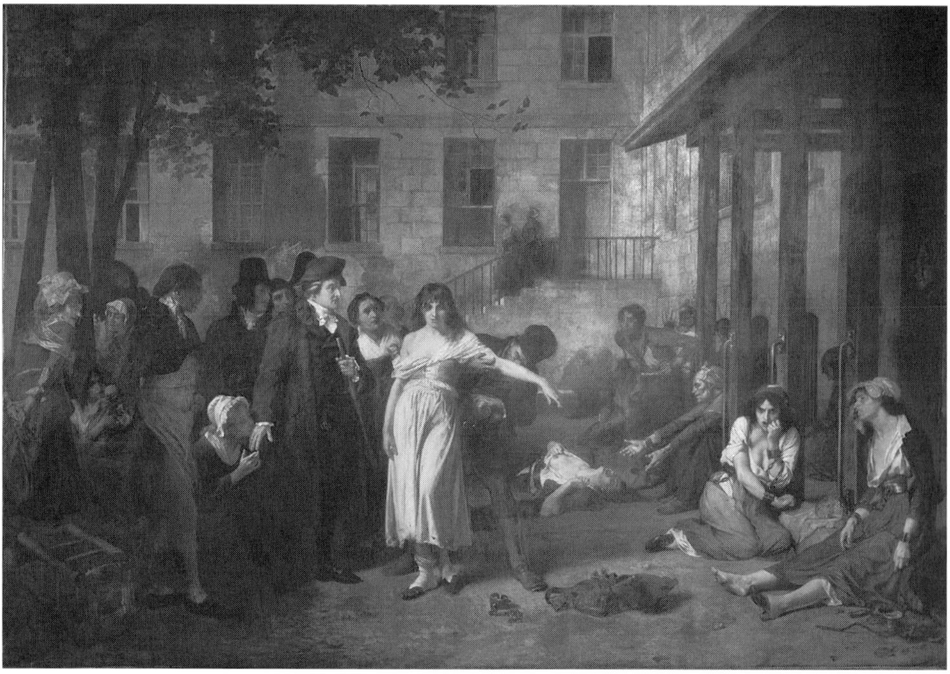

53 Tony Robert-Fleury, *Pinel, Médecin en chef de la Salpêtrière en 1795 (Pinel Freeing the Insane)* (1876), oil on canvas, 33.4 x 41.7cm.

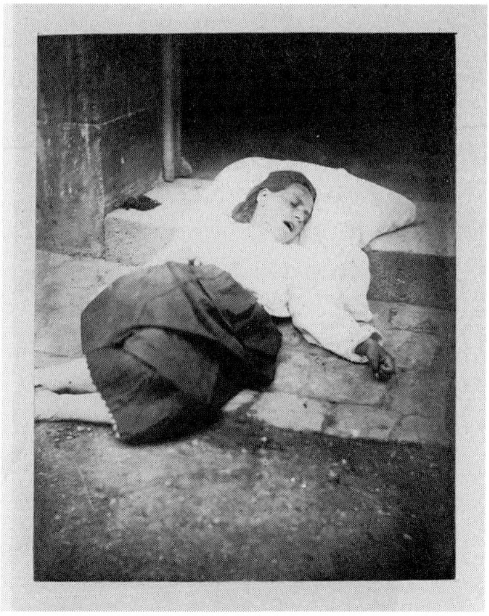

54 Paul Régnard, 'Hystéro-Épilepsie: Attaques', from Bourneville and Régnard, *Iconographie Photographique de la Salpêtrière* (1875), photograph.

dirt of the Salpêtrière courtyard, though in Robert-Fleury's the woman tears at her shirt, exposing her breasts. In both works, female sexuality is shown as primitive, submissive, and dirty. Yet in Robert-Fleury's work, only the young hysterics have bare chests and revealing clothing; the older patients are fully clothed and their hair is covered. Hysteria is only portrayed as sexually alluring when it belongs to a young body.[93]

Brouillet's Wittman is fabricated out of the standing and horizontal young hysterics in Robert-Fleury's work. Like Robert-Fleury's standing hysteric, she is youthful, has bare shoulders, unfastened white undergarments, and unsteady feet. Like the horizontal woman, she has an exposed and twisted neck, clenched fists, and contorted arms. The old hysteric reaching out to the young one in Robert-Fleury's work parallels the old nurse's gesture rendered by Brouillet and also refers back to the arched bodies in earlier religious iconography reproduced in *Les Démoniaques dans l'art*. By drawing on previous art forms as well as medical iconography, Robert-Fleury's realism, like Brouillet's, is manufactured out of other realistic representations: religious, medical, and artistic. The similarities between Brouillet's and Robert-Fleury's paintings suggest that Brouillet created an updated version of life at the Salpêtrière. He replaced the courtyard with a modern amphitheatre, Pinel with Charcot, and the humane act of unchaining with medical hypnosis. Brouillet, however, continued to show hysteria as a female illness, and the Salpêtrière as an anticlerical space. It was well known that during the 1790s Pinel was an active republican, who, like Charcot, sought to free medicine from the chains of clerical and royal influence.[94] There is no evidence of the Church in either of these works.

Unlike Robert-Fleury's painting, Brouillet's never hung at the Salpêtrière. Documents show that Brouillet offered the painting to the State, which bought it for 3,000 francs and sent it to a municipal museum in Nice.[95] Thuillier and Signoret suggested that Gérôme, Brouillet's teacher, spoke to Charcot about having his young student paint the scene and that Charcot had a role in deciding what and who was painted, but no documents exist to support these claims, nor are there any records of Charcot's views of the work. Although it is likely that a photographic reproduction of the painting was on display at the Salpêtrière, when it appeared is unknown. Significantly, it was the print of the work that popularised the painting. The print's wide distribution publicised Charcot's central role in hysteria studies and his identity as a prominent leader. Freud famously kept a reproduction in his office.

Representations of naked or semi-covered women next to clothed men were common in Salon painting, be it in images of artists with their models, doctors with patients, or owners with slaves. Such narratives displayed the power differences between clothed and unclothed, particularly since the naked body was usually female and often non-European. The staging of Brouillet's Salpêtrière scene recalls Gérôme's *The Slave Market in Rome* (1884) where women are shown as exotic, available, and under the control of clothed men (Figure 55).[96] In both paintings, women's vision is blocked, their flesh exposed, and their

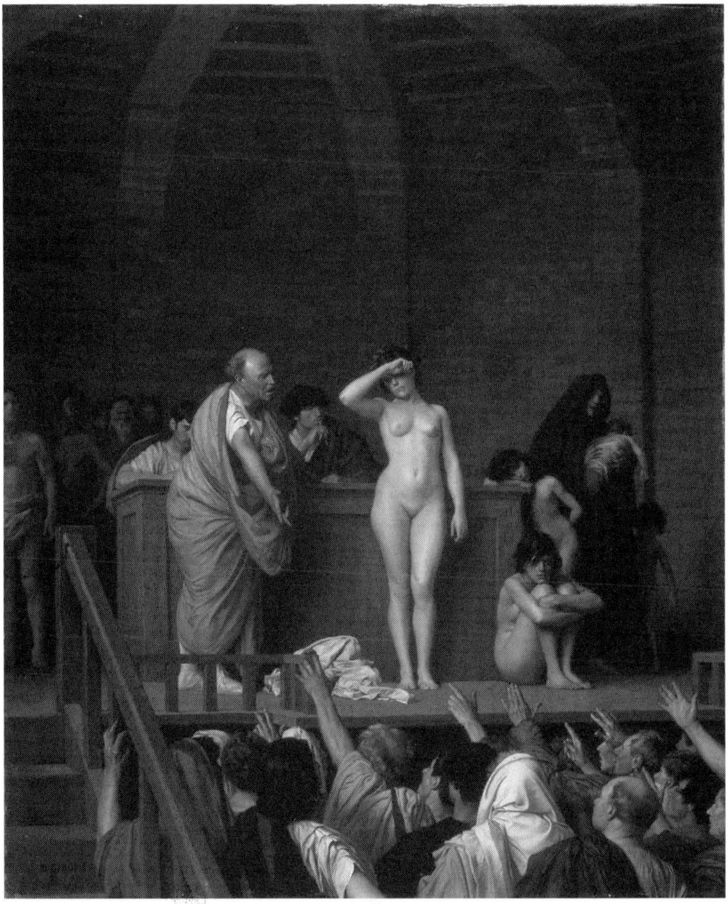

55 Jean-Léon Gérôme, *The Slave Market in Rome* (c.1883–84), oil on canvas, 92 x 74cm.

bodies displayed on stages before male audiences. 'Oriental' and hypnotised women were sensational spectacles in Paris: both were on display at exhibition venues like the Exposition Universelle.[97] The 'otherness' of foreign bodies was aligned with the diseased body, since both were positioned in opposition to the healthy bodies of European men. As is evident in Gsell's 1887 portrait of Pasteur, foreigners, particularly those from the French colonies in North Africa, 'needed' saving. In *Une leçon clinique*, Brouillet transformed Gérôme's idealised nude slave into a sickly and modern *Parisienne*.

Brouillet's work required a hysterical body that was visibly ailing because the legibility of the patient's illness was integral to the painting's narrative and to the identity of the professional men depicted. Yet, his desire to be noticed at the Salon demanded that he show hysteria as sensational and sensuous. The body could not be too sick or too naked (it could not assault bourgeois taste). Therefore, Brouillet did not portray the woman fully undressed, as Charcot often examined patients, nor did he create a nude or idealised Odalisque. Rather, his image of a hysterical woman fluctuates between the real and the ideal, the rational and the spectacular. This fluctuation in realist representations of women in medical contexts is also present in Gervex's painting, in which the artist faced the problem of how to render a sick female body realistically while simultaneously making it pleasurable and suitable for Salon audiences.

For contemporary critics, the dishevelled attire of the hysteric in *Une leçon clinique* symbolised a female body out of control, falling outside the rigid structures of proper femininity, while the male bodies signified knowledge and health. Unlike the bourgeoisie portrayed in the scientific arena as mothers who turn to science as a means to raise healthy families in Gsell's 1887 painting of Pasteur, the woman in Brouillet's canvas is a hysteric in need of saving. Identified by Salon critics as a hysteric, a neurotic, and a cataleptic, this woman was simultaneously described as being hypnotised, in nervous contractions and as going through a phase of the *grande attaque hystérique*. Critics' descriptions of Wittman's body demonstrate the art world's fluency with the medical language of hysteria and show how they read the disease from the body's exterior. They saw hysteria and hypnosis in the woman's state of undress, the arch of her back, the flexing of her wrists, and the turn of her ankle – poses that were familiar to them because of their representation in nineteenth-century literature, photography, and popular medical journals as well as in Charcot and Richer's *Les Démoniaques dans l'art*. In *Une leçon clinique*, Brouillet fixed multiple characteristics of hysteria onto one body. Rather than show it in a single pose or gesture, or as belonging to various bodies – male or female, rich or poor – Brouillet located the illness on the body of one young woman.

Blanche Wittman occupies a central position in Charcot's studies: she was the patient most discussed and photographed in the 1879 volume of the *Iconographie photographique*. In this book, patients are photographed in various stages of

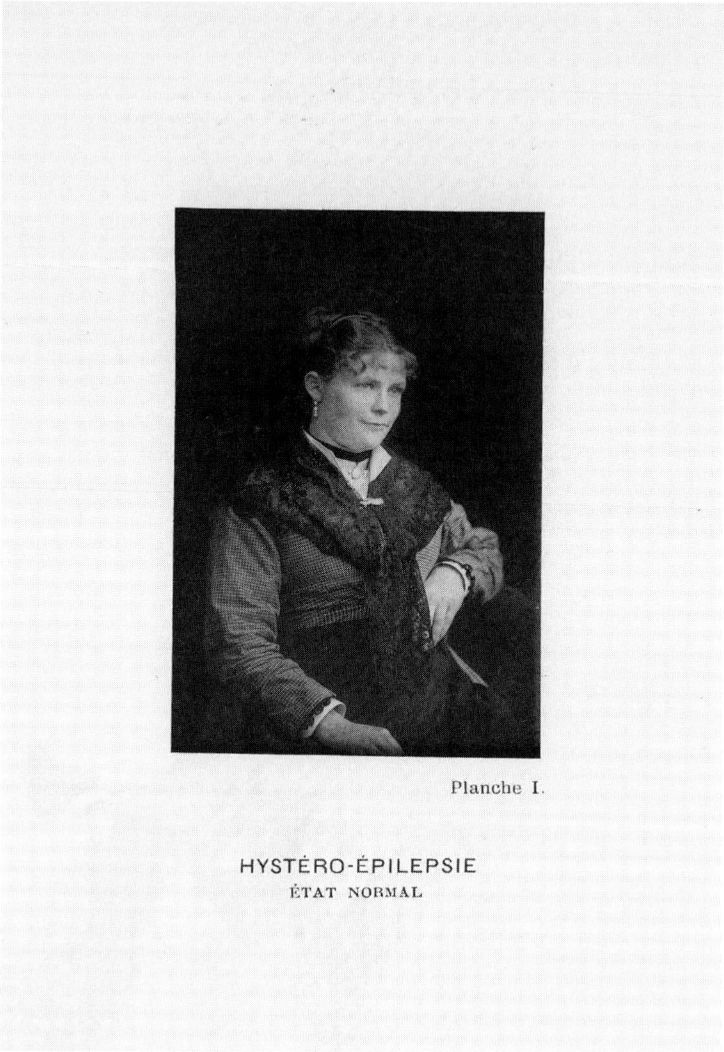

56 Paul Régnard, 'Hystéro-Épilepsie: Attaques', from Bourneville and Régnard, *Iconographie Photographique de la Salpêtrière* (1879), planche I, photolithograph.

attacks while the accompanying text describes their symptoms and treatments. In its Figures 1–10 and 33–35, Wittman was photographed in multiple hysterical states and undergoing various experiments. She was shown in an *état normal*, conservatively dressed and manicured, as well as dishevelled, asleep, and in an

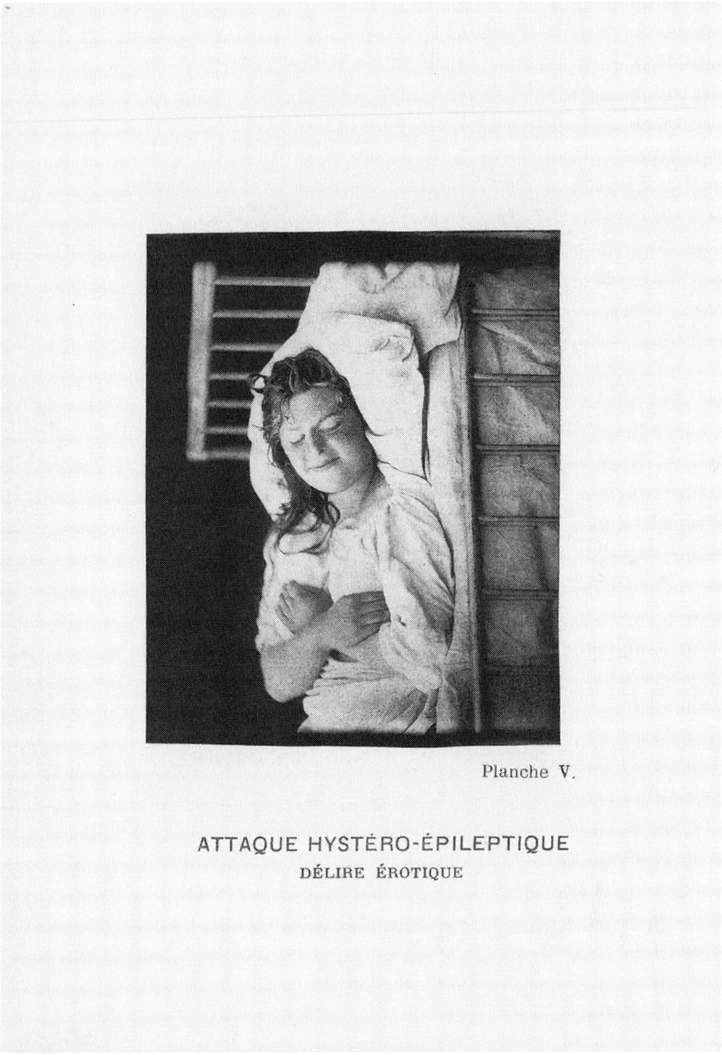

Paul Régnard, 'Attaque Hystéro-Épileptique', from Bourneville and Régnard, *Iconographie Photographique de la Salpêtrière* (1879), planche V, photolithograph. 57

arc en cercle (Figures 56 and 57). Looking through the photographs of Wittman, visual similarities between her and Brouillet's hysteric become apparent.

The visual ties between Brouillet's painting and these medical photographs endorsed the documentary status of *Une leçon clinique*. Yet the face of Brouillet's hysteric is more beautiful than the photographed Wittman, and her body much thinner. These adjustments demonstrate how Brouillet added to and omitted from visible reality to produce an image of hysteria that satisfied conventions of beauty and Salon painting, yet could nonetheless be categorised as a truthful recording of modern medical life. Brouillet imbued his hysterical woman with the sense of the real through its juxtaposition with his rendition of Richer's drawing on the back wall. Unlike Brouillet's copy of Richer's drawing, which is simple and monochromatic, his Wittman is meticulously detailed, modelled, and coloured. Although the inclusion of Richer's drawing – and Richer himself – showcases the artist's awareness of cutting-edge medicine, it also suggests that his painting has an equal – or perhaps even greater – claim to reality than Richer's simple sketch.

When examining Brouillet's depiction of the hysteric in comparison to that of the men, it is evident that the artist spent more time and effort painting Wittman: she has a smoothly painted surface and detailed clothing, light and shadow play across her bare chest, and her expressive features are meticulously observed. In contrast, the male figures look one-dimensional and stiff, and the paint that creates their skin is rough and flat. Despite the recognisable men, others become mere types: their beards, suits, and roughly painted features erasing all signs of individuality. Perhaps men, as creators and cataloguers of images and illnesses, did not require the realistic rendering that sick female bodies demanded, or perhaps Brouillet did not want to spend his time 'touching them up'. Ollendorf's review references the criticism that Brouillet received for his representation of the audience: 'these are not living, clothed individuals that we see before us; this is clothing enveloping forms that are unrelated to anatomy and instead closely akin to studio mannequins'.[98] Realism was considered an essential element of portraiture, yet it was in the likeness of the portraits that Brouillet failed. In contrast to his sketchy execution of healthy men, his portrayal of Wittman demonstrates the labour required to produce a lifelike image. His depiction of her body reveals an attention to detail that was not extended to the men.

Brouillet's failure to create convincing male portraits of the seated crowd was attributed by some critics to the belief that the painting was rushed. 'Monsieur Brouillet, no doubt pressed for time, seems not to have had the opportunity and leisure to study in depth the individual physiognomy of his models', wrote Mantz. 'Some are not convincing likenesses. Sometimes his paintbrush moved too hastily, and my sense is that some of the portraits – those that will be of future interest – should have been revisited and enhanced with some more realistic touches.'[99] Ollendorf and Merson agreed that Brouillet had rushed. The painting did not fulfil its intended realism. Despite the verisimilitude invoked by the painting's narrative and the detailed rendering of the hysteric's body and daylight, the sense of urgency produced by the hurried portraits of the audience belied the documentary impulse of realist rhetoric. How could it stand as a historical document for future viewers with all these faults?

The desire for painting to be quick, contemporary, and realistic exposes the conflicts between the demands of realism in paint and the relative immediacy provided by photography. Unlike the comparatively quick click of the camera, painterly realism was time-consuming and slowed down by the human hand. The smooth surface of a photograph appeared to erase all signs of human interaction, thus emphasising its understanding as a mechanically objective recording. Brouillet's realism in paint required hours of touching to create a similar sense of detachment. He could never entirely erase his touch. The strokes of his brush remain obvious signs of his bodily involvement and subjectivity. Although these signs contributed to the image's identification as a sincere document because they indicated his status as witness, they also exhibited an overt subjectivity that was not as blatant in photography. As Mantz's criticism attests, the painting's unreliability as a historical document for the future was caused by Brouillet's failure to provide the painting with '*accents plus vrais*'.[100]

Brouillet turned to photography to imbue his painting with a sense of the real. Ollendorf suggested that 'The background and the entire left part [of the painting] are filled with such carefully grouped figures that one would think that the artist, having spent a day observing the illustrious practitioner, had left the hospital taking with him an invaluable instantaneous photograph, no doubt courtesy of the capable director of the art department at the Salpêtrière',[101] and Fernand Levillain confirmed in 1891 that, 'The artist copied, without modification, the print made by Monsieur Londe, the capable head of the photography department at the Salpêtrière'.[102] Levillain substantiated this claim by reproducing Londe's photograph with his article. Although Brouillet's use of photographs was praised, his painting's similarity to photography was also considered one of its downfalls. 'For me, *Une leçon clinique à la Salpêtrière* is spoiled by its resemblance to a large painted photograph', Charles Ponsonhaille wrote in *L'Artiste*. '[T]he composition is mediocre, and many of the figures seem to be glued to each other.'[103] The critics' contradictory attitudes towards photography reflect broader nineteenth-century debates surrounding its status. Similar comments were made about Bonnat's portrait of Pasteur in 1886. Although the intricate details, smooth surface, and exactness of photography was certainly commendable, not all of photography's characteristics were considered desirable in paint.

Photography at the Salpêtrière: scientific pictures and procedures

Tissandier dedicated a whole chapter of his book *La Photographie* (1882) to the relationship between art and photography, outlining the different roles of artists and photographers as well as offering ways in which artists could use photography to their own benefit. Significantly, Tissandier believed that a partnership between painter and physician would raise the status of photography to art: 'There is no denying that the photographic apparatus, manipulated by an operator who has both the physician's deftness and the painter's taste, gives birth to works stamped with the seal of art'.[104] Photography was a meeting place for art and medicine, as medical and art students alike used photographs to improve their skills and their knowledge of the human body.

In 1882, Charcot appointed Albert Londe to head the Salpêtrière photography department. This highlighted the essential role of photography in the study of hysteria and located the hospital as a site of photographic advances, particularly since Londe was known for developing new photographic techniques and apparatuses.[105] It also portrayed Charcot as an innovative leader who promoted technological advances. Londe was not a doctor but a leader in the newly formed society of amateur photographers and an organiser of the 1889 Congrès International de la Photographie held in Paris. Londe's invention of the *appareil à douze objectifs* enhanced both medical and artistic investigations of the body, particularly when Richer, who took over from Mathias Duval as chair of anatomy at the École des Beaux-Arts, introduced these new photographic processes and results to the art school.[106]

Historians of photography have noted how photography claimed to offer a universal language of truth that appealed to nineteenth-century positivists.[107] The conscious desire for it to be scientific persisted well into the 1880s and beyond, as was expressed by M. Janssen in his opening remarks at the 1889 international congress when he claimed that the medium 'still awaits its scientific foundation. Thus we must endeavour to give it, and make it accept, its rank among the sciences'.[108] The integration of photography into the Parisian hospital system demonstrates the continued legitimacy medical practitioners gave to the medium and its role in the scientific arena. Burais's 1896 doctoral thesis on the medical applications of photography outlines its 'perfection' over other media, as its ability to produce exacting images allowed for diagnoses based on viewing a photograph rather than the patient:

> Photography allows for the simplification of things. In experienced hands, photographic reproduction achieves such perfection that in many cases, diagnosis can be made just by seeing the image, and a few lines accompanying the photograph are sufficient, where previously four tedious pages of text would have given but an approximate idea of what the author was trying to describe.[109]

The examination of medical photographs, like moulages, did not depend on the availability of patients nor was it confined by social restrictions on viewing naked bodies. Burais stressed the relationship between the visual and textual in medical diagnosis. Although a photograph could speed up diagnosis because its visual details were considered more comprehensible on quick viewing than pages of detailed writing that required concentrated reading, medical images were tied to explanatory texts and labels. Photographs were regularly used to illustrate, and their literalness was praised as necessary for medical use, unlike Salon paintings where literal realism was criticised by French critics as a negative trait typical of nineteenth-century English art.[110] Text filled in the details that photography lacked to ensure that the reader/viewer linked the signs and symptoms of diseases with the appropriate body. Similarly, photography stood in when textual analysis was not enough, or when it was too time-consuming.

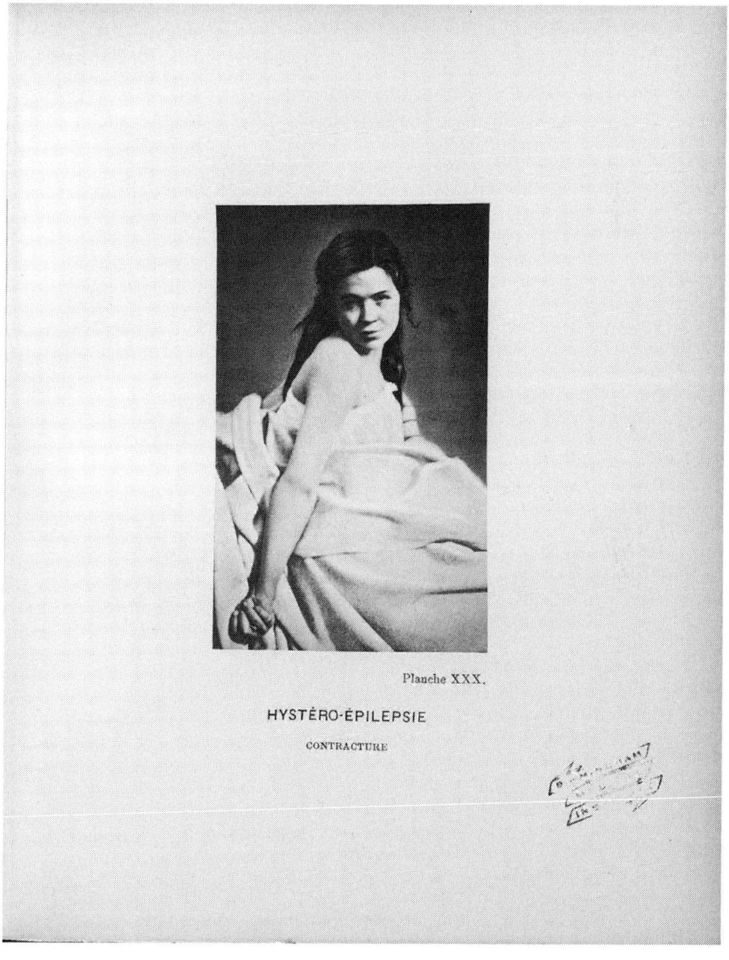

Paul Régnard, 'Hystéro-Épilepsie', from Bourneville and Régnard, *Iconographie Photographique de la Salpêtrière* (1878), planche XXX, photolithograph, Paris. 58

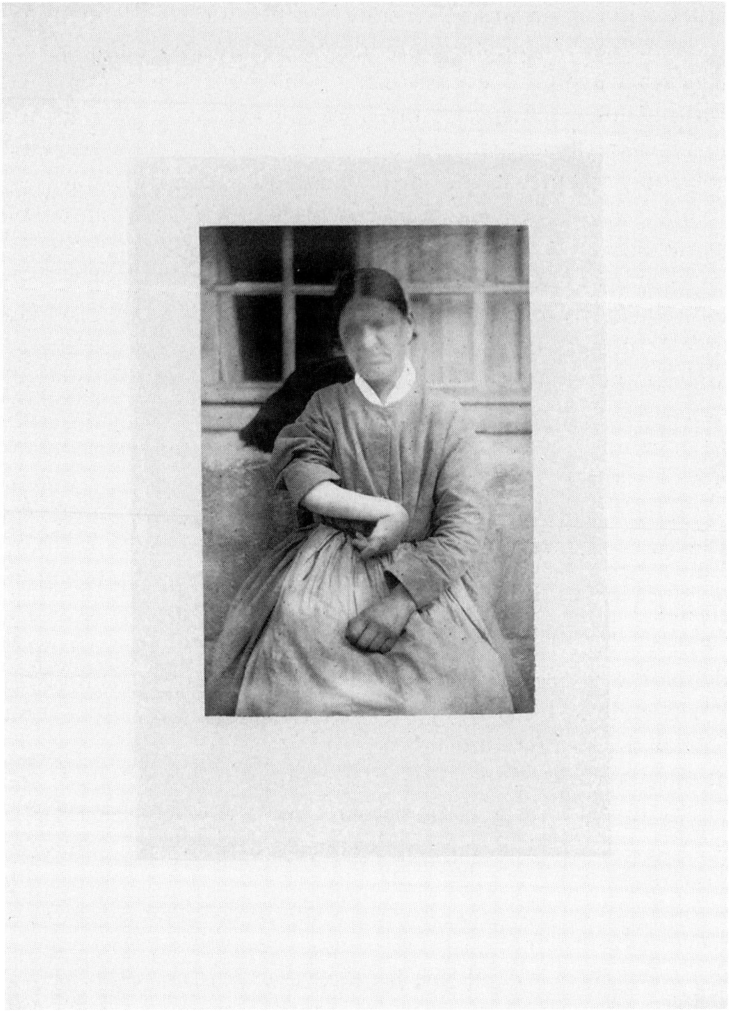

59 Paul Régnard, 'Atrophie cérébrale: Hémiplégie – épilepsie', from Bourneville and Régnard, *Iconographie Photographique de la Salpêtrière* (1875), photograph.

The competing claims of different realist methods and media, as well as their varying abilities to represent the real, are evident in the *Iconographie photographique* series, where photographs, texts, drawings, etchings, and charts work together to produce Charcot's conception of hysteria. The photographs in this series hold a prominent place in twentieth-century discussions of hysteria, particularly those of Augustine in volume 2 (Figure 58). As many twentieth-century scholars, including Charles Bernheimer, Didi-Huberman, and Janet Beizer argue, the photographs of Augustine are highly sexed, contrived images that exhibit a scantily clad female body posed for visual pleasure. Augustine's come-hither stare and cascading hair in the photographs transform her from ailing patient into seductress. Yet, these photographs should not be unquestionably accepted as the norm for studies on the iconography of hysteria. Although they are the most easily accessible to scholars (they are by far the most reproduced images), these photographs must be studied in relation to the plethora of images and objects that were created, commissioned, and displayed at the Salpêtrière and in its publications. Since they are all products of a historical moment, an institution, and a particular series, they must be read in relation to one another and to their accompanying texts. Together the works constructed hysteria as Charcot and his followers wished it to be understood. They produced a taxonomy of the disease that secured and promoted Charcot's reputation as the leading specialist. The variety of women portrayed in Salpêtrière iconography contributed to the scientific character of the photographic project at the hospital and, consequently, to Charcot's scientific persona. The photographs captured different forms of hysteria that were classified by specific symptoms, to aid education. While many of the photographs in the *Iconographie photographique* show women in nightgowns and tangled in sheets, there are also photographs of fully clothed women with shrunken and twisted arms and hands, women with crippling physical deformities, an obese woman with her hair pulled tightly back, and a young girl with blank eyes (Figure 59).

Many studies of hysteria, particularly since 1980, have overlooked the photographs in the first edition of the first volume (1875). These photographs are primarily of older, unattractive women with physical deformities. A number of the photographs are blurred, and the faces are hard to read because the patients' movement 'ruined' the photographs. Some were taken outdoors for brighter light. When comparing these earlier photos with those of Augustine from volumes 2 and 3, it is evident that the staged and still poses of young hysterics in these later volumes avoided the technical photographic problems produced by a moving and agitated patient to create legible photographs that were better for learning.

The Salpêtrière books and photographs were an important part of Charcot's taxonomic project; they enriched medical knowledge and spread Charcot's beliefs internationally. Behind the façade of scientific objectivity, however, Charcot's works demonstrate an obsession with hysterical female bodies as doctors meticulously observed and unrelentlessly experimented on patients, often focusing on the *grande hystérie* and the progression of the attack towards the orgasmic *arc en cercle*. Although photography presented the Salpêtrière project as documentary, the iconographic concentration on the *grande hystérie* contradicts the textual accounts that present a different picture of reality at the hospital. The textual records explain that few patients qualified as *grandes hystériques* and only a few bodies hit the hysterical climax. The numerous photographs and drawings of this state contradict the texts, which suggests that the focus on eroticised images of hysteria fulfilled the personal desires of medical men who conceived of the pathological state. These pictures exceeded the requirements of professional duty and medical representation. The salaciousness of the female patients' poses was noted by Brouillet, who used it to create Wittman's seductively arched body.

Texts were also full of sexual content; they could describe what was considered obscene in photography: defecating, urinating, and masturbating. Although photography could capture naked and unconscious female bodies in orgasmic poses under the guise of scientific respectability, there were limits; when removed from their context, medical photographs could slip into the world of pornography. Such an example shows the ways in which realism, whether textual or visual, was dependent on social expectations and allowances as some forms had more leeway than others.

The books emerging from the Salpêtrière and those produced by the hospital's doctors are filled with multiple realistic representations of hysteria. Explanatory texts, accounts of experimental procedures, photographs, prints, charts, and drawings construct hysteria as a disease that required documentation through all available means. The books contain accounts of what hysterical bodies did, how they were diagnosed as hysterical, how they were tamed and cured, and how they reacted to medical experimentation. They are historical records that demonstrate how the hysterical body was displayed, photographed, drawn, cast, electrified, drugged, and hypnotised. The process of creating realistic representations of hysteria was as important as the final products. By documenting these procedures, medical professionals framed the production of visual records and their relentless experimentations on patients as sensible pursuits. Significantly, Brouillet depicted and symbolised a variety of these processes in his work in order to emphasis their import to the production of medical knowledge, and, notably, their centrality to Charcot's identity.

The medical subject of the Salpêtrière photographs of women, their production within the hospital milieu, and their publication in medical books appeared to rid these images of the implicit sexual nature of photographs of semi-naked young women. There is no doubt that many nineteenth-century physicians celebrated what they believed to be 'photography's inherent guarantees of truthfulness', as Bourneville described it in his preface to the 1878 volume of *Iconographie photographique*.[111] Yet, as Erin O'Connor and others have argued, clinical photographs cannot simply be understood as 'misguided attempts at an obviously impossible objectivity'.[112] Rather, they must be considered in relation to other photographic forms because their conceptual foundation is linked to the early clinical uses of the camera. Medical photography utilised artistic conventions. The aesthetic and diagnostic were closely aligned. Medical photography's claim to record reality accurately was relatively unharmed by its lack of focus, grainy texture, and black-and-white surface, while abstraction in paint appeared to reinforce artistic subjectivity and the distance between image and reality.

The photographs of Wittman, for example, blur the boundaries of traditional portraiture and medical photography: they are simultaneously portraits of a specimen, a person, and a disease.[113] In the first image in the series of photographs of Wittman in *Iconographie photographique* (1879), she is shown in a three-quarter pose with her seated body turned slightly away from the camera (Figure 56). She is fully clothed, wearing a chequered-print shirt neatly tucked into her dark skirt, and a knitted shawl is wrapped primly around her shoulders and secured with a pin. Her blonde hair is meticulously arranged, as evidenced by her straight centre parting, the evenly manicured curly fringe on her forehead, and the orderly sections of hair twisted and fastened on her head. Shown with demure dangling earrings and a closed-mouth smile, this photograph portrays Wittman as a composed working-class woman. The photograph's composition, the sitter's conventional pose, and the flattering frontal light source that softens Wittman's facial features classifies the photograph as a portrait; it is visually similar to the thousands of portraits taken in the newly affordable photographic studios in Paris. Yet, as is indicated by the text below the photograph, this picture depicts Wittman in an '*état normal*'. The text transforms the portrait into a medical example for the taxonomy of hysteria. The photograph's function was to show Wittman before the onslaught of a hysterical attack and was to serve as the healthy template from which all other representations of her sick body were to be compared. The following photographs show Wittman in, amongst other poses, an 'erotic frenzy', 'muscular hyperexcitability', and a 'state of arousal' (Figure 57). Her poses in the photographs mimic those drawn by Richer of Charcot's conception of the different stages of a hysterical attack and reiterate the gestures from the religious iconography analysed by Richer and Charcot.

The numerous photos of Wittman attest to her popularity as a medical case study and the associated texts demonstrate an obsession with the documentation and control of her body. As if the photographic records were not detailed enough, the text produces an account of her every inch and action:

> W … is tall (1m, 64) … she is blonde with a lymphatic complexion. Her skin is white. Her breasts are quite voluminous … She is of barely average intelligence. Her memory is fairly good … She is glassy eyed: the sight and presence of men produces in her a particular sort of excitement.[114]

Wittman's attacks were defined, timed, and monitored, her words and personal history recorded, her taste, sight, vaginal secretions, and vomit studied. Her treatments were documented: Wittman was given ether, chloroform, ovarian compressions, and nitrite amyl, and was hypnotised, electrocuted, and written upon with needles. Such experiments were justified not only by their use in the medical realm, but also by the suggestion that Wittman was excited by medical male attention.

In fact, the production of portraits at the Salpêtrière became a joke played on sick women by medical men. The promise of having one's picture taken was used to lure hysterical women into the photographic studio. As Londe explained, '[t]he hysterics were led before the camera under the pretext of having their portrait taken. At that moment, a gong was struck, and they all fell into cataleptic seizures'.[115] Unlike portraiture, a genre that privileged status and was used to create flattering images, these photographs degraded patients because they put their diseases on display.

Frenzied realisms: competing claims to truth

Paintings, drawings, prints, and photographs were used interchangeably at the Salpêtrière. *Une leçon clinique*, Charcot's medical museum, and the *Iconographie photographique* series all demonstrate that multiple media and stylistic techniques were used in tandem to visualise hysteria. Photographs were drawn on, etchings were made after photographs, and photographs after paintings. Didi-Huberman's analysis of Richer's drawing of a hysteric in the tetanic phase in *Études cliniques* of 1881 reveals how it was based on an earlier photograph taken by Regnard for the *Iconographie photographique* of 1878. In Richer's drawing, the hysterical body is more expressive, the white sheets covering the patient in the photograph are removed to reveal naked and twisted legs, the foam dripping from her mouth is more pronounced, and the restraining belt is removed.[116] Such alterations allowed Richer to make hysteria more visible, animated, and obvious. Richer's turn away from photography, in this instance, reveals how it was not always able to provide enough, or the right, details. Despite its precise character, photography failed to draw out the symptoms of hysteria that Richer wished to expose nor could it construct the reality he wished to show.

There was an established link between photography and drawing in these books. Bourneville and Regnard claimed that photographs (referred to in the books as *planches*) and drawings (*figures*) were both needed to provide exact recordings.[117] Although some realistic media were considered better than others for certain tasks, drawing and photography could work together, each performing a certain role. Nevertheless, there are drawings in these books that, at first glance, seem to undermine the realism demanded by medical professionals, such as the printmaker Jean-François Badoureau's image of a woman in an attack, reproduced in both the 1877 *Iconographie photographique* and the first volume of Charcot's *Œuvres complètes* (Figure 60). This work is cartoon-like and drawn out of proportion: the woman has exaggerated and monstrous facial features. Although such rough sketches seem to be the antithesis of photographic records, their context in a medical book and their relationship to other realistic images secured their position as relevant for medical study. While it may seem ridiculous to assume that these drawings were considered trustworthy, the evidence of the doctor/artist's hand in these works attested to his first-hand experience of hysteria and his role in its diagnosis and documentation; subjectivity – when belonging to a member of the medical or artistic elite – was an essential part of producing realist images. These drawings contributed to the accuracy of hysteria's representation, filling in the details that photography was unable to provide. The exaggerated and fluid character of the drawings mimicked the overstated symptoms of hysteria, producing images that portrayed the look of hysteria in a way that photography could not. Movement in photography created blurred images. Furthermore, hysterical poses, like the infrequent *arc en cercle,* were hard to catch photographically, and thus needed to be staged or reproduced by hand from memory or experience.

Hysterical hands were also rendered through various modes and media as the state of the hand came to signify the whole hysterical body. Brouillet used this potent symbol of hysteria in *Une leçon clinique* by showing Wittman with a turned wrist and clamped fist. The clenched hand was a symbol of illness that allowed for an attractive body – there was no drooling, no open eyelids revealing upturned eyeballs, and no tongue hanging out. The numerous representations of hysterical hands are another example of the medical fixation on hysteria.[118] The first half of the photographs and drawings in the 1878 volume of *Iconographie photographique* are of women with their hands in fists, their arms and wrists deformed and bent. Richer's drawings and engravings of hysterical hands provide further evidence of this focus. Nineteenth-century criminology also studied hands; fingerprints were taken so that identities could be catalogued and hands of different workers were compared to ostensibly determine their intellectual abilities (Londe reproduced his photograph of workers' hands in *Photographie médicale* in 1893). For Pierre Janet, the paralysed hysterical hand was a symbol of ignorance.[119] In contrast to the skilled hands

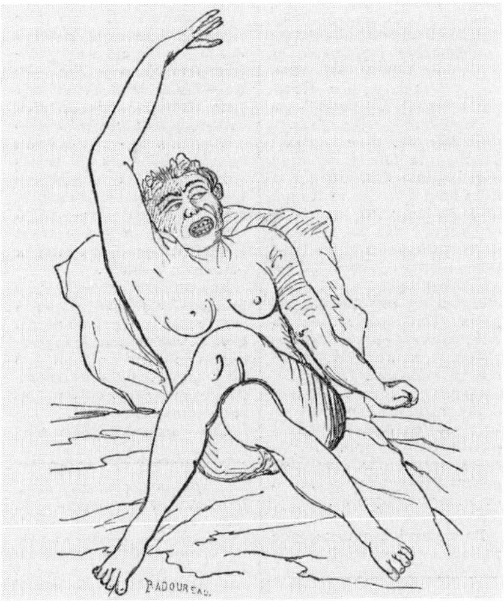

60 Badoureau, 'Hystéro-Épilepsie', from Bourneville and Régnard, *Iconographie Photographique de la Salpêtrière* (1877), figure 1, drawing.

of physicians, some hysterical hands were unable to touch, manipulate, or feel. The hysteric was denied touch while doctors' haptic explorations were essential to medical study.

Didi-Huberman argues that the immobile state of the hysterical 'dead hand' not only stood in as the ultimate gesticulation of the hysterical body, but also provided the material for waxes, photographs, and drawings. Tetanism was a 'godsend' for the doctors, he claimed, because it literally froze the body part, allowing it to be photographed without blurred results, examined easily, and set into plaster without difficulty.[120] Like photography, casting was able to produce an indexical mould of the body, making the resulting object seem like an impartial recording. Like photography, casting was a process that could portray commonalities and rarities. The Salpêtrière casts, like the photographs and wax models at Hôpital Saint-Louis, built a visible taxonomy to be studied by doctors and students. Furthermore, they 'proved' the existence of hysteria as a disease and strengthened Charcot's claims. Like the casts made from the hands of famous artists and writers, such as those of Auguste Rodin, Adolph Menzel, and the entwined hands of Elizabeth and Robert Browning, the cast hands produced at the Salpêtrière are portrait-like.[121] Yet, unlike the narratives invoked by the cast hands of lovers and artists, where professional identities and personal intimacies are on display, the cast hands produced at the Salpêtrière are portraits of illness, deformity, and disease.

Plaster and wax casts of hysterical bodies and body parts were shown in Charcot's medical museum. Jules Claretie described the space in his novel *Les Amours d'un interne* as

> a bizarre workshop, evocative of the amphitheatre and the medical museum, where human remains lie alongside the heads of criminals, cast after they died on the gallows. A singular ground floor where copies of the Venus de Milo and Michelangelo's slaves provide consoling antitheses to the atrocious deformities that the caster preserved or modelled for the vitrines of the hospital.[122]

A photograph of the museum was published in the popular press, showing the variety of objects that were commissioned by Charcot and on display at the hospital. Although the objects were exhibited in a medical setting, it was also a site of entertainment and fear, as Claretie's statement attests. Claretie's novel, Fernand Levillain's 1891 article 'Charcot et l'école de la Salpêtrière' in *Revue encyclopédique* and Maurice Guillemot's 1887 commentary about the museum in *Paris illustré*, describe how medical *moulages* and casts were shown alongside real skeletons, artistic models, and portrait busts. The museum was a venue for the creation and exhibition of pathological bodies, as representations of hysterical bodies were confirmed as diseased and deformed not only by their display in a medical museum, but also by their difference to such faultless bodies as the Venus de Milo. The idealised figures created within the world of art acted as foils against which medical pathologies could be made obvious. Although the majority of casts on display were of fragmented forms, a full wax model of a naked woman described as suffering from ataxia was also on show (Figure 61). As Maurice Guillemot wrote in 1887:

> A vitrine that fully occupies the centre of the room holds our attention. Inside, laid out on its back, is a full body cast of a hysteric who died at the Salpêtrière. She is hideous in her realism and misery, with her scrawniness, her crooked legs, her deformed shoulders, her hollowed chest, her torso furrowed at the sides, the ribs piercing the skin.[123]

For Guillemot, realism was associated with deformity, monstrosity, illness, and death. Unlike the idealised bodies of marble and plaster Venuses that lured viewers in by their beauty, this wax woman enticed them by her disfigured hips, bony skeleton, and sagging skin.

The desire to portray this hysterical body realistically is evident through the hyper-realism of the wax figure – a realism that provided so many details that it was considered hideous – and by its photographic imaging (Figure 62). In the photograph, the woman is alive, her face is in a crooked grin, her hands are at her side, and a bonnet is on her head. In contrast, the wax model shows a sleeping or dead body, eyes closed and head turned to the side. Although the wax body's nakedness, uncovered hair, and deformed body suggest that this is an unaltered representation, the woman's wax hand is placed over her genitals, suggesting that this inanimate body retains the modesty of a young Venus, who simultaneously hides and draws attention to her sex by the placement of her hand. The artistic conventions used here create a bizarre vision of deformity in an idealised yet deathly pose.

In 1889, Brouillet's painting was reproduced next to a photograph of the Salpêtrière museum in *Revue encyclopédique* (Figure 47). This juxtaposition linked Brouillet's canvas and the Salpêtrière museum as sites for the display of realistic representations of hysteria. A comparison of these two images invites us to draw a connection between the young hysteric depicted by Brouillet and the emaciated wax woman in the centre of the photograph: the old patient portrayed in wax foreshadows the eventual state of women at the Salpêtrière. Fixed into wax, this corpse-like sculpture brings to mind the spectacle of dead bodies on display at the Paris Morgue and recalls the importance of autopsies in the confirmation and discovery of diseases.[124] Wax, like photography, could contain and objectify the body, making it still for study and documentation. However, such renderings could never replace the human body, which was filled with organs, blood, neurological matter, and bones. They could not be cut open to reveal the source of illness. As indexical media that provided mimetic recordings of the body's exterior, wax and photography prioritised surface.

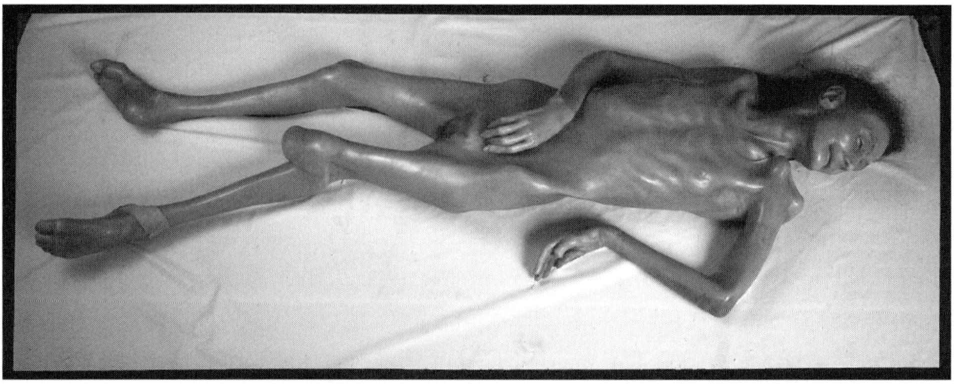

61 Wax model of 'Ataxic Venus', from the Salpêtrière, Archives de l'Assistance Publique.

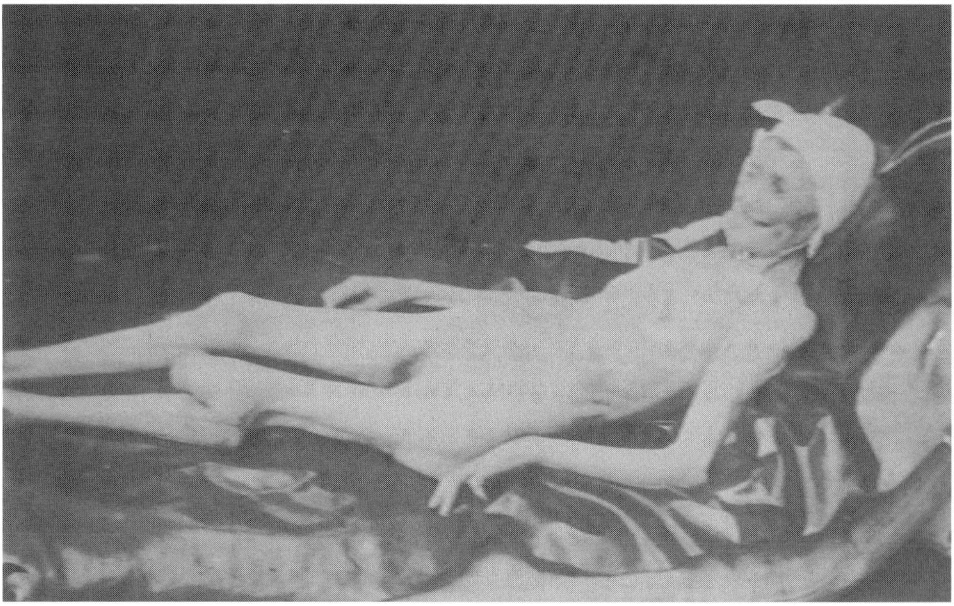

62 Photograph of 'Ataxic Venus', from Charcot's clinical dossiers, Archives de l'Assistance Publique.

Despite their claims to the real, they could never fully replace the real body because they did not have 'insides'.

The casts and photographs at the Salpêtrière ultimately invoked the absence of living bodies by their presence. Like Pasteur's death mask and commemorative photographic portraits, and Péan's wax models, they had historical links to death. Only through the symbolic death of the subject by realistic rendering could the hysterical body be real enough to prove the existence of hysteria. Similarly, only through actual death could hysteria potentially be confirmed, as probing the body to find the organic cause of the disease would have ultimately killed the patient. The 'reality' of hysteria was 'proven' by death and realist representation: both were required in order to confirm a hysterical diagnosis.

In the bedroom: touching the hysterical body

Lascivious tales of hysteria fascinated the public; Brouillet's dishevelled Wittman was certainly popular, as was Claretie's *Les Amours d'un interne.* Hysterical women's supposed sexual availability was emphasised by their frequent portrayal next to young doctors. Medical texts emerging from the Salpêtrière claimed that hysterical women seduced medical men with their charisma and physical attributes. Even though Charcot clearly stated that hysteria did not produce overtly sexual women ('[W]e protest against the opinion universally adopted by the public that all hysterical women have a tendency to hypersexuality, almost bearing on nymphomania'), the eroticism of hysterics remained of great popular and medical interest.[125] In his overview of *Une leçon clinique*, Javel wrote: 'We seem to see her tremble and quiver, this unfortunate young woman whose half-closed eyes have, ironically, retained something of a smile'.[126] Although Wittman is posed under the focused gaze of Charcot's audience, trapped on the Salpêtrière stage, Javel saw a smile, perhaps a mischievous grin, in her semi-closed eyes. Depictions of hysterical women with slight smiles and suggestive glances (exemplified by the photographs of Augustine and sleeping women in the *Iconographie photographique* series), staged hysterical female sexuality as pathological yet seductive. The grins presented medical procedures at the hospital as pleasurable acts since the women in the photographs stare teasingly out at the viewer, showing no signs of pain.

Brouillet and Gervex depicted semi-clothed unconscious women to lure Salon viewers to their canvases. Both paintings contain a sub-narrative of a young doctor's intimate contact with a bare-chested female patient. In Gervex's portrait, one of Dr Zacharian's hands lingers near the patient's pink nipple while his other hand, holding a chloroformed cloth, waits to touch her mouth. In Brouillet's work, Dr Babinsky supports the hysteric's body, his hand beneath her breast, fingers pressed against the boning of her loosened corset while his eyes focus on her exposed bust. Both works highlight a moment of touch that threatens professional conduct, yet is rationalised by the medical context and the painting's realist effects. Brouillet justified medical touch and exhibited his medical knowledge by showing Babinsky's hand under the hysteric's left breast; Charcot claimed that three main hysterogenic points were on the back, leg, and under the left breast.[127] Brouillet and Gervex hinted at the intimate connection between sexual desire and medical experimentation in their works as medical observation and touch are focused on stripped, inert women. The medical settings, the piercing eyes of the audiences and the suited professional men cannot hide the sexual narratives that lurk within the painted images. While the works' medical contexts prohibit the intimate physical contact between young doctor and patient to progress, its presence, and promise, remains.

In contrast to Brouillet's painting and the prints in the popular press, medical men were not usually photographed with their female patients at the Salpêtrière. Their role in the production of visual images was paramount even though Charcot claimed distance: 'Behold the truth. I've never said anything else; I'm not in the habit of advancing things that aren't experimentally demonstrable … I am nothing more than a photographer; I inscribe what I see.'[128] Paradoxically, physicians' desire to have camera-like mechanical objectivity was encouraged while patients' camera-like behaviour was a symptom of hysteria. A case study in *Nouvelle iconographie* from 1889 describes hysterics whose eyes winked like camera shutters and who saw only in black and white; they were diagnosed as 'photophobic' and their vision understood as impaired.[129]

Physicians and photographers prepared patients for photographic recording: clothing was removed to expose signs of disease and bodies were manhandled into pathological poses. In Poyet's engraving, *Photography at the Salpêtrière*, the photographer and patient are in close proximity (Figure 63). A handheld device allowed the photographer to simultaneously adjust the patient and take a photograph since he did not need to be behind or next to the camera in order to take a shot. The intimate contact between patient and photographer is exemplified in a photograph of Londe holding a hysterical body (Figure 64). He stands behind the patient while the camera's mechanical attachment hangs over the bedpost, thus demonstrating the connection between touching (posing) a patient to make a coherent photograph and the touch required to activate the camera. However, the physical relationship between the patient and photographer was problematic. The patient's body had to be legible as a pathological body in an identifiable hysterical pose and therefore often needed doctors and photographers to mould it into the desired position. Yet, the body's natural pathological contortions were required to show its disease. Londe described the problems encountered when posing a body and using supports:

> These apparatuses have the great disadvantage of placing the models in poses that are stiff and contrived. In Medicine, this subterfuge must be completely avoided, for in addition to variations in form, one often encounters postures that are specific to the individual patient, having been imprinted on him by the disease with which he is afflicted. These postures are extremely valuable from a diagnostic point of view, and they must be represented in a rigorous manner.[130]

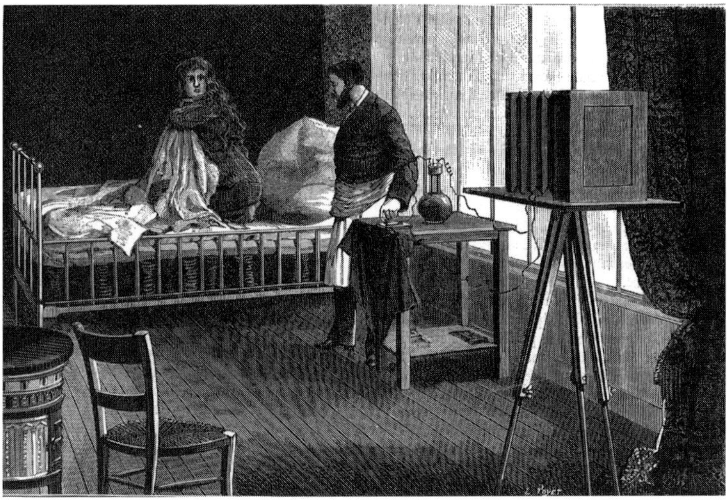

Poyet, 'Photography at the Salpêtrière', from *La Nature*, 1 September 1883 (no. 535, t. 2), pp. 215–218, engraving. 63

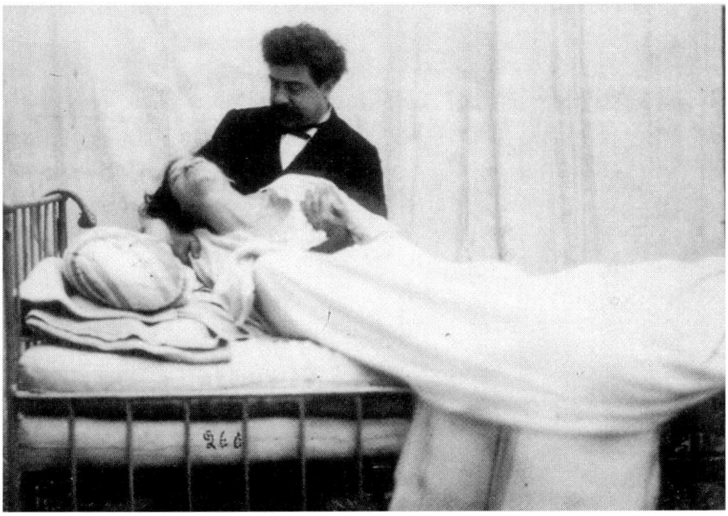

Albert Londe, 'Melle Mabillon, attaque hystérique' (1882), photograph from a Salpêtrière album. 64

Londe's job required balancing the production of accurate visual records for medical learning with the technological limitations of photography. His expert involvement was crucial. There are, however, no photographs of doctors or photographers in any of the *Iconographie photographique*. The posing of bodies is never illustrated – the patients' contorted forms and dramatic expressions appear detached from any manipulation or studio setting.

Photography at the Salpêtrière was considered a method of clinical and objective documentation even though the main prop in the photographic studio was a bed. Pushed against the wall and cornered by the steadfast gaze of a camera, the bed was a site of hysterical documentation. In the majority of photographs, particularly those published in the *Iconographie photographique* series, the bed's location in the photographic studio is not depicted (as it is in Poyet's print). For example, Regnard's photographs of Augustine and Blanche in a series of *attitudes passionnelles* reveal nothing more than the fact that the women are in a bed. Devoid of a medical setting or further visual contextualisation, these photographs provide an unrestricted access to a horizontal female body. In one plate from the 1878 *Iconographie photographique*, Augustine is wrapped in sheets, staring out at the viewer seductively (Figure 58).[131] Her 'come hither' pose, exemplified by her intense gaze and raised bare shoulder, recalls precedents from the mid-century, such as Félix Jacques Moulin's photographic series of a woman in bed, surrounded by draped sheets, suggestively looking out at an implied viewer (Figure 65). The rotation of Augustine's arm and her twisted wrist identify her as hysterical seductress. Removed from a medical setting and displayed within a 'bedroom', the female patients in Salpêtrière photography are similar to those in studio photographs, where reclining naked women are shown in stages of unconsciousness and undress for viewers' pleasure. Whereas

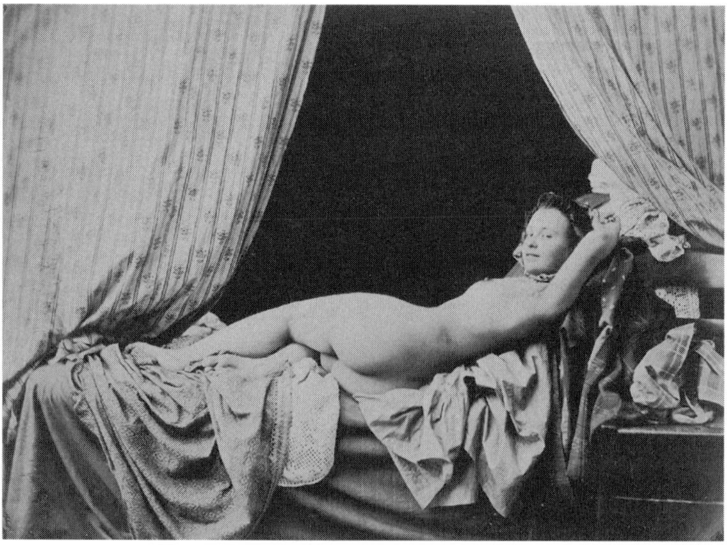

65 Felix-Jacques Moulin, *Female Nude* (1856), albumen silver print, 16.51 x 21.9cm.

pornographic recordings of the female body often promised an orgasmic outcome, Salpêtrière photography focused on the journey to the *arc en cercle.*

In contrast to the number of photographs of women in bed at the Salpêtrière, few exist of men. Photographs of naked male patients became more popular during the 1880s, when Charcot became interested in studying male hysteria. The increase in photographs of men may be attributed to Londe's interest in recording movement since male bodies, with their pronounced muscularity, produced better accounts of the human figure in motion. In 1885, Londe took a series of photographs of a naked male patient in various stages of a hysterical attack (Figure 66). The man is captured in a series of contortions with his arms tied to bedposts. These photographs differ from those of women: there are men standing around the patient's bed, while in the photographs of women, the patient is often alone or with nurses. Like similar photographs by Londe and his contemporaries, Étienne-Jules Marey and Eadweard Muybridge, these sequential photos of a male hysteric emphasise technological progress. Londe

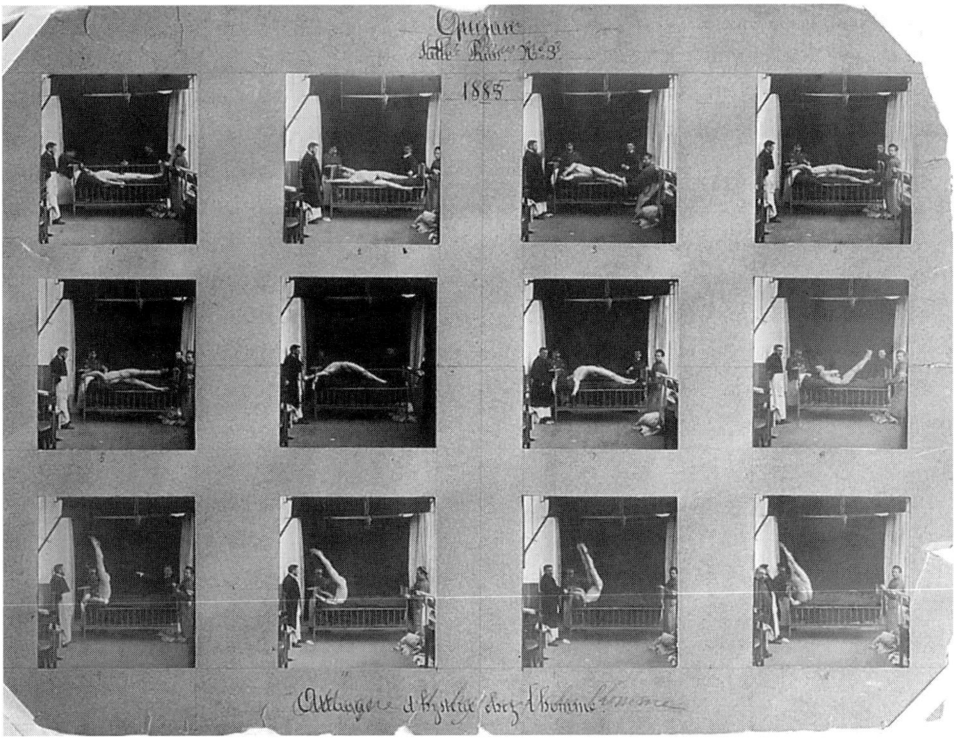

Albert Londe, 'Male Hysteric' (late nineteenth century), photograph from a Salpêtrière album. 66

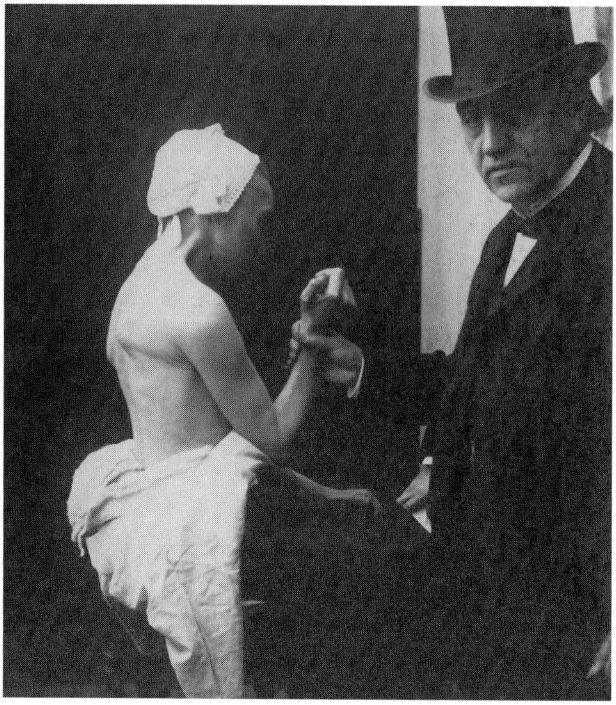

67 Anonymous, *Jean Martin Charcot with female patient suffering from locomotive ataxia* (c.1885), photograph.

achieved his desire to take photographs in quick succession in 1893, when he created a camera that could take twelve photographs at speedy intervals.[132]

Despite the absence of physicians in most Salpêtrière photographs, their presence is evident. Londe wrote, 'Depending on the case, the patient will be photographed from the front, from the back, in three-quarter and profile views; standing or seated. It is the doctor who will determine the positions in which the subject should be represented.'[133] The photographs implicated the physician by their very creation. The format and size of photographs catered to medical learning ('prints must be produced in a format suitable for study by the doctor').[134] The fingerprints of male professionals linger on the slick surface of Salpêtrière photographs, confirming physicians' roles in the visual fabrication of hysteria.

Two photographs exist of Charcot gripping the wrist of an old ataxic woman (Figure 67). These were discovered in the archives of Hôpital Saint-Louis in 1985 and were not reproduced in Charcot's publications. In the photographs, Charcot is wearing a formal suit and top hat. He is staring out at the viewer, his assertive stance enhanced by his compositional dominance in the photograph.

In contrast, the hysteric is shown from the side, wearing a white hospital bonnet, and the top of her dress is pulled down to her waist, exposing a naked upper body. Her bare skin reveals sharp shoulder bones and toned arms. Her face looks down. Could this patient be the woman who was photographed and later ended up dead and depicted in wax? The scribbled notes on the side of the photograph indicate that the woman was suffering from ataxia – a disorder known for the production of uncontrollable, paralysed, and confused bodies. The woman's ill state in the photograph is indicated by her undress and proximity to clothed medical men, as it is in *Une leçon clinique*. The two photographs show the ways in which ataxia, as embodied by the female hysteric, was defined and handled by Charcot. His grip attests to the disease's reality; he holds on to its host and prepares her for the photographer. The cuffed hand of a male professional – physician or photographer – that is shown touching the woman's knee, indicates that close physical contact with semi-clothed female patients was necessary to produce images of hysteria. This photograph shows a moment when the woman and her disease are pinned down and prepared for representation through the touching of male hands and the steady gaze of the camera.

Critics at the 1887 Salon saw Charcot's touch in *Une leçon clinique*. Javel wrote that the doctor 'underscores, with a very natural gesture of his right hand, the line of reasoning he is developing, while with his left hand he holds the arm of the subject, a young hysteric who is being propped up by an intern'.[135] Similarly, Hippolyte Devillers described Charcot as 'holding a hypnotised woman upright with one hand'.[136] Upon examination of the painting, it is evident that Charcot's left hand is not shown: his lower left arm disappears behind the bodice and full skirt of the hysterical woman. Unquestionably, it is the young doctor who holds the patient. Perhaps these two critics did not examine the painting closely enough or perhaps they saw Charcot's touch in all that concerned the hysterical body, particularly his role in the multiple realist representations and performances that are depicted in Brouillet's canvas.

'From the moment she is hypnotised she belongs to us':[137] hypnosis as realist performance

Charcot's role in producing visual representations of hysteria went beyond drawing, wax, and photography. The medical acts and visualising processes that he performed on his patients presented hysteria as a disease of performance and visualisation in which both doctor and patient had starring roles. The visuality of hysteria that Charcot insisted on turned the disease into a spectacle, and returned hysteria to what Elisabeth Bronfen calls 'a malady of or by representation'.[138] Charcot's contemporaries noted the drama of his experiments: Dr Henry Meige termed them 'theatrical performances'[139] and Platel criticised his 'full-blown scientific showmanship'.[140] Charcot was not the only medical man associated with performance. Descriptions of the oratory skills of doctors and scientists were regularly recorded, as performance was a key component of professional success. All innovations, discoveries, and new technologies had to be brought up before the Académie de Médecine and Académie de Sciences for approval. These debates and their delivery were analysed in the popular press, as well as in medical and scientific journals. Physicians, surgeons, and scientists were responsible for presenting their work and defending others. For example, Charcot assertively and publicly defended Pasteur's rabies vaccine. A performative culture culminated in triumphant events in Paris, such as Pasteur's jubilee, Bernard's funeral, hospital openings, Expositions Universelles' pavilions for science, and international conferences on medical innovations. Banners, speeches, and parades celebrating medicine brought new discoveries to the public, and fulfilled the republican desire to educate the masses and commemorate the nation.

As part of his participation in visualising the hysterical body, Charcot applied a modern method of performance – hypnosis – to his armoury of realistic forms of representation. Like hysteria, hypnosis implicated mimesis in the rendering of reality: the hysterical patient acted out the symptoms of hysteria as they were suggested to her by medical men. Hypnosis was Charcot's realist technique and the hysterical body – an actual living being – his most realistic medium. Hypnosis allowed him to 'freeze' the body into specific gestures that corresponded to his conception of the *grande attaque* and its set poses. Charcot and his colleagues used an assortment of lights, metals, large tuning forks, clocks, and drums to set hysterical women into semi-unconscious states. The multiple modes of making women unconscious are reproduced in the *Iconographie photographique* series and in the images that accompanied Regnard and Bourneville's article in *La Nature* (Figure 68). Like anaesthetics, these tools and procedures gave medical men control of consciousness.

In his lecture on metallotherapy and hypnosis, Charcot explained that when a body was made to assume a specific gesture, the face corresponded with an appropriate expression. The patient is, Charcot wrote:

> transformed into a kind of expressive statue, an immobile model representing the most varied expressions with striking truth, and which artists can most certainly, turn to the best account. The immobility of attitudes obtained in this way is highly favourable to photographic reproduction. With the assistance of Monsieur Londe, responsible for the photographic service of the Salpêtrière, we have obtained a series of photographs, the most interesting of which we have reproduced here, and which, we note, were taken during the earliest experiments attempted in this domain.[141]

Hypnosis, like photography, could make a body still for medical study. Cartaz described medical men's mastery over hypnotised bodies:

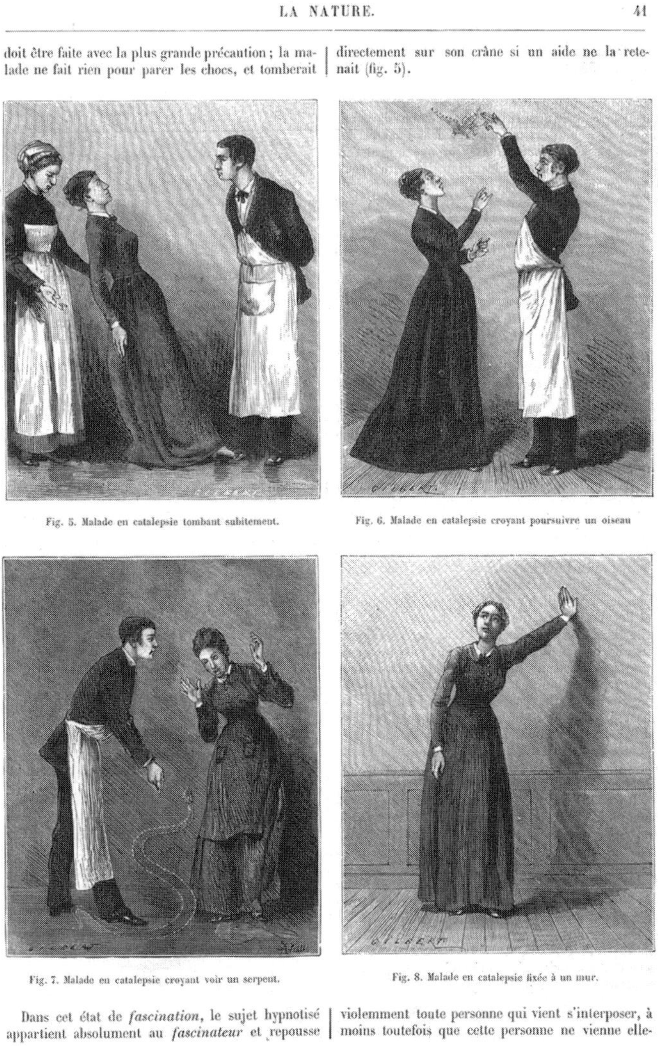

LA NATURE. 41

doit être faite avec la plus grande précaution ; la malade ne fait rien pour parer les chocs, et tomberait directement sur son crâne si un aide ne la retenait (fig. 5).

Fig. 5. Malade en catalepsie tombant subitement.

Fig. 6. Malade en catalepsie croyant poursuivre un oiseau

Fig. 7. Malade en catalepsie croyant voir un serpent.

Fig. 8. Malade en catalepsie fixée à un mur.

Dans cet état de *fascination*, le sujet hypnotisé appartient absolument au *fascinateur* et repousse violemment toute personne qui vient s'interposer, à moins toutefois que cette personne ne vienne elle-

'Les Phénomènes d'hypnose', from *La Nature*, 9: 2 (1881), p. 41, engravings. **68**

First, let us say that this lethargic state – somnambulism, if you will – ceases as suddenly as it appeared, and with the greatest of ease. It suffices, for example, to blow upon the subject's face. The lethargy vanishes, there is a look of slight confusion, and the patient emerges from her dream without the slightest memory of what has happened.[142]

Through hypnosis, Charcot created a body that was presumably detached from consciousness, a blank slate put to sleep and woken with a simple breath. It allowed him to display the workings of the unconscious – the relationship between mind and body – on a malleable 'expressive statue'.[143] Young artists were also interested in taking advantage of the expressive potential of hypnotised bodies. Gérôme's students hypnotised a female model after frequenting a lecture by Charcot; she almost died, so the story goes, and Gérôme's atelier was closed for a month (it is unknown if Brouillet was a part of this class).[144] For Charcot, hypnosis was the process through which hysteria was confirmed; it brought symptoms to the surface to 'prove' its organic roots. Photographing these hypnotised moments allowed him to further fix these symptoms on the body's exterior since recording these instants 'verified' their reality. Whereas the living patient would wake from hypnosis, the photographic image kept her locked in a cataleptic trance. Significantly, the still poses held by hypnotised women simplified their photographic representation. Their fits were slowed down for the camera so they did not cause blurring, making it easier to capture the hypnotised hysteric one move at a time.

Charcot's studies on hypnosis began in the late 1870s. In 1882, he presented his famous paper 'On the various nervous states determined by hypnotisation in hysterics' to the Académie des Sciences as part of his bid for membership. He argued that hypnosis was a pathological condition and a manifestation of hysteria. He believed that it could be a diagnostic tool and argued that only hysterics, or those with hysteric predispositions, could be hypnotised.[145] Charcot's works contributed to the public fascination with hypnosis during the 1880s. Max Dessoir's *Bibliographie des Modernen Hypnotismus* (1888) calculated that between 1840 and 1880 less than 30 publications on hypnosis were made per decade in relevant European publications while 1,030 publications appeared during the 1880s alone.[146] During the 1889 Exposition Universelle, both the International Congress on Physiological Psychology and the first International Congress on Experimental and Therapeutic Hypnotism met to discuss hypnosis. Furthermore, the first issue of *Revue de l'hypnotisme expérimental et thérapeutique* appeared in 1887, claiming that '[h]ypnotism is the order of the day. Its study has become scientific'.[147] Concurrently, hypnosis was being explored as a means to fortify the country. In 1891, Alfred Fouillé wrote that the whole of France could improve if everyone concentrated on the country's strength.[148]

Despite the medical use of hypnosis and Charcot's desire to safeguard it from abuse outside the medical realm, it remained a form of public entertainment that was often scrutinised. Drs Bourneville and Regnard linked hypnotism to charlatanism and fraud, claiming that anyone involved was deceiving or deceived.[149] Outside of the medical sphere, anyone could take part in hypnosis to momentarily free themselves from social constraints, or take pleasure in viewing the spectacle of hypnotised bodies performing outlandish poses and pranks. Depictions

28 LA NATURE.

LA SCIENCE AU THÉATRE

IMITATION DE PHÉNOMÈNES D'HYPNOTISME A LA SALLE ROBERT HOUDIN A PARIS

Tous les soirs on donne, à la mignonne salle du boulevard des Italiens, à Paris, une grande scène de magnétisme simulé. Ce divertissement, qui obtient un grand succès, a été composé par M. Méliès, directeur de l'établissement fondé il y a bien des années par le célèbre prestidigitateur dont il porte le nom encore populaire. Ce spectacle n'est pas sans porter son enseignement, car il montre combien facilement peuvent être simulés les phénomènes les plus surprenants de l'état pathologique.

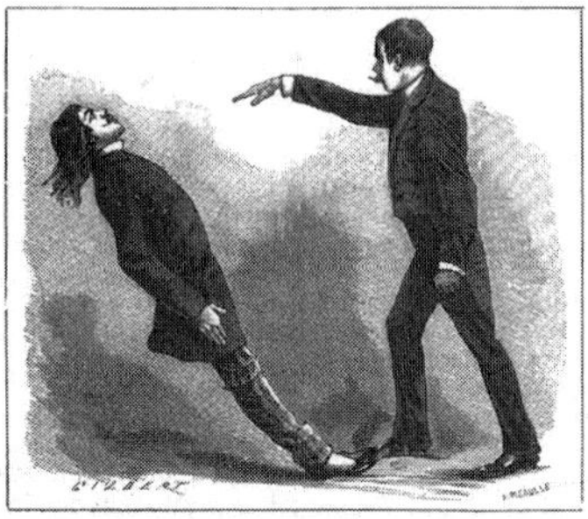

Fig. 1. — Raideur cataleptique.

Plusieurs scènes sont figurées chaque soir dans ce but.

M. Harmington, disciple convaincu de Mesmer, demande un sujet, et il en trouve dans la salle. Un jeune artiste, nommé Marius, se présente. M. Harmington lui fait exécuter toute espèce d'extravagances, accompagnées d'un feu roulant de lazzis, rendus plus piquants par l'état de sommeil supposé. Au moment où Marius termine ses exercices les plus extraordinaires, un gendarme fait irruption sur la scène pour faire exécuter les ordonnances récentes relatives à l'hypnotisme. Mais il est lui-même subjugué par M. Harmington et terrassé par les vibrations dont l'encéphale de ce terrible magnétiseur est le centre. Quand le rideau tombe, le représentant de l'autorité se débat contre la catalepsie qui l'envahit.

Tous les phénomènes de sommeil provoqué sont successivement simulés avec beaucoup de naturel par M. Jules David qui joue le rôle de Marius, dans cette charmante petite pièce.

A un certain moment, après des passes habilement simulées par le magnétiseur, M. Jules David devient tout d'un coup aussi raide qu'un morceau de bois. Il tombe en pivotant sur ses talons (fig. 1). Si M. Harmington ne se hâtait d'accourir à son aide, il se briserait infailliblement le crâne sur le plancher, mais le magnétiseur se trouve juste derrière lui pour recevoir son sujet dans ses bras. Alors il le soulève et le pose sur deux chaises convenablement espacées comme il le ferait d'une simple planche : sur le siège de l'une, il place l'occiput de son sujet, et sur le siège de l'autre, il fait reposer ses talons. M. Jules David reste alors dans une parfaite immobilité. On ne voit pas un seul de ses muscles broncher, aucun mouvement ne trahit chez lui la persistance de la vie. La simulation est complète.

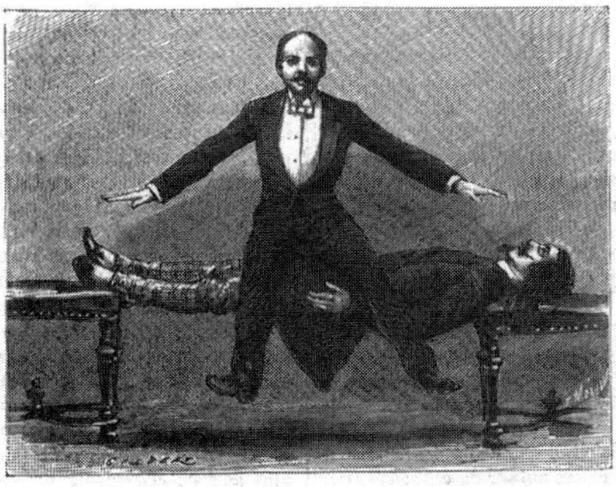

Fig. 2. — Expérience sur le même sujet.

Afin de mettre le comble à l'étonnement du public, M. Harmington se place triomphalement sur le ventre de M. Jules David. Il soulève lentement ses pieds qu'il tient suspendus en l'air, de manière à bien montrer que c'est uniquement le patient qui le soutient, sans qu'il ait besoin d'autre point d'appui que les deux chaises (fig. 2.)

Il ne manque pas d'ordinaire de personnes assez naïves pour croire que M. Jules David est réellement endormi d'un sommeil cataleptique dont un des caractères est la rigidité cadavérique.

Le cou de M. Jules David, étant complètement dégagé de vêtements, il n'est pas possible de supposer que le simulateur de la catalepsie porte un corset

69 'La Science au Théâtre – Imitation de Phénomènes d'hypnotisme à la salle Robert Houdin à Paris', from *La Nature*, 19:1, (1891), p. 28, engravings.

of hypnosis as public performances were very similar to those at the Salpêtrière. For example, in the non-medical images in *La Nature*, which show a hypnotist performing on a clothed male subject, the acts performed by hypnotic victims are similar to those demanded from hysterical subjects (Figure 69). In both, hypnotised bodies fall down, lie across chairs, and are pricked with needles. Emmanuel Arène described in his 1887 article in *République française* (which appeared on the same page as the paper's criticism of Brouillet's painting at the Salon), how his friends took part in hypnosis for entertainment, but that the experience left them 'troubled, agitated; some of them appeared to suffer greatly'.[150] Hypnosis provoked anxiety because people feared that it could be applied without consent. The largely publicised 1888 trial of Henri Chambige contributed to this fear – he declared his innocence by claiming that he was hypnotised when he killed a married woman. Medico-legal experts were called upon in such cases, including those who were past students of Charcot. Gilles de la Tourette's *L'Hypnotisme et les états analogues au point de vue médico-légal* (1887) and J. Liégeois's 1889 *De la suggestion et du somnambulisme dans les rapports avec la jurisprudence et la médecine-légale* (1889) are examples of Charcot's direct influence over these new laws and policies.[151]

The support of Charcot's theories by his followers into the last years of the 1880s was crucial for his reputation. In a publicised debate following the publication of Dr Bernheim's book *De la suggestion dans l'état hypnotique* in 1884, Bernheim and the medical school of Nancy argued that Charcot's understanding of hypnosis was wrong.[152] Bernheim argued that hypnotism was culturally cultivated because most humans were hypnotisable; it was, therefore, based on suggestion.[153] If Bernheim was right, Charcot's theories (and the laws based upon them) were bogus, and hypnosis could no longer confirm a hysterical diagnosis. Furthermore, it would suggest that hypnosis was used at the Salpêtrière for sinister purposes, particularly since public debates focused on the ways in which hypnotisers, medical or otherwise, took advantage of women who were under their trance. For example, Liégois's book references a story about a dentist who was jailed for ten years for having sex with a young patient while she was hypnotised for a tooth operation. Tourette's published account of hypnosis in 1887 describes how interns at the Salpêtrière tried to get Wittman to undress and take a bath in front of them while she was still under a hypnotic trance. Despite being under their spell and having just performed for an audience, Wittman refused.[154]

Charcot fought back against the opposition by claiming that he was only interested in *grand hypnotisme*, and therefore did not argue that *petit hypnotisme* could be found in others, particularly those with hysterical susceptibilities. He sought to redeem his reputation by discussing how his 'scientific' use of hypnosis protected the public from the dangers of hypnosis when used by unqualified men. He explained that the Salpêtrière used hypnotism to cure a young woman who had been hypnotised at a town fair.[155] Charcot further legitimated hypnosis as a valuable medical technique when he allowed Dr Dumontpallier to borrow Wittman in 1888. Dumontpallier used Wittman in his own studies, as well as during his speech at the *Congrès international de l'hypnotisme* in 1889. Wittman's performance as star hysteric was confirmed at the Exposition Universelle where she not only performed for Dumontpallier, but was also portrayed on the walls of the art exhibition in Brouillet's painting and in the medical photographs at the photographic exhibition. By showing the benefits of hypnosis when used by qualified experts, Charcot justified a medical process that was often associated with taking sexual advantage. It also allowed him to defend his fixation on making people unconscious. His 'medicalisation' of hypnosis was considered a key component of his legacy in his obituaries, yet these medical breakthroughs did not maintain their status for long. On the occasion of the doctor's death, there were differing views on the status of hypnosis. *Journal de médecine et de chirurgie pratique* wrote that it was Charcot's interest in the 'occult sciences' that struck the public's imagination,[156] while *Revue de l'hypnotisme expérimental et thérapeutique* claimed that, 'Thanks to the authority of his word, hypnotism and its related studies immediately gained acceptance within official science'.[157]

Hypnosis at the Salon

The paintings of hypnosis, particularly *Une leçon clinique*, did not go unnoticed at the 1887 Salon: 'at this time, [hypnosis] is one of the most current and attractive subjects', declared Merson.[158] Brouillet indicated Wittman's hypnotic state by her comatose body, semi-closed eyes and repose in Dr Babinsky's arms. Babinsky, Charcot's *chef de clinique*, was well known for his experiments with hypnosis. In January 1887, *L'Illustration* published an article about how he was able to transfer hysterical symptoms from one patient to another while they were under his hypnotic trance.[159] Furthermore, Brouillet's inclusion of M. Duval, biologist and Professor of Anatomy at the École des Beaux-Arts, pointed to hypnosis as well: Duval was an expert, having published an article about hypnosis in *Nouveau dictionnaire de médecine et chirurgie pratique* in 1874.[160]

Roger Ballu, who ultimately praised Brouillet's painting, nonetheless prefaced his discussion of *Une leçon clinique* with 'let us return to the hospital; it will not be for long, I assure you ... Good God, what sort of medicine is this?! Hypnotism – what a nightmare!'[161] Other newspapers, such as *Gazette de France*, objected to the painting's subject matter because they thought that hypnosis was cruel. Alexis Martin wrote in *Guide du visiteur – la peinture et la sculpture au Salon de 1887*, published as a supplement to *La gazette des femmes*:

> For our part, we cannot approve of the current trend among artists to reproduce these tedious surgical scenes; to see a woman suffering, being operated on, being hypnotised in the midst of fifteen men dressed in black is a spectacle that, for all the talent on display, will always be of mediocre interest.[162]

Unlike the majority of critics who praised paintings with medical themes as historical documents for future generations, Martin expressed 'profound antipathy' for these works with 'unpleasant subjects'. After considering Gervex's *Avant l'opération*, Martin advised that 'we run quickly towards those with more modesty'.[163] Despite Martin's stated dislike for medical narratives, he nonetheless described them in detail. The fact that this publication was targeted at women makes it apparent that such themes were deemed more socially suitable for a male audience and that these works were considered less welcoming to female viewers. Had Brouillet and Gervex not illustrated this in their paintings where women are objects of male experimentation? Female audiences may also have had trouble with the depiction of Charcot and of hypnosis itself, understood as an act that made women vulnerable to male sexual appetites and also diagnosed them as hysteric. Platel acknowledged a gender divide in reactions to Charcot's work when he wrote that Charcot 'stunned men. He terrified women'.[164]

Significantly, women, whether hysterical or not, were considered to be more susceptible to hypnosis than men, thus implying that all women were potential hysterics. Bourneville and Regnard claimed that 'there are few women who cannot be hypnotised', [165] but that hypnosis 'will go more quickly and more surely if performed on a hysteric—preferably a young one, as they are more sensitive, more impressionable'.[166] Arène's article on hypnosis also described in detail how a *hypnotiseur* took advantage of women by having them kiss him and sit on his lap,[167] and *Le Courrier français* published the article 'Ce que l'hypnotisme peut faire' with drawings of women undressing while under a hypnotic trance.[168] Therefore, it is likely that bourgeois women chose not to subject themselves to a process that could possibly undo the proper comportment of femininity that they had worked so hard to fabricate.

There was another canvas at the Salon depicting hypnotism, in the same room as *Une leçon clinique*, but this painting received less mention in contemporary reviews. The Swedish artist Richard Bergh's *La Séance d'hypnose* (referred to as *Suggestion* by M. le Roux in *Le Temps* and *Somnambule* by Fourcaud) represents three men and a woman watching as a *magnétiseur* hypnotises a seated woman (Figure 70).[169] This work was described by Fourcaud as a 'medical painting' along with those by Brouillet and Gervex. Yet unlike the other two images, the scene in Bergh's painting is not a hospital room. In contrast to the bare walls and institutional settings rendered by Gervex and Brouillet, Bergh depicted a room with flowered wallpaper, covered chairs, and a sofa. Ponsonailhe described the painting as showing 'an experiment among intimates'.[170] The four figures watching the hypnosis seem to be onlookers and part of a domestic séance rather than medical students. Although they are all dressed similarly in black and stare at the hypnosis taking place, there are no instruments or medical paraphernalia included. Their identities are not referred to in the painting's title nor in contemporary reviews, thus diminishing the potential of Bergh's painting to be seen as a historical document or significant portrait within a French context. Although the absence of celebrity sitters could have contributed

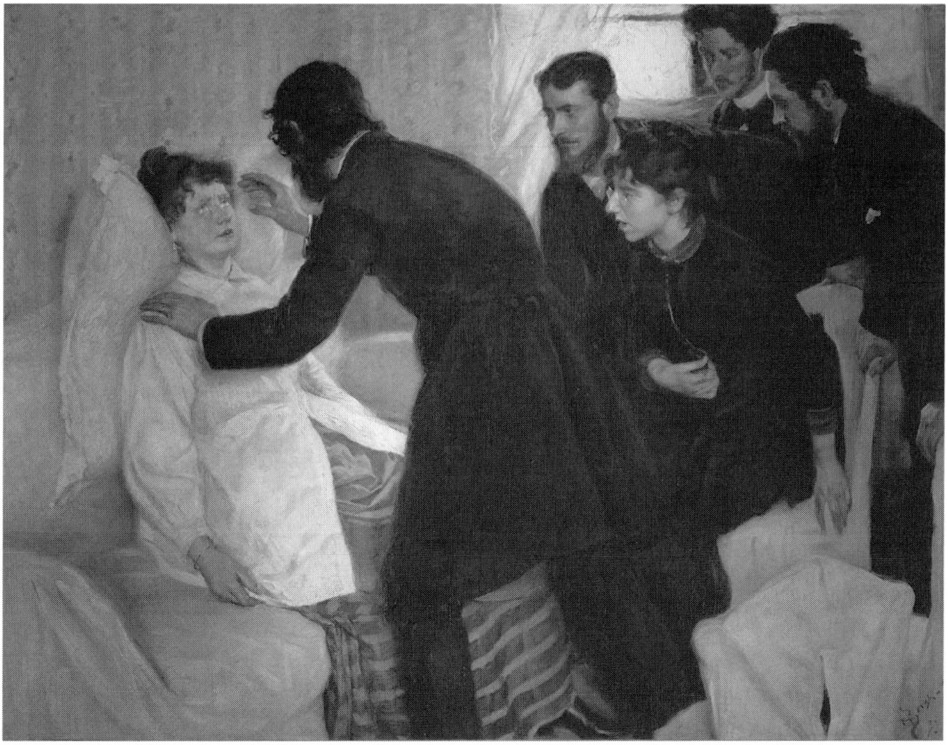

Richard Bergh, *La Séance d'hypnose* (1887), oil on canvas, 153 x 195cm. 70

to the painting's lack of notice by Salon critics, its subject matter was certainly fashionable. The lack of attention given to Bergh's work was likely caused by the way in which he depicted a hypnotised woman: she is fully clothed, her body is slumped and as shapeless as the sofa on which she sits. Unlike the unconscious young women painted by Brouillet and Gervex, this woman is not undressed, nor is she beautiful. Her hypnotised condition makes her less, not more, attractive: her brow is furrowed, her body is lumpy, and her blank eyes roll back into her head. Whereas Wittman's curved back, unfastened dress, and position next to a stretcher symbolised the promise of her horizontal hysterical climax, the woman in *La Séance d'hypnose* is devoid of sexual appeal because she is seated, supported by pillows, and conservatively dressed. Although she is no doubt hypnotised, she is not necessarily a hysteric: she is not shown in a medical setting, nor does she bear any overt signs of hysteria. Did her lack of overt illness contribute to the critic's lack of admiration for this picture?

Women in unconscious states fascinated men at the Salpêtrière. The majority of photographs in the first volume of *Iconographie photographique* are of unconscious hysterical women, sleeping, yawning, and in the various stages of hysterical attacks (particularly the moments in which the female body goes unconscious). Hypnosis allowed medical men to control the stages of hysteria because under hypnosis they could put the body to sleep, make it perform an *attitude passionelle* or *état normal*, wake it up, put it back to sleep again, sometimes for days. The hypnotised body mimicked hysterical symptoms as they were suggested by the physician – hypnosis, like hysteria, could never be fruitful without the intervention of the doctor.

Studies of hysteria since the 1970s have often focused on the ways in which physicians, particularly Charcot, and hysterical women worked together to perform – women could act out the symptoms while men directed.[171] The hysterical woman's performance has also been understood as a rebellion against patriarchal culture, and a result of her entanglement in a world in which she has no control. As Janet Beizer argues, the inarticulate language expressed by the hysterical body is in fact the language of hysteria created by Charcot, mapped onto the female body. Hysterical women, for Beizer, are 'ventriloquised bodies' and Charcot the puppet master. Sander Gilman claims that hysterical women learned to perform hysterical behaviour by mimicking the images produced at the Salpêtrière.[172] The performances at the Salpêtrière, therefore, must be understood as a multifaceted network of both mutual participation and individual rebellion. By reading Brouillet's painting from left to right, it is evident that the iconography of hysteria produced at the Salpêtrière, symbolised in *Une leçon clinique* by Richer's drawing, provided visual depictions of hysterical bodies that patients could emulate and doctors could use as diagnostic templates. Yet reading the painting from right to left illustrates how the female body is simultaneously pathologised and transformed into art as it is filtered through the male audience, whose occupations demanded the study and creation of realistic representations of hysteria. Although the hysterical patient could participate in the performance, it was only through male bodies and realist modes and methods that the hysteric and hysteria were made 'real'.

Hypnosis promised to uncover the 'real' hysterical body and prepare it for observation while it also produced a theatrical setting in which the female body could remain hidden behind its hypnotic trance. While Wittman's state of partial undress in *Une leçon clinique* parallels the clinical striptease she was made to perform, she was also clothed by the symptoms fashioned by medical iconography. Although hypnosis had the realist medium *par excellence* – an actual living body – hypnosis, like the hysteric, could never be fully trusted to reveal the truth. The patients' subjectivities, agencies, and identities always threatened to emerge, thus exposing the frailty of hysteria and hypnosis as stable medical conditions and procedures. Although the physical presence of a patient's body was seen to attest to hysteria's reality and, in turn, the physical manifestations of hysteria (produced by the physician's practice of hypnosis) attempted to fix the malady on the body's surface, this 'unseeable' disease could never be pinned down regardless of the multiple realist modes and mediums of representation that sought it out. The historical and cultural connotations of hypnosis and hysteria constantly threatened to erode the seemingly rational façade of modern scientific medicine and realist formal strategies. The sexual lure of observing and manipulating the body tied it to the world of fantasy and pleasure. The hysterical female body was ultimately a realist trope. Despite the desire to secure and 'prove' hysteria's presence through realist representations, the multiplicity of these modes of recording ultimately pointed to hysteria's transience and absence of the real.

Electrotherapy as realist brush

An electrotherapy machine is depicted in the centre of Brouillet's canvas in order to contain the sense of desire invoked by hypnosis and the rendering of a semi-nude woman in close proximity to clothed men. Placed on the table to Charcot's proper right, the machine and its brushes are the only obvious medical instruments depicted. Like hypnosis, electrotherapy was believed to prove that hysteria existed by producing visible evidence on the body's surface. It was famously used by Duchenne de Boulogne in the mid-nineteenth century to link physiological expressions and gestures with emotions.[173] His photographs show how he touched the patient's face with an electrical probe or brush. The current caused the facial muscles to contract, making the patient assume an expression. Charcot's manipulation of hypnotised hysterical bodies evolved from Duchenne's procedures. The religious poses held by Duchenne's patients are iconographic predecessors to the Salpêtrière's photographs. Duchenne believed his experiments and photographs could provide artists with a means of realistically recording human emotion. He wrote:

> The masters of Art were not always able to capture the essential lines … after instinctively drawing them very accurately in a sketch, they lost sight of them in the process of finishing their work and were not able to find them again. Localised electroshock … reveals the physical cause of all of these folds and wrinkles by inducing partial or multiple muscle contractures … allows us to formulate with certainty the rules that must guide the artist.[174]

Duchenne's belief in the future possibilities of drawing and painting through electricity are evident when he used a metaphor of painting when referring to his rheophore brush. In 1862, he claimed that '[a]rmed with a rheophore brush, one can, as nature herself has done, paint the expressive lines of the soul's emotions on the face of a man'.[175] Duchenne's interest in unifying art and medicine culminated in the donation of his personal collection of medical photographs to the École des Beaux-Arts in 1875. The use of these photographs by artists suggests how photography became heir to the *tête d'expression*.

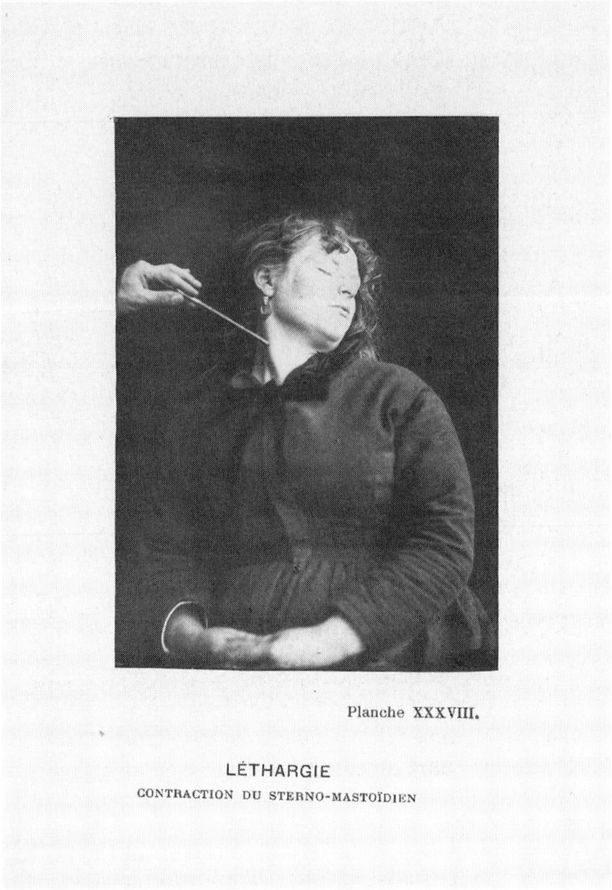

71 Paul Régnard, 'Léthargie', from Bourneville and Régnard, *Iconographie Photographique de la Salpêtrière* (1879), planche XXXVIII, photolithograph.

Electricity was used at the Salpêtrière for therapeutic and experimental purposes.[176] The 1879 volume of the *Iconographie photographique* and Charcot's *Œuvres complètes* are filled with photographs that are similar to those made by Duchenne. Significantly, Wittman was often the woman photographed undergoing electrotherapy. In the 1879 volume, an unknown male hand is holding a metal stick to Wittman's throat (Figure 71). Although her neck muscle is exposed and rigid, she appears to be in little pain. Such photographs contradict electrotherapy as it was discussed in the adjoining text: 'W … received the electrical current; the delirium nevertheless continued. Feeding via esophageal tube. She vomited up part of the ingested liquids. Insomnia; incessant chatter. She was placed on a night-commode; she urinated.'[177] The

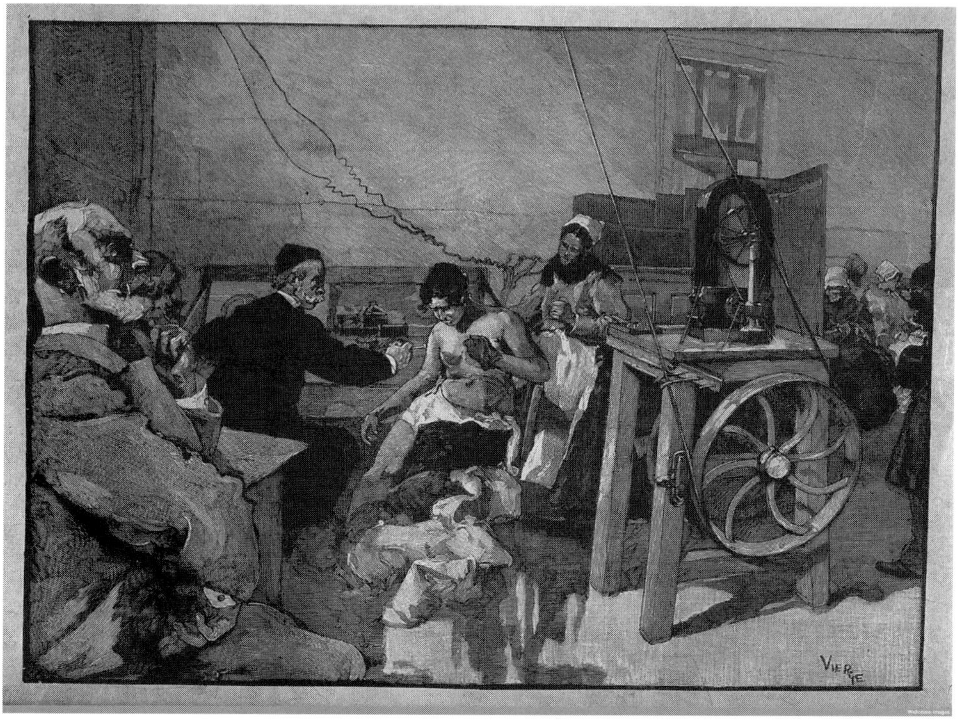

G.D.I. after Daniel Vierge's watercolour, *Examen d'un malade à la table d'électrothérapie, électro-diagnostique par le Dr Vigouroux* (1887), process print of wood engraving, 20.2 x 27.3cm. **72**

violence of electrical experimentation is absent from the photographs as is the individual who is in charge of its application. Although the text refers to Dr Vigouroux, head of the electrical unit at the Salpêtrière, he is not fully present in the photographs. Similarly, Brouillet did not depict him in close contact with the machine with which he was associated. Rather, Brouillet portrayed Vigouroux in the front row of the crowd, recognised by his aged face, black cap, and bushy white moustache. The distance between practitioner, patient, and the tools of experimentation implies that Vigouroux had already performed, or shortly would. Although Brouillet showed Charcot as Wittman's co-star, the inclusion of an empty chair and full glass of water suggests that Charcot will eventually sit down and let others have a turn.

The use of electrotherapy at the Salpêtrière was widely known. In 1885, *La Nature* published an illustrated article about the electrotherapy room at the Salpêtrière that describes how patients were attached to a machine that produced electrical currents. Patients received different types of electrotherapy depending on their illness: in the illustration in *La Nature*, a group of male and female patients line up for treatment, while in another corner a woman is dealt with privately. The electrotherapy procedure shown on the right was performed on an average of 180 people per day, while that on the left tended 200 people.[178] A few months after the 1887 Salon, *Le Monde illustré* published a series of prints of the gouaches by Daniel Vierge of various rooms at the hospital, including the electrotherapy area. In one, Vigouroux touches the arm of a bare-chested woman with his electrical brush, and in another, women, men, and children receive electrotherapy in the Salpêtrière's *bains électriques* (Figure 72).[179] Electrotherapy rooms, like photography studios, laboratories, and operating theatres, were modern scientific spaces supported by republican policies. The electrotherapy machine was a new apparatus that symbolised technology and science, thus making it an ideal tool of modern medicine.

As with hypnosis, Charcot was more interested in electrotherapy as an investigatory tool than a therapeutic method.[180] He, like Duchenne, saw the rheophore as an electric paintbrush that could visibly illustrate the relationship between mind and body.[181] Yet, unlike hypnosis, which was riddled with controversy, electrotherapy was considered mechanically objective and beyond personal exploitation. It manipulated the hysterical body in the same way that hypnosis did, but under a technical guise since it contained the elements of science and modernity that hypnotism lacked. The visible presence of the rheophore in *Une leçon clinique* helped make hypnosis appear more technical and therefore more rational, thus masking the obsessive observations and clinical experimentations Charcot and his colleagues performed on scantily clad women. Furthermore, the depiction of a cutting-edge medical apparatus contributed to *Une leçon clinique*'s status as contemporary while also attesting to its realism. The electric brush of the electrotherapy machine, which is perched over the corner of the wooden table, symbolically refers to Brouillet's paintbrush. This instilled the act of painting with the mechanical modernity of electricity, thus symbolically aligning the painting with the assumed technological sincerity and abilities of photography. Gervex used a similar artistic convention by aligning his paintbrush with Péan's new surgical tools. Electricity was modern and non-human, and therefore appeared void of subjectivity. Yet, behind the technical façade of such procedures, touch remains. Vigouroux's brush touched the patient, transforming her into the medium of his electrical performance, while Brouillet's brush touched the canvas in order to create an image of her body. Touch in representation threatens to rupture the objectivity attributed to realism as it alludes to desire and physical contact. However, touch is also needed to confirm the presence of the real.

Conclusion: 'Triste archive de l'humanité souffrante'

Painting, photography, casting, hypnosis, and electrotherapy all require touch. Although the opticality and meticulous detailing of realistic representations produces a sense of distance and neutrality between doctor and patient – as well as artist and model – the close scrutiny involved in their production confirms bodily presence. The required intimacy of touching and observing bodies threatens the assumed detachment of realist practice and the objectivity of scientific medicine. The multiple forms of realism, compounded by the excessive number of depictions of hysteria produced at the Salpêtrière, demonstrate a madness that goes beyond the requirements of medical practice and also defines the creating and collecting practices of the Salpêtrière. The insanity of the hospital's collection was noted by Maurice Guillemot, who claimed that

> Although fascinating, Doctor Charcot's practice leaves a painful impression, like the memory of a museum of horrors, of a reunion of gnomes, of monsters, of fantastic and illusory beings, of nightmarish visions borrowed from Dante's infernal cycles or from Poe's macabre œuvre. A sad archive of suffering humanity, a horrible ossuary of the hospice and the clinic.[182]

For Guillemot, the realistic images and objects commissioned by Charcot were distressing and painful, sad archives for the future. In contrast, Salon critics celebrated Brouillet's painting as a trustworthy document that offered the spectacle of hysteria in the form of an unconscious young woman with bare skin. Brouillet's realism was more palatable and appealing than the realist depictions, performances, and procedures produced at the Salpêtrière – perhaps this is why Brouillet's painting, rather than a scene from 'real life', was used as the model for Spitzner's wax version of Charcot's lecture. Created for an entertainment venue, hysteria needed to be shown as spectacular in order to draw a crowd.[183] Perhaps this is also the reason why Brouillet's painting was never bought by Charcot or the Salpêtrière.

Une leçon clinique demonstrates the ways in which representations of the hysterical female body involved a process of inclusion and exclusion in an attempt to construct the most real image of hysteria. Its verisimilitude was grounded – and guaranteed – by its relationship with the Salpêtrière networks of the real.[184] However, the hysterical woman, as the embodiment of this disease, was the site on which realism fought to prove the reality of hysteria. Although the correspondence between different discourses of verisimilitude aided in the formulation of a shared definition and iconography of hysteria, the layering and appropriation of realistic depictions, from fifteenth-century miniatures to photographic *académies*, ultimately exposed the lack of evidence to prove that the disease existed. How could realism portray a body that was simultaneously sentient and unconscious, controlled and chaotic, seductive and repulsive, real and unreal? Nineteenth-century hysteria and realist modes of representation were mimetic performances and processes that mimicked the 'reality' defined and demanded by male professionals. Fluctuating between order and disorder, presence and absence, similarity and difference, realism as a mimetic agent could never pin down and secure 'the wandering womb'. Rather, it veiled the hysterical body, providing yet another layer to an empty shell.

Notes

1 Charcot taught at the Salpêtrière, a hospital in Paris that specialised in the study and treatment of the elderly and mentally ill. For a history of the Salpêtrière and its impact on French culture and society, see Mark S. Micale, 'The Salpêtrière in the Age of Charcot: An Institutional Perspective on Medical History in the Late Nineteenth Century', *Journal of Contemporary History*, 20:4 (1985), 703–701.

2 Le Roux, 'La Vie à Paris: A travers le Salon', n.p.: 'le succès du Salon'.

3 'Le Salon', *Le Journal des arts*, 3 (1887), p. 2: 'une des œuvres les plus importantes du Salon'.

4 De Fourcaud, 'Le Salon de 1887', p. 325.

5 Merson, 'Salon de 1887 – II', p. 282: 'pourrait bien être la toile à sensation du Salon de 1887'.

6 Meurville, 'Le Salon – La nature au Salon', p. XII; and Mantz, 'Le Salon – I', n.p.

7 Audiences at Charcot's lectures were as large as 500. For a discussion of the popularity of Charcot's lessons, see Elaine Showalter, *Hystories: Hysterical Epidemics and Modern Culture* (London: Picador, 1997), pp. 30–37.

8 Jean-Martin Charcot, 'Leçon d'ouverture', *Œuvres complètes III* (Paris: Bureaux du Progrès Médical, 1890), p. 4: 'musée pathologique vivant'.

9 In 1922, Léon Daudet recalled the popularity of Brouillet's painting when he wrote in *Les Hommes*, 'Un tableau célèbre (et dont les photographies courent les rues) a popularisé ces séances de la Salpêtrière, dont tout Paris s'entretenait il y a trente-cinq ans et auxquelles assistaient mêlés aux médecins, des écrivains, des artistes, des hommes politiques'. A celebrated painting (reproduced in photographs on every street corner) popularised the sessions at the Salpêtrière, which were the talk of all Paris thirty-five years ago, and which were attended by a mixed audience of doctors, writers, artists and even politicians.) L. Daudet, *Les Œuvres dans les hommes* (Paris: Nouvelle librairie nationale, 1922), as cited in Philippe Bata, Marie-Véronique Clin, Catherine Duffault *et al.*, *André Brouillet 1857–1914*, exhibition catalogue (Poitiers: Musées de la ville de Poitiers, 2000), p. 104.

10 De Fourcauld, 'Le Salon de 1887', p. 325: 'il serait difficile de consacrer par un tableau plus sincère le souvenir des mémorables expériences du docteur Charcot et de l'affluence spéciale qu'elles ont attirée durant ces dernières années, à son cours'.

11 Ollendorf, *Salon de 1887*, pp. 62–63. 'La composition conforme à la vérité, est claire et bien comprise; elle met en valeur, sans grossissement et sans artifice, le sujet principal, qui est le docteur Charcot'.

12 Ballu, 'Salon de 1887', n.p.: 'une certaine réalité vous saisit'.
13 Meurville, 'Le Salon – la nature au Salon', p. XII: 'une minute suffit pour admirer la vérité des personnages et de la lumière; il ne reste aucune découverte à faire après cela'.
14 I concentrate on the female body because, although 40 per cent of Charcot's cases concerned working-class men, the majority of visual representations of hysterical patients were of women. For hysteria's connection to the female body, see Helen King, 'Once upon a Text: Hysteria from Hippocrates', pp. 3–90; and G.S. Rousseau, '"A Strange Pathology": Hysteria in the early modern world, 1500–1800', pp. 92–224, both in Gilman *et al.*, *Hysteria Beyond Freud.*
15 For an account of the secondary literature on hysteria up to 1989, see Mark S. Micale, 'Hysteria and Its Historiography: A Review of Past and Present Writing', *History of Science,* 27 (1989), 223–261. See also Bronfen, *The Knotted Subject: Hysteria and Its Discontents*, pp. 101–138.
16 For a discussion of hysteria in men, see Vernon A. Rosario, 'Pointy Penises, Fashion Crimes, and Hysterical Mollies: The Pederasts' Inversion', in Jeffrey W. Merrick and Bryant T. Ragan (eds), *Homosexuality in Modern France* (New York: Oxford University Press, 1996), pp. 146–176; and Mark S. Micale, 'Charcot and the Idea of Hysteria in the Male', *Medical History*, 34:4 (1990), 363–411.
17 Didi-Huberman, *Invention of Hysteria,* pp. 74–75.
18 Sander L. Gilman, Helen King, Roy Porter *et al.*, *Hysteria Beyond Freud* (Berkeley: University of California Press, 1993).
19 For a discussion of the relationship between Freud and Charcot, see Sander L. Gilman, *The Case of Sigmund Freud: Medicine and Identity at the Fin de Siècle* (Baltimore: Johns Hopkins University Press, 1993).
20 This is evident in work by many feminist writers and artists. For example, Cixous conceptualised hysteria as a form of feminist rebellion, Mary Kelly's project *Interim* (1985) disallowed any overt objectification of women while simultaneously making reference to Charcot and Salpêtrière, and Beth B's artwork *Hysteria 2000* criticised medical constructs of hysteria through a feminist appropriation of medicalised images of women. See Elaine Showalter, 'Hysteria, Feminism and Gender', in Gilman *et al.*, *Hysteria Beyond Freud*, pp. 286–344; Showalter, 'Politics, Patients and Feminism', in Showalter, *Hystories*, pp. 49–61; Mary Kelly, *Interim* (New York: New Museum of Contemporary Art, 1990); Margaret Iversen, Douglas Crimp and Homi K. Bhabha, *Mary Kelly* (London: Phaidon Press, 1997); Kemp and Wallace, *Spectacular Bodies*, pp. 176–183.
21 Both authors disagree with Didi-Huberman's view of the hysterical woman as a desiring subject rather than object of the medical gaze. See Carol Armstrong, 'Probing Pictures: Carol Armstrong on Georges Didi-Huberman – *Invention of Hysteria: Charcot and the Photographic Iconography of the Salpêtrière*', *Artforum Online* (September 2003); and Judith Surkis, 'Review of Didi-Huberman', *H-France Review*, 4 (4 January 2004).
22 Showalter, *Hystories,* pp. 115–201.
23 Showalter, *Hystories*, p. 15.

24 Jules Claretie, *Les Amours d'un interne* (Paris: E. Dentu, 1881), p. 122. 'C'est plutôt un détraquement général du système nerveux. Ça peut être érotique – pour donner raison au vulgaire, – ça peut être sombre, ça peut être mystique, ça peut être religieux, ça peut être tout. L'hystérique mange trop ou ne mange rien, dort trop ou ne dort pas assez, semble absorbée comme une idiote ou exaltée comme une folle; elle aime le tapage, les couleurs violentes, les inventions romantiques, veut qu'on s'occupe d'elle, et qu'on ne s'occupe que d'elle; elle est en dehors de la règle de commune, et le monde et le demi-monde; le théâtre, les salons, tout Paris est plein d'hystériques, dont la maladie parfaitement caractérisée aurait besoin des soins du docteur Charcot … C'est même la grande maladie moderne, l'hystérie! La société souffre d'une névrose ou d'une névrite gigantesque'.

25 Charcot asked the Assistance Publique for funding a museum on 15 September 1878. For further information, see Nadine Simon-Dhouailly, *La Leçon de Charcot – voyage dans une toile* (Paris: Imprimerie Tardy Querey, 1986), pp. 63–66.

26 Daston and Galison, *Objectivity*.

27 For a full list of the audience memembers, see Simon-Dhouailly, *La Leçon de Charcot*, pp. 4–5.

28 Mantz, 'Le Salon – I', n.p. 'Tous les visages sont des portraits, et les journaux ne se sont pas fait faute de nommer les personnages qui ont posé devant le jeune peintre.'

29 Ballu, 'Salon de 1887', n.p.: 'aura du succès, et il ne le devra pas seulement à l'intérêt des portraits qu'on cherchera à reconnaître'.

30 All biographical information on the people depicted in *Une leçon clinique* is from J. L. Signoret, '*Une leçon clinque à la Salpêtrière* (1887) par André Brouillet', *Revue neurologique*, 139:12 (1983), 696–699; Jean Thuillier, *Monsieur Charcot de la Salpêtrière* (Paris: R. Laffont, 1993), p. 227; and Simon-Dhouailly, *La Leçon de Charcot*, pp. 4–5, 20–21.

31 Richer's influence on French art was celebrated. For a nineteenth-century discussion of his interest in the arts, see Raphaël Blanchard, *Hommage à M. le Dr Paul Richer, membre de l'Académie de Médecine, professeur d'anatomie à l'école des Beaux-Arts, à l'occasion de son élection à l'Académie des Beaux-Arts, 22 Juillet, 1905* (Paris: Renouard, 1906), p. 10: 'on ferait le diagnostic sur ces dessins!'

32 For a discussion of the relationship between doctors and the École des Beaux-Arts, see Callen, 'The Body and Difference', 23.

33 Blanchard, *Hommage à M. le Dr Paul Richer,* p. 12: 'une source précieuse de documents pour l'histoire médico-artistique … l'Art et la Science, si longtemps étrangers l'un à l'autre, y fraternisent étroitement et vous êtes le principal auteur de cette union féconde'.

34 For a discussion of Duval's role in artistic and medical representations, see Callen, 'Doubles and Desire', 669–699.

35 Georges Guinon, *Les Agents provocateurs de l'hystérie* (Paris: Progrès Médical, 1889), p. 208. For an account of Blanche, see Asti Hustvedt, *Medical Muses: Hysteria in Nineteenth-Century Paris* (New York: W.W. Norton & Co., 2011), pp. 35–141.

36 For a discussion of Charcot's popularity, see Christopher Goetz, Michel Bonduelle and Toby Gelfand, *Charcot: Constructing Neurology* (Oxford: Oxford University Press, 1995), pp. 235–237.

37 Henri Ellenberger, 'Charcot and the Salpêtrière School', in Mark S. Micale, *Beyond the Unconscious: Essays of Henri F. Ellenberger in the History of Psychiatry* (Princeton: Princeton University Press, 1993), p. 139.

38 Doctor A. Cartaz, 'Du somnambulisme et du magnétisme à propos du cours du Dr Charcot à la Salpêtrière', *La Nature*, 7:1 (1879), 102. 'La presse s'est occupée dans ces derniers temps d'expériences et de démonstrations sur le somnambulisme et le magnétisme, faites par M. le docteur Charcot à la Salpêtrière. Depuis plusieurs années, l'éminent professeur a inauguré … une série de leçons cliniques sur les maladies nerveuses dont son service est si abondamment pourvu. Ces leçons qui on lieu chaque dimanche à neuf heures et demie, dans une salle de plus en plus insuffisante pour le grand nombre d'auditeurs, portent, comme je viens de dire, sur la démonstration des principaux types de névroses.' (Lately the press has been filled with accounts of the experiments and demonstrations on somnambulism and magnetism conducted by Doctor Charcot at the Salpêtrière. Several years ago the eminent professor inaugurated … a series of clinical lessons on the nervous afflictions found in such abundance in his department. These lessons, which take place every Sunday at nine thirty, in a lecture hall that is increasingly insufficient to handle the large audiences, focus, as I have said, on demonstrating the main types of neurosis.)

39 Gaston Tissandier, 'J.M. Charcot', *La Nature*, 21:2 (26 August 1893), 193–194. 'Depuis de longues années, les leçons du maître, pratiquées à la Salpêtrière sur la grande névrose, sur l'hypnotisme, sur les différentes formes de l'hystérie ont attiré l'attention universelle'. (For many years, the master's teaching sessions at the Salpêtrière, on acute neurosis, hypnotism, and the different forms of hysteria have attracted widespread attention.)

40 Félix Platel (Ignotus), *Les Hommes de mon temps* (Paris: Victor-Harvard, c.1889), p. 378. 'M. Charcot est devenu surtout célèbre par ses exhibitions de la Salpêtrière. Le public entre là'. (Monsieur Charcot owes his fame chiefly to his performances at the Salpêtrière, which are open to the public.)

41 Jean-Martin Charcot, *Œuvres complètes* (Paris: Bureaux du Progrès Médical, 1892), pp. 389–390. 'Dessinée par P. Richer, d'après un croquis fait sur nature par M. Charcot'.

42 Doctor P. Dubray, 'Promenades au Salon', *Union médicale* (14 May 1887), 755: 'MM. Jules Claretie, Alfred Naquet et Paul Arène ne suivent pas normalement, que je sache, les leçons de M. Charcot.'

43 Weisberg, 'The Representation of Doctors at Work in Salon Art of the Early Third Republic in France', pp. 439–441. Weisberg also claims that many of the interns who attended the majority of Charcot's lectures, including Blocq, Hillemand, Valet, Thibault, Achard, and Poulalio, are not depicted.

44 Richard Brilliant suggests that group portraits should not be understood as random groupings, but as deliberate constructions that display professional personalities as unified. He writes that group portraits 'make ideological statements about

the values, attitudes and practices shared by their members, and by the portrait painter as well'. Brilliant, *Portraiture* (London: Reaktion Books, 1991), pp. 92–99.

45 M. Joffroy, 'Jean Martin Charcot (1825–1893)', *Archives de médecine expérimentale et d'anatomie pathologique*, 5 (1893), 27–28. 'Quant à l'hystérie on peut dire qu'il l'a créée presque de toutes pièces.'

46 Henri Meige, 'Charcot artiste', *Nouvelle iconographie de la Salpétrière*, 11 (1898).

47 Sigmund Freud, 'Charcot', in James Strachey (ed.), *The Standard Edition of the Complete Psychological Works of Sigmund Freud*, volume III (London: Hogarth Press, 1962).

48 For a brief discussion of how Charcot and other nineteenth-century practitioners' procedures and processes were considered scientific, see Bynum, *Science and the Practice of Medicine in the Nineteenth Century*, pp. 92–95, 109, 217.

49 As cited in Didi-Huberman, *Invention of Hysteria*, pp. 22–23.

50 As quoted in Tissandier, 'J.M. Charcot', p. 194. 'Charcot a mis de l'ordre et de la précision dans une foule de questions médicales qui n'étaient que désordre avant lui'.

51 Bianchon, *Nos grands médecins d'aujourd'hui*, p. III: 'elle seule, l'école de Charcot – car c'est lui le rénovateur, le grand initiateur à la méthode moderne – compte par centaines ces victoires scientifiques; et les meilleures, en Allemagne, dérivent de Charcot ou de notre Pasteur'.

52 For an in-depth account of Charcot's personal interest in art, see Debora Silverman, *Art Nouveau in Fin-de-Siècle France: Politics, Psychology and Style* (Berkeley: University of California Press, 1989), pp. 75–106.

53 The first volume was published in 1875, with a second edition coming out in 1877. Volumes 2 and 3 were published in 1878 and 1879–80, respectively.

54 For an account of the original purpose of the books, see Bourneville's preface to *Iconographie photographique de la Salpêtrière* (Paris: Progrès Médical, 1877), pp. iii–iv.

55 Albert Londe, *La Photographie médicale* (Paris: Gauthier-Villars et fils, 1892), p. 343. 'Admirons en passant ces artistes scrupuleux qui ne craignaient pas de reproduire la nature même dans ses laideurs et ses difformités, et nous ont laissé ainsi des documents de la plus haute valeur. Ce rôle qu'ils ont rempli appartient désormais aux médecins, qui peuvent maintenant, grâce à la Photographie, laisser aux siècles futurs des documents iconographiques d'un prix inestimable.'

56 Jan Goldstein, 'The Hysterical Diagnosis and the Politics of Anticlericalism in Late Nineteenth-Century France', *Journal of Modern History*, 54:2 (1982), 209–239.

57 Paul Richer and Jean-Martin Charcot, *Les Démoniaques dans l'art* (Paris: Delahaye et Lecrosnier, 1887), p. 307.

58 Charcot praised Richer's methodological investigation of hysteria in his preface to Richer's *Études cliniques sur la grande hystérie ou hystéro-épilepsie* (Paris: Delahaye et Lecrosnier, 1881). He commended Richer for his 'talent d'artiste' and his 'qualité d'observateur conscencieux et sagace' (ability as a wise and conscientious observer).

59 Mantz, 'Le Salon – I', n.p.: 'le volume sur les *Démoniaques dans l'art*, un livre dont nous avons été profondément touchés, car il nous a appris que, même en un passé fort lointain, les artistes ont connu les maladies du système nerveux et

les convulsions et la grande attaque, et que, si quelques-uns en ont donné des représentations amendées ou chimériques, notre ami Rubens a été l'un des plus exacts à traduire par le pinceau le terrible spectacle du phénomène sincèrement observé'.

60 For a discussion of the anticlerical politics in the Parisian hospital system, particularly the role of nursing in its formation, see Schultheiss, *Bodies and Souls*, Goldstein, *Console and Classify*, pp. 363–364; and Bertrand Taithe, *Defeated Flesh*, pp. 151–154.

61 Mme Bottard, who worked as a nurse for forty-eight years, received the Légion d'honneur in 1898. Weisberg, 'The Representation of Doctors at Work in Salon Art of the Early Third Republic in France', pp. 441–442.

62 Archives nationales, côte F/21*7655.

63 Hamel wrote, 'M. Gervex a fait une Œuvre de bonne peinture en traitant une donnée moderne … alors que sur un thème analogue M. Brouillet n'a produit qu'une illusion médiocre' (Monsieur Gervex has created a good painting that treats a modern subject, whereas using an analogous theme Monsieur Brouillet has produced only a mediocre illusion). Hamel, 'Le Salon de 1887', p. 479.

64 Firmin Javel, 'Le Salon', *L'Art français* (1 May 1887), n.p. 'il a vu la scène poignante qu'il retrace avec une réelle émotion'.

65 Mantz, 'Le Salon – I', n.p. 'qu'avant de peindre, il s'est informé. C'est à la Salpêtrière, c'est en suivant les leçons du maître qu'il a étudié la disposition de la scène, noté les détails de l'expérience, précisé l'attitude de la malade'.

66 Mantz, 'Le Salon – I', n.p. 'M. Brouillet reste ce qu'il a été dès le début, un amoureux de la lumière'.

67 Mantz, 'Le Salon – I', n.p. 'Dès que la science intervient, la vraie lumière envahit la maison'.

68 Ollendorf, *Salon de 1887*, p. 61. 'En entrant chez les savants, la lumière s'apaise cependant et se refroidit poliment. Elle prend le ton de la maison. Elle se fait austère et scientifique. Elle ne confond pas la fantaisie avec la science.'

69 Olmer, *Salon de 1866*, p. 62: 'tableaux documentaires avec une méticuleuse exactitude et une parfaite méthode … Du laboratoire à la clinique, la distance est courte et la lumière que nous voyons dans le tableau de M. Brouillet ne diffère pas sensiblement de celle que nous venons d'admirer dans le tableau de M. Gueldry.'

70 Merson, 'Salon de 1887 – II', p. 282.

71 Platel, *Les Hommes de mon temps*, p. 385. 'La longue salle est aménagée comme une salle de spectacle. Il est dix heures du matin – et le gaz éclaire ce théâtre fermé avec soin au soleil. Le spectacle commence sans musique, comme au Théâtre-Français. Au fond, sur la scène, par le *côté jardin*, entre le grand Charcot. Ses clients le suivent.'

72 For an account of Felix Platel's critiques of Charcot, most of which were written under his pseudonym Ignotus, see Goetz, Bonduelle and Gelfand, *Charcot: Constructing Neurology*, pp. 234–235.

73 Tissandier, 'J.M. Charcot', pp. 193–194: 'brillait avec le plus d'éclat … a éclairé, d'une nouvelle lumière, tout un domaine d'investigation jusque-là confiné dans

les ténèbres', 'brille d'un vif éclat par les travaux qu'elle a produits et par le nombre des hommes éminents qui la composent'.

74 Meurville, 'Le Salon – la nature au Salon', n. p.: 'quelques médecins répondent que la lumière est toujours profitable'.

75 Hirschler, *Nos docteurs*, pp. 12–13: 'la trouvaille lumineuse qui conduira les générations futures vers l'absolue vérité'.

76 Callen, *The Spectacular Body*, pp. 111–137.

77 Javel, 'Le Salon', n.p. 'C'est le docteur et son sujet qui attirent et retiennent tout d'abord le regard du spectateur. Le drame est là.'

78 Javel, 'Le Salon', n.p. 'Les personnages qui écoutent sont posés avec une vérité d'attitude qui dénote, chez M. Brouillet, une sûreté de vision absolument remarquable'.

79 Merson, 'Salon de 1887 – II', p. 282.

80 Javel, 'Le Salon', n.p.

81 Mantz, 'Le Salon – I', n.p. 'Dans ce savant auditoire, chacun reconnaît un ami'.

82 Darcours, 'Beaux-Arts et Théâtre', p. 146: 'tous nos médecins de notoriété'.

83 Doctor Dubray, 'Promenades au Salon', as translated in Weisberg, 'The Representation of Doctors at Work in Salon Art of the Early Third Republic in France', pp. 403–404.

84 Javel, 'Le Salon', n.p.: 'respire l'intelligence et la bonté … il est bien rare que la bonté ne soit pas le complément du génie'.

85 Platel, *Les Hommes de mon temps,* p. 384. 'Les cheveux qu'il a tous et presque dans leur première teinte, disent la force de volonté, indiquée d'ailleurs par le nez. Il a besoin de ses cheveux pour ressembler à Bonaparte – et il ne veut pas que ses cheveux tombent, comme à nous autres, pourtant bien moins âgés que lui! Son regard a des airs mystiques, étonnants de la part d'un matérialiste. Ce regard est oblique, – ce qui surprend dans un masque de Bonaparte. Le sommet du crâne est moins large que la partie basse de la face, ce qui veut dire que l'homme aime les jouissances matérielles. La bouche a ce pincement qui indique que l'homme est plus apte à la haine qu'à l'amour. Le nez est puissant et particulier. Toute la force de M. Charcot est là. Le nez romain est bien attaché et bien dessiné – c'est comme l'extrémité d'une proue de galère romaine, destinée à fendre les flots, malgré vents et marée.'

86 Charcot was often aligned with Bonaparte. This is most evident in the number of profiles of the doctor that look very similar to those of the French leader.

87 Merson, 'Salon de 1887 – II', p. 315: 'la seule variété introduite dans cette vaste uniformité'.

88 Jules Falret, *Études cliniques sur les maladies mentales et nerveuses* (Paris: Baillière, 1890), p. 502.

89 For a discussion of how Charcot's performances influenced French theatre, and of how they continue to do so today, see Showalter, *Hystories*, pp. 100–112.

90 Pierre Janet, *The Mental State of Hystericals,* trans. Caroline R. Corson (New York: Putnam, 1901), pp. 151–155. Hysteric patients had an 'extraordinary attachment to their physician. The doctor who attends them is no longer an ordinary man. He assumes a preponderant position, against which no other influence can prevail.

For him they will do everything; for they have once and for all made up their mind to obey him blindly; they think of him all the time and regulate their whole conduct after that thought. But in return they are extremely exacting; they claim him altogether, are jealous of his interest in others, make constant calls upon him, want him to stay with them, and take it really to heart if he shows the least indifference.'

91 Officially titled *Pinel, médecin en chef de la Salpêtrière en 1795* in the Salon catalogue of 1876, this painting was bought by the State and hung in the main lecture hall of the Salpêtrière. Sander Gilman refers briefly to Robert-Fleury's painting in his chapter 'The Image of the Hysteric', in Gilman *et al.*, *Hysteria beyond Freud*, p. 345.

92 Jane Kromm, '"Marianne" and the Madwoman', *Art Journal*, 46:4 (1987), 299–304.

93 Kromm claims that this is a Marianne figure because the woman is shown with dark hair, in a peasant dress and has a bare chest. Kromm, '"Marianne" and the Madwoman', p. 300.

94 Weisberg suggests that this image is as much about the unchaining of patients as it is about medical separation from the church. Weisberg, 'The Representation of Doctors at Work in Salon Art of the Early Third Republic in France', p. 231.

95 Archives Nationales, côte F/21*2059.

96 The connection between these two paintings has also been made by Thuillier, *Monsieur Charcot de la Salpêtrière,* pp. 225–226, and Signoret, '*Une leçon clinque à la Salpêtrière* (1887) par André Brouillet', p. 690.

97 In his discussion of spectacle and modern culture, Jonathan Crary draws connections between the spectacle of colonised people on display at the Exposition Universelle of 1889 and the display of hypnotised bodies at the First International Congress on Hypnosis, which was occurring simultaneously. He points out that both were linked by their understood connections to child-like and regressive states, which were seen as fundamentally opposed to Western rationalism. Crary, *Suspensions of Perception: Attention, Spectacle and Modern Culture,* pp. 230–236.

98 Ollendorf, *Salon de 1887*, pp. 63–66: 'ce ne sont pas des personnages vivants et habillés que nous avons devant nous: ce sont des vêtements enveloppant des formes étrangères à l'anatomie et proches parents des mannequins de l'atelier'.

99 Mantz, 'Le Salon – I', n.p. 'Nous devons dire toutefois que M. Brouillet, pressé sans doute par la fatalité des dates, ne semble pas avoir eu la possibilité et le loisir d'étudier à fond la physionomie particulière de ses modèles. Quelques-uns ne sont pas d'une ressemblance bien avérée … Parfois le pinceau a couru trop vite, et mon sentiment est que certains portraits, ceux auxquels s'intéressera l'avenir, devraient être repris et soulignés par quelques accents plus vrais.'

100 Mantz, 'Le Salon – I', n.p.

101 Ollendorf, *Salon de 1887*, p. 63. 'Le fond de la toile et toute la partie gauche sont remplis par des personnages si bien groupés, qu'on croirait que l'artiste, passant un jour dans la salle de l'illustre practicien, a quitté l'hôpital emportant avec lui une précieuse photographie instantanée due sans doute à la bienveillance de l'habile chef des travaux artistiques de la Salpêtrière'.

102 Fernand Levillain, 'Charcot et l'école de la Salpêtrière', *Revue encyclopéeique*, 78:4 (1891), 113. 'L'artiste a copié sans modifications l'épreuve qu'avait faite M. Londe, l'habile directeur du service photographique de la Salpêtrière'.

103 Charles Ponsonhailhe, 'Le Salon', *L'Artiste* (July 1887), 48–49. '*Une leçon clinique à la Salpêtrière* m'est gâtée par sa ressemblance avec une grande photographie peinte, la composition est médiocre, beaucoup de personnages sont collés les uns aux autres'.

104 Gaston Tissandier, *La Photographie* (Paris: Hachette, 1882), p. 523. 'Mais on ne peut nier que l'appareil photographique manœuvré par un opérateur ayant tout à la fois l'adresse du physicien et le goût du peintre, donne naissance à des épreuves marquées au sceau de l'art'.

105 For a history of Londe's technological contributions to photography, see Denis Bernard and André Gunthert, *L'Instant rêvé: Albert Londe* (Nîmes: J. Chambon, 1993).

106 For interesting studies on the relationship between art, science, and photography, and the influence of Londe and Richer on this work, see 'Mutations de l'académie par la photographie scientifique', in Sylvie Aubenas, *L'art du nu au XIXe siècle: le photographe et son modèle* (Paris: Hazan: Bibliothèque nationale de France, 1997), pp. 152–183.

107 Alan Sekula shows that photography appeared to fulfil the Enlightenment desire for a universal language. He argues that the mimetic language of the camera provided a 'truth that could be uttered in the universal abstract language of mathematics'. Alan Sekula, 'The Body and the Archive', in Richard Bolton (ed.), *The Contest of Meaning* (Cambridge, MA: MIT Press, 1989), p. 352.

108 M. Janssen, *Congrès international de photographie* (Paris: Imprimerie Nationale, 1889), p. 6. 'Messieurs, l'art photographique, malgré … l'admirable ensemble de méthodes dont il s'est enrichi, attend encore ses bases scientifiques. Aussi devons-nous nous efforcer de lui donner et de lui faire prendre son rang parmi les sciences.'

109 Burais, 'Applications de la photographie à la médecine', p. 2. 'La Photographie permet de simplifier les choses. Entre des mains expérimentées, la reproduction photographique arrive à être d'une perfection si grande que, dans nombre de cas, le diagnostic s'impose à la vue de l'épreuve, et qu'une notice de quelques lignes accompagnant la planche suffit où quatre pages de texte pénible à lire n'eussent donné qu'une idée approximative de ce que l'auteur voulait décrire.'

110 French critics described James Tissot's realism as literal and 'English'. For a brief account of the traits of English realism from a French perspective, see Larousse, *Grand Dictionnaire universel du XIXe siècle*, p. 754.

111 Bourneville and Regnard, *Iconographie photographique de la Salpêtrière* (1878), p. II: 'garanties de véracité inhérentes à la photographie'.

112 Erin O'Connor, 'Camera Medica: Towards a Morbid History of Photography', *History of Photography*, 23:3 (1999), 232–233.

113 For a discussion of the relationship between portraiture and medical specimens, see Ruiz-Gómez, 'The "Scientific Artworks" of Doctor Paul Richer', p. 9; and Mechthild Fend, 'Portraying Skin Disease: Robert Carswell's Dermatological

Watercolours', in Kevin Siena and Jonathan Reinarz (eds), *A Medical History of Skin* (London: Pickering and Chatto, 2013), pp. 147–164.

114 Bourneville and Regnard, *Iconographie photographique de la Salpêtrière* (1879), p. 7. 'W … est grande (1m ,64) … elle est blonde, avec un teint lymphatique. La peau est blanche. Les seins sont très volumineux … Son intelligence atteint à peine la moyenne. La mémoire est assez bonne … Son regard est brillant: la vue et le contact des hommes produisent chez elle une espèce d'excitation particulière.'

115 Londe, *La Photographie médicale*, p. 90. 'Les hystériques ont été amenées devant l'appareil sous le prétexte de faire faire leur portrait. A ce moment, un coup de gong a été donné et elles sont toutes tombées en catalepsie'.

116 Didi-Huberman, *Invention of Hysteria*, p. 126.

117 Bourneville and Regnard, *Iconographie photographique de la Salpêtrière* (1877), pp. 16–17. 'Les attaques, dans ce cas, offrent des formes assez nombreuses et qu'il serait bien difficile de décrire clairement et d'une manière très exacte, si nous nous aidions des figures et des planches. Bien que les unes et les autres soient en partie connues, nous les produirons afin de mieux réaliser le but que nous poursuivons, à savoir la représentation fidèle des différentes phases des attaques convulsives.' (The attacks, in this case, occur in many different manifestations, and it would be extremely difficult to describe them clearly and precisely without the aid of drawings and photographs. Although both of these are to some extent familiar, we will produce them to further our goal of providing a faithful representation of the different phases of convulsive attacks.)

118 For an analysis of hysterical hands, see Natasha Ruiz-Gómez, 'A hysterical reading of Rodin's *Gates of Hell*', *Art History*, 36:5 (2013), 1009–1010.

119 Pierre Janet, *Psychological Healing: A Historical-Clinical Study II* (New York: The Macmillan Company, 1925), pp. 712–714.

120 Didi-Huberman, *Invention of Hysteria*, pp. 123–126.

121 For a discussion of nineteenth-century casts, see Papet, Feeke *et al.*, *À fleur de peau – Le moulage sur nature au XIX*[e] *siècle.*

122 Claretie, *Les Amours d'un interne,* p. 112. 'Un atelier bizarre, sentant l'amphithéâtre et le musée de médecine, où des débris humains traînaient à côté de têtes de criminels, moulées sur nature après échafaud. Rez-de-chaussée singulier où des copies de la Vénus de Milo et des captifs de Michel-Ange faisaient comme des anti-thèses consolantes aux difformités atroces que le mouleur conservait ou modelait pour les vitrines de l'Hôpital'.

123 Maurice Guillemot, 'À la Salpêtrière II', *Paris illustré* (1 October 1887), 371. 'Une vitrine, qui tient tout le milieu de la pièce, retient l'attention; elle contient, étendu sur le dos, le moulage sur nature du corps entier d'une hystérique morte à la Salpêtrière, hideuse de réalisme, de misère, avec sa maigreur, ses jambes torses, ses épaules déformées, son buste raviné, son ventre sarclé du côté, les os crevant la chair'.

124 For a discussion of the public display of dead bodies in Paris, see Schwartz, *Spectacular Realities*, pp. 45–88.

125 Charcot and Pierre Marie Janet, *Dictionary of Psychological Medicine* (London, 1892), p. 629.

126 Javel, 'Le Salon', n.p. 'Il semble qu'on la voit trembler et frémir, cette malheureuse jeune femme dont les yeux à demi-clos ont, singulière ironie, conservé quelque chose de souriant'.

127 Bourneville and Regnard, *Iconographie photographique de la Salpêtrière* (1879), p. 58.

128 Jean-Martin Charcot, *Leçon du mardi* (Paris: Bureaux du Progrès Médical, 1887–88), as translated in Didi-Huberman, *Invention of Hysteria*, p. 29.

129 For a discussion of hysterics' eyesight, see Didi-Huberman, *Invention of Hysteria*, pp. 129–135.

130 Londe, *La Photographie médicale* (Paris: Gauthier-Villars et fils, 1893), p. 317. 'Ces appareils ont le grave inconvénient de donner aux modèles des poses raides et empruntées. En Médecine, il faut éviter ce subterfuge d'une manière absolue, car, outres modifications de la forme, on rencontre souvent des attitudes particulières qui ont été imprimées au malade par l'affection dont il est atteint. Ces attitudes ont une grande valeur au point de vue du diagnostic, et la représentation doit en être faite d'une manière rigoureuse.'

131 Other images from this series suggest that Augustine was photographed sitting on a chair. Importantly, all signs of the chair are cropped out of the image, thus making it look like the photographs are of hysterical women in bed.

132 For a discussion of Londe's camera, see Albert Londe, 'La photographie dans les sciences médicales', *La Nature*, 21:2 (1893), 370–374.

133 Londe, *La Photographie médicale*, p. 68. 'Suivant les cas, on prendra des épreuves de face, de dos, de trois quarts, de profil; debout ou assis. C'est au médecin qu'il appartiendra d'indiquer les positions dans lesquelles le sujet devra être reproduit.'

134 Londe, *La Photographie médicale*, p. 332. 'Il est nécessaire d'obtenir des épreuves d'un format convenable pour être étudiées par le médecin'.

135 Javel, 'Le Salon', n.p. 'souligne, d'un geste très naturel de la main droite, le raisonnement qu'il est en train de développer, tandis que, de la main gauche, il tient l'un des bras du sujet, une jeune hystérique soutenue par un interne'.

136 Devillers, 'Salon de Paris', p. 234. 'Soutenant d'un bras une femme hypnotisée'.

137 Georges Gilles de la Tourette, as cited in Martha Noel Evans, *Fits and Starts: A Genealogy of Hysteria in Modern France* (Ithaca, NY: Cornell University Press, 1991), p. 37.

138 Bronfen, *The Knotted Subject*, p. 175.

139 Meige, 'Charcot Artiste', p. 493. 'Il n'en fallut pas d'avantage pour qu'on traitât d'exhibitions théâtrales les séances qu'il consacra à l'étude des manifestations de la grande hystérie'.

140 Platel, *Les Hommes de mon temps*, p. 383. 'Pratiqua en grand le cabotinage scien--tifique'.

141 Charcot, 'Leçons sur la métallothérapie et l'hypnotisme', in *Œuvres complètes*, IX, p. 443, as translated in Didi-Huberman, *Invention of Hysteria*, appendix 17, p. 294.

142 Cartaz, 'Du somnambulisme et du magnétisme à propos du cours du Dr Charcot à la Salpêtrière', p. 105. 'Disons d'abord que cet état léthargique, somnambulique, si l'on veut, cesse aussi subitement qu'il est apparu et cela avec la plus grand facilité; il suffit, par exemple, de souffler sur le visage du sujet. La léthargie s'efface, il y a

une apparence de confusion légère et la malade sort de son rêve sans le moindre souvenir de ce qui s'est passé.'

143 Charcot, *Œuvres complètes IX*, p. 443.
144 Showalter, *Hystories*, p. 35.
145 For a discussion of Charcot's approach to hypnosis, see Andreas Mayer, *Sites of the Unconscious: Hypnosis and the Emergence of the Psychoanalytic Setting* (Chicago: University of Chicago Press, 2013); Didi-Huberman, *Invention of Hysteria*, pp. 184–185; and Derek Forrest, *Hypnotism: A History* (London: Penguin, 2000), pp. 213–253.
146 Forrest, *Hypnotism*, p. 228.
147 Edgar Berillon, *Revue de l'hypnotisme expérimentale et thérapeutique* (Paris: Redaction, 1887), introduction: 'L'hypnotisme est à l'ordre du jour. Son étude est devenue scientifique.'
148 See Silverman, *Art Nouveau in Fin-de-Siècle France*, pp. 78–91 for a discussion of how hypnosis infiltrated various parts of nineteenth-century life.
149 Bourneville and Regnard, 'Les phénomènes d'hypnotisme', *La Nature*, 9:2 (1881), 542.
150 Emmanuel Arène, 'Chronique: de l'hypnotisme', *La République française*, 30 April 1887, p. 2. 'Troublés, agités; quelques-uns avaient l'air de souffrir beaucoup'.
151 Gilles de la Tourette, *L'Hypnotisme et les états analogues au point de vue médico-legal* (Paris: Plon, Nourrit et Cie, 1887); and J. Liégeois *De la suggestion et du somnambulisme dans les rapports avec la jurisprudence et la médecine-légale* (Paris: Doin, 1889).
152 For an account of the rivalry between the Salpêtrière and the school at Nancy, see A.R.G. Owen, *Hysteria, Hypnosis and Healing: The Work of J.M. Charcot* (London: Dobson, 1971), pp. 182–206; and Forrest, *Hypnotism*, pp. 228–253.
153 As cited in Alain Lellouch, *Jean Martin Charcot et les origines de la gériatrie* (Paris: Payot, 1992), p. 267. 'L'hypnotisme de la Salpêtrière est un hypnotisme de culture'.
154 De la Tourette, *L'Hypnotisme et les états analogues*, p. 203.
155 Jean-Martin Charcot, 'Accidents hystériques graves survenus chez une femme à la suite d'hypnotisations pratiquées par un magnétiseur dans une baraque de fête', *Revue de l'hypnotisme et de psychologie physiologique* (1 July 1889), 3–11.
156 'La mort de Charcot', *Journal de médecine et de chirurgie pratique* (September 1893), 642.
157 'La mort de M. le Professeur Charcot', *Revue de l'hypnotisme expérimental et thérapeutique*, 8 (1894), 34 (Salpêtrière Archives, Charcot obituaries). 'Grâce à l'autorité de sa parole, l'hypnotisme et les études qui en dérivent acquéraient immédiatement droit de cité dans la science officielle'.
158 Merson, 'Salon de 1887 – II', p. 282: 'à cette heure, est des plus actuels et des plus attrayants'.
159 'L'influence de l'aimant dans l'hypnotisme', *L'Illustration* (22 January 1887), 66–67.
160 Weisberg, 'The Representation of Doctors at Work in Salon Art of the Early Third Republic in France', p. 425.
161 Ballu, Salon de 1887', n.p. 'Rentrons à l'hôpital; ce ne sera pas pour longtemps, je vous assure … Que de médecine, bon Dieu! L'hypnotisme, oh, le cauchemar!'

162 Martin, *Guide du visiteur – la peinture et la sculpture au Salon de* 1887, p. 34. 'Nous approuvons peu, pour notre part, la tendance des artistes à reproduire ces pénibles scènes chirurgicales; voir souffrir, opérer, hypnotiser une femme au milieu d'une quinzaine de messieurs en vêtements noirs est un spectacle qui, malgré tout le talent déployé, sera toujours d'un médiocre intérêt'.

163 Martin, *Guide du visiteur – la peinture et la sculpture au Salon de 1887*, pp. 41–42. 'Nous fuyons vite vers des plus modestes'.

164 Platel, *Les Hommes de mon temps*, p. 383. 'Étonna l'homme. Il effraya la femme'.

165 Bourneville and Regnard, *Iconographie photographique de la Salpêtrière* (1881), p. 408. 'Il est peu de femmes que l'on ne puisse hypnotiser'.

166 Bourneville and Regnard, 'Les phénomènes d'hypnotisme', p. 408. 'Ira plus vite et plus sûrement en prenant une hystérique. De celles-là, les jeunes seront préférables, elles sont plus sensibles, plus impressionnables.'

167 Arène, 'Chronique: de l'hypnotisme', p. 2.

168 'Ce que l'hypnotisme peut faire', *Le Courrier français* (29 May 1887), 6–7.

169 For an overview of this work, see Michelle Facos, 'Richard Bergh: Natural Science and National Art in Sweden', *Interdisciplinary Science Reviews*, 35 (2010), 39–50. Facos points out that Bergh was attempting to capture the moment of becoming unconscious.

170 Ponsonailhe, 'Le Salon', pp. 48–49. 'Une expérience entre intimes'.

171 This is one of Didi-Huberman's main points. For an account of the varying views on the role of patient and doctor in performances at the Salpêtrière, see Bronfen, *The Knotted Subject*, particularly Chapter 4, 'Jean-Martin Charcot's Vampires', pp. 174–239.

172 Gilman, 'The Image of the Hysteric', in Gilman *et al.*, *Hysteria Beyond Freud.* Although I agree with Gilman's argument, I do not see, as Gilman does, that the representation of Wittman in Brouillet's painting is looking at the Richer drawing in order to learn how to perform. Wittman's eyes are closed, or partially so, and her head is turned away from Richer's drawing.

173 Duchenne's book, *De l'électrisation localisée et de son application à la pathologie et à la thérapeutique*, first published in 1855 and re-edited and reprinted in 1862 and 1872, exemplifies the popularity of his work. For a discussion of Duchenne de Boulogne's studies and corresponding photographs, see Jean-François Debord, 'Le mécanisme de la physionomie humaine: la vie et l'œuvre de Duchenne de Boulogne', in Clair (ed.), *L'Âme au corps: arts et sciences, 1793–1993*, pp. 412–419.

174 Duchenne de Boulogne as cited in Debord, 'Le mécanisme de la physionomie humaine', pp. 416–419. 'Les maîtres de l'Art n'ont pas toujours su trouver les lignes fondamentales … après les avoir instinctivement dessinées avec une grande vérité dans une esquisse, ils les ont perdues en finissant leur travail sans pouvoir les retrouver. L'électrisation localisée … fait connaître la cause physique de tous ces plis, de toutes ces rides en provoquant la contraction des muscles partiellement ou par groupes … permet de formuler à coup sûr les règles qui doivent guider l'artiste.'

175 Duchenne de Boulogne as cited in Debord, 'Le mécanisme de la physionomie humaine', p. 416. 'Armé de rhéophores, on pourrait, comme la nature elle-

même, peindre sur le visage de l'homme les lignes expressives des émotions de l'âme'.

176 Doctor Z, 'L'électricité à la Salpêtrière', *La Nature* 13 (17 October 1885), 305–306.

177 Bourneville and Regnard, *Iconographie photographique de la Salpêtrière* (1879), p. 15. 'W … a été électrisée: le délire n'en a pas moins continué. Alimentation par la sonde œsophagienne. Elle a vomi une partie des liquides ingérés. Insomnie; bavardage incessant. On l'a placée sur la chaise-percée, elle a uriné.'

178 Doctor Z., 'L'électricité à la Salpêtrière', 305.

179 The article was published in *Le Monde illustré*, 7 August 1887.

180 Forrest suggests that Charcot didn't turn to hypnosis as a therapeutic method because he was sceptical about psychological methods that he believed lacked precision and clarity. Forrest, *Hypnotism*, p. 227.

181 Charcot referred to the machine as a 'coup de pinceaux', which Didi-Huberman has translated to 'electric paintbrush'. For a further discussion of this tool, see Didi-Huberman, *Invention of Hysteria*, pp. 199–203.

182 Guillemot, 'A la Salpêtrière II', p. 371. 'Bien que fort intéressant, le cabinet du docteur Charcot laisse une impression pénible, comme le souvenir d'un musée des horreurs, d'une réunion de gnomes, de monstres, d'êtres fantastiques, chimériques, de visions de cauchemars empruntées aux cycles infernaux du Dante ou à l'œuvre macabre de Poe. Tristes archives de l'humanité souffrante, horrible ossuaire de l'hospice et de la clinique.'

183 In 1908, Spitzner produced a wax model of the right section of Brouillet's *Une leçon clinique*.

184 This reading is indebted to Crary's 'Géricault, the Panorama, and Sites of Reality in the Early Nineteenth Century', 5–25.

Conclusion

The 1886 and 1887 Salon paintings of Pasteur, Péan, and Charcot were once again on display to thousands of visitors during the 1889 Exposition Universelle in Paris. They were hung in different buildings and rooms – according to subject matter and the artists' status and nationality – and were used to exhibit France's international authority in art, medicine, and science. In the large illustrated catalogue of the exhibition that reproduced prints of the works by Bonnat, Gervex, and Brouillet, the art critic William Walton argued that the main motivation behind these paintings was to satisfy contemporary human interest, to show the attitudes of intelligent men confronting 'old problems by new methods', and to present 'the mere recording of new triumphs of science.' He wrote that it was:

> the intelligent presentation of these unpictorial things that gives the modern works a greater general interest than mere good paintings alone would do, – suffering humanity (potential and actual) stops to regard these scenes with a quickness of apprehension that would not be evoked by any excellence of *facture*.[1]

For Walton, subject matter was more significant than painterly prowess. As he pointed out, the works' lack of admirable facture was key to their understanding. Facture – as visible evidence of painterly touch and subjectivity – seemed to have no place in depictions of clinics or operating rooms.

The Face of Medicine has demonstrated how the scientific and medical personae and narratives depicted in these artworks shaped artistic decisions regarding style, composition, genre, and medium. Like objects in medical museums, they required 'objective' aesthetic strategies. Despite this desire for neutrality, representations of bodies in artistic and medical spheres entertained, educated, repulsed, and delighted viewers – be they Salon paintings, photographic portraits, or medical wax models. These images and objects did not always fit easily into the seemingly separate categories of art and science, subjectivity and objectivity, or irrationality and rationality. In fact, as I have argued, they embody the complexities of realism, and point to the contradictory claims to truth made by particular occupations, discourses, styles, histories, and artistic practices. Although Walton argued that these 'most carefully and judiciously rendered' works were 'conceived soberly – without any undue straining for effect', the 1886 and 1887 Salon criticism shows that pleasure and fear were felt when viewing paintings with contemporary scientific and medical themes, especially when spectacular elements, such as naked female flesh or exotic foreign patients, took centre stage.[2]

Artists and doctors worked together to produce images and objects that were considered as truthful as possible. Realist formal practices emerging from the art world merged with modern medicine's authoritative claim to neutrality in order to construct the 'truth' of bodies, diseases, and sexualities. The desire to represent reality and identity was at the heart of the paintings by Edelfelt, Bonnat, Gsell, Gervex, and Brouillet. It was also a primary concern of the men they portrayed, who wanted their masculinity, nationalism, social status, collectivity, and occupational skills and discoveries to be on display through the images and objects they commisioned. In order to manufacture a sense of sincerity, the Salon portraits had to appear somewhat 'unpictorial'; theatrical lighting, fantastical compositions, and blatant brushwork would have threatened the structured objectivity of the clinical scenes and men portrayed. The paintings, however, also had to delight viewers, draw the attention of Salon critics, and encourage future commissions. Similarly, the images and objects commissioned by Pasteur, Péan, and Charcot required learned artistic skills, expert input, and often 'mechanically objective' media and technologies to produce ostensibly trustworthy educational tools, scientific proof, and historical documents. Yet, as shown in this study, they too were marked by individual ambition, competitive cultures, and subjective desires.

In the medically themed Salon review that began this book, Chamillac addresses the close but often contradictory relationship between art, medicine, and science, claiming that despite the pain provoked by the 'pictorial virus', one cannot live without it:

> It is very good that annually the harsh vaccine from the Palais de l'Industrie – terrible but indispensable – anaesthetises us with one quick shot to the eyes and brain; without it, what would become of us miserable inhabitants of the Paintrapole without the perpetual avalanche of the pictorial virus scattered in our atmosphere?[3]

Chamillac's review unites the themes of vaccination, anaesthetics, and madness, positioning the Salon, like the Pasteur Institute, the Hôpital Saint-Louis, and the Hôpital de la Salpêtrière, as sites where art and scientific medicine converged. While medicine drew upon artistic conventions in order to depict bodies and sexualities as healthy or sick, Chamillac used scientific medical themes as a rhetorical filter through which modern paintings could be understood. Paintings anaesthetised and vaccinated viewers; they were indispensible yet addictive; they surrounded and infected. The contradictory metaphor of vaccination – one must be infected in order to be cured – demonstrates the conflicting and multifaceted attitudes nineteenth-century society had towards scientific medicine, its practitioners, and its visual culture. Science and medicine were integral to a sucessful modern nation – they contributed to economic stability, military strength, colonial power, and the future health of populations, but they also contained elements that threatened bodily and social thresholds, expectations, and relationships.

The paintings of Pasteur, Péan, and Charcot, along with the other depictions of bodies in these men's collections, forged boundaries of difference between sickness and health, femininity and masculinity, reason and insanity, truth and deceit, reality and fiction. However, the binaries addressed in this book also point to the fluidity and contradictory nature of mimetic representations, and show how processes of inclusion and exclusion were integral to the visualisation of sexualities, histories, identities, realities, and physical states. Although medical men and artists emphasised the objectivity and reason of their realistic objects, whether in paint, wax, photography, or print, pleasure and subjectivity were a vital component of creating and collecting bodies.

Notes

1 Walton, *Chefs-d'œuvre de l'exposition universelle de Paris, 1889*, p. 88.
2 Walton, *Chefs-d'œuvre de l'exposition universelle de Paris, 1889*, p. 88.
3 Chamillac, 'Le Virus pictural', p. 350. 'Il est vraiment heureux qu'annuellement la rude vaccine du Palais de l'Industrie terrible, mais indispensable, nous anesthésie d'un seul coup les yeux et le crâne; sans cela, que deviendrions-nous, misérable habitants de la Peintrapole, sans la perpétuelle avalanche du virus pictural éparpillé dans notre atmosphere?'

Select bibliography

Ackerknecht, Erwin Heinz. *Medicine at the Paris Hospital, 1794–1848*. Baltimore, MD: Johns Hopkins Press, 1967.

Adamson, Natalie and Toby Norris (eds). *Academics, Pompiers, Official Artists and the Arrière-garde: Defining Modern and Traditional in France, 1900–1960*. Newcastle-upon-Tyne: Cambridge Scholars Publishing, 2009.

Agulhon, Maurice. *Marianne into Battle: Republican Imagery and Symbolism in France 1789–1880*. London: Cambridge University Press, 1981.

Aisenberg, Andrew Robert. *Contagion: Disease, Government, and the 'Social Question' in Nineteenth-Century France*. Stanford, CA: Stanford University Press, 1999.

Alberti, Samuel J.M.M. *Morbid Curiosities: Medical Museums in Nineteenth-Century Britain*. Oxford: Oxford University Press, 2011.

Alberti, Samuel J.M.M. and Elizabeth Hallam (eds). *Medical Museums: Past, Present, Future*. London: Royal College of Surgeons, 2013.

Alsdorf, Bridget. *Fellow Men: Fantin-Latour and the Problem of the Group in Nineteenth-Century French Painting*. Princeton, NJ: Princeton University Press, 2012.

Aubenas, Sylvie. *L'Art du nu au XIXe siècle: le photographe et son modèle*. Paris: Hazan/Bibliothèque nationale de France, 1997.

Auerbach, Erich. *Mimesis: The Representation of Reality in Western Literature*. Translated by Willard R. Trask. Princeton, NJ: Princeton University Press, 1953.

Auerbach, Nina. *Woman and the Demon: The Life of a Victorian Myth*. Cambridge, MA: Harvard University Press, 1982.

Balducci, Temma, Heather Belnap Jensen and Pamela Warner (eds). *Interior Portraiture and Masculine Identity in France, 1789–1914*. Aldershot: Ashgate, 2011.

Bann, Stephen. *Parallel Lines: Printmakers, Painters and Photographers in Nineteenth-Century France*. New Haven, CT: Yale University Press, 2001.

Barthes, Roland. *Camera Lucida: Reflections on Photography*. Translated by Richard Howard. New York: Hill and Wang, 1981.

Barthes, Roland. *The Rustle of Language*. Translated by Richard Howard. Oxford: Basil Blackwell, 1986.

Bata, Philippe, Marie-Véronique Clin, *et al*. *André Brouillet 1857–1914*. Poitiers: Musée de la ville de Poitiers, 2000.

Beizer, Janet. *Ventriloquized Bodies: Narratives of Hysteria in Nineteenth-Century France*. Ithaca, NY: Cornell University Press, 1994.

Bernard, Denis and Andre Gunthert. *L'Instant rêvé: Albert Londe*. Nîmes: J. Chambon, 1993.

Bernheimer, Charles. *Figures of Ill Repute: Representing Prostitution in Nineteenth-Century France*. Cambridge, MA: Harvard University Press, 1989.

Bernheimer, Charles and Claire Kahane (eds). *In Dora's Case: Freud, Hysteria, Feminism*. London: Virago, 1985.

Brauer, Fae and Barbara Larson (eds). *The Art of Evolution: Darwin, Darwinism, and Visual Culture*. Hanover, NH: University Press of New England, 2009.

Braun, Marta and Elizabeth Whitcombe. 'Marey, Muybridge, and Londe: The Photography of Pathological Locomotion', *History of Photography*, 23:3 (1999), 218–224.

Brilliant, Richard. *Portraiture*. London: Reaktion Books, 1991.

Bronfen, Elisabeth. *Over Her Dead Body: Death, Femininity and the Aesthetic*. Manchester: Manchester University Press, 1992.

Bronfen, Elisabeth. *The Knotted Subject: Hysteria and Its Discontents*. Princeton, NJ: Princeton University Press, 1998.

Brooks, Peter. *Body Work: Objects of Desire in Modern Narrative*. Cambridge, MA: Harvard University Press, 1993.

Brooks, Peter. *Realist Vision*. New Haven, CT: Yale University Press, 2005.

Bryson, Norman, Michael Ann Holly and Keith Moxey (eds). *Visual Theory: Painting and Interpretation*. Cambridge: Polity/Blackwell, 1991.

Burgess, R. *Portraits of Doctors and Scientists in the Wellcome Institute of the History of Medicine*. London: Wellcome Institute of the History of Medicine, 1972.

Butler, Judith. *Gender Trouble: Feminism and the Subversion of Identity*. New York: Routledge, 1989.

Butler, Judith. *Bodies That Matter: On the Discursive Limits of 'Sex'*. New York: Routledge, 1993.

Bynum, W.F. *Science and the Practice of Medicine in the Nineteenth Century*. Cambridge: Cambridge University Press, 1994.

Callebat, Louis (ed.). *Histoire du médecin*. Paris: Flammarion, 1999.

Callen, Anthea. *The Spectacular Body: Science, Method and Meaning in the Work of Degas*. New Haven, CT: Yale University Press, 1995.

Callen, Anthea. 'The Body and Difference: Anatomy Training at the École des Beaux-Arts in the Later Nineteenth Century', *Art History*, 20:1 (March 1997), 23–60.

Callen, Anthea. 'Masculinity and Muscularity: Dr Paul Richer and Modern Manhood', *Paragraph*, 16:1 (July 2003), 17–41.

Callen, Anthea. 'Doubles and Desire: Anatomies of Masculinity in the Later Nineteenth Century', *Art History*, 26:5 (November 2003), 669–699.

Camille, Michael and Adrian Rifkin (eds). *Other Objects of Desire: Collectors and Collecting Queerly*. Oxford: Blackwell, 2001.

Canchy, Jean-François de (ed.). *Henri Gervex, 1852–1929*. Paris: Paris-Musées, 1992.

Cartwright, Lisa. *Screening the Body: Tracing Medicine's Visual Culture*. Minneapolis, MN: University of Minnesota Press, 1995.

Celebonovic, Aleksa. *The Heyday of Salon Painting: Masterpieces of Bourgeois Realism*. Translated by Peter Willis. London: Thames and Hudson, 1974.

Challons-Lipton, Siulolovao. *The Scandinavian Pupils of the Atelier Bonnat, 1867–1894*. Lewiston, NY: Edwin Mellen Press, 2001.

Chodorow, Nancy. *Femininities, Masculinities, Sexualities: Freud and Beyond*. Cambridge: Cambridge University Press, 1991.

Chu, Petra ten-Doesschate. *French Realism and the Dutch Masters: The Influence of Dutch Seventeenth-Century Painting on the Development of French Painting between 1830 and 1870*. Utrecht: Haentjens Dekker & Gumbert, 1974.

Clair, Jean (ed.). *L'Âme au corps: arts et sciences 1793–1993*. Paris: Réunion des musées nationaux, 1993.

Clark, T.J. *Image of the People: Gustave Courbet and the 1848 Revolution*. London: Thames and Hudson, 1973.

Clark, T.J. *The Painting of Modern Life: Paris in the Art of Manet and His Followers*. Princeton, NJ: Princeton University Press, 1984.

Clayson, Hollis. *Painted Love: Prostitution in French Art of the Impressionist Era*. Los Angeles, CA: Getty Publications, 2003.

Clin, Marie-Véronique. *Le Musée d'histoire de la médecine de Paris*. Paris: Musée d'histoire de la médecine de Paris, 1994.

Comar, Philippe (ed.). *Figures du corps: une leçon d'anatomie à l'École des Beaux-Arts*. Paris: Beaux-Arts de Paris les éditions, 2008.

Connell, R.W. *Masculinities*. Berkeley, CA: University of California Press, 2005.

Connell, R.W. and James W. Messerschmidt. 'Hegemonic Masculinity: Rethinking the Concept', *Gender and Society*, 19:6 (December 2005), 829–859.

Corbin, Alain. *Women for Hire: Prostitution and Sexuality in France after 1850*. Translated by Anne Sheridan. Cambridge, MA: Harvard University Press, 1990.

Crary, Jonathan. *Techniques of the Observer: On Vision and Modernity in the Nineteenth Century*. Cambridge, MA: MIT Press, 1990.

Crary, Jonathan. *Suspensions of Perception: Attention, Spectacle and Modern Culture*. Cambridge, MA: MIT Press, 1999.

Crary, Jonathan. 'Géricault, the Panorama, and Sites of Reality in the Early Nineteenth Century', *Grey Room*, 9 (2002), 5–25.

Crissey, John Thorne, Lawrence Charles Parish, and Karl Holubar. *Historical Atlas of Dermatology and Dermatologists*. Carnforth: Parthenon, 2001.

Cunningham, Andrew and Perry Williams (eds). *The Laboratory Revolution in Medicine*. Cambridge: Cambridge University Press, 1992.

Curtin, Philip D. *Disease and Empire: The Health of European Troops in the Conquest of Africa*. Cambridge: Cambridge University Press, 1998.

Curtin, Philip D. *Death by Migration: Europe's Encounter with the Tropical World in the Nineteenth Century*. Cambridge: Cambridge University Press, 1989.

Dahlberg, Laurie. *Victor Regnault and the Advance of Photography: the Art of Avoiding Errors*. Princeton, NJ: Princeton University Press, 2004.

Darmon, Pierre. *Le Médecin parisien en 1900: la vie quotidienne*. Paris: Hachette littératures, 2003.

Daston, Lorraine and Peter Galison. *Objectivity*. New York: Zone Books, 2007.

Daston, Lorraine and H. Otto Sibum. 'Scientific Personae', *Science in Context*, 16:1–2 (2003), 1–8.

Dawkins, Heather. *The Nude in French Art and Culture, 1870–1910*. Cambridge: Cambridge University Press, 2002.

Debré, Patrice. *Louis Pasteur*. Paris: Flammarion, 1994.

Delaunay, Albert and Hilda Benichou. *Pasteur Institute: the Museum, the Main Library, the Funeral Chapel*. Paris: Institute Pasteur, 1972.

De Witt, Anne. *Moral Authority: Men of Science and the Victorian Novel*. Cambridge: Cambridge University Press, 2013.

Didi-Huberman, Georges. 'Wax Flesh, Vicious Circles', in Petra Lamers-Schütz and Yvonne Havertz (eds), *Encyclopaedia Anatomica – A Complete Collection of Anatomical Waxes*. Köln: Taschen, 1999, pp. 64–74.

Didi-Huberman, Georges. *Invention of Hysteria: Charcot and the Photographic Iconography of the Salpêtrière*. Translated by Alisa Hartz. Cambridge, MA: MIT Press, 2003.

Didi-Huberman, Georges. *Confronting Images: Questioning the Ends of a Certain History of Art*. Translated by John Goodman. University Park, PA: Pennsylvania State University, 2005.

Dixon, Laurinda S. *Perilous Chastity: Women and Illness in Pre-Enlightenment Art and Medicine*. Ithaca, NY: Cornell University Press, 1995.

Downing, Lisa. *Desiring the Dead: Necrophilia and Nineteenth-Century French Literature*. Oxford: European Humanities Research Centre, 2002.

Doy, Gen. *Women and Visual Culture in Nineteenth-Century France, 1800–1852*. New York: Leicester University Press, 1998.

Dubos, René J., and Thomas D. Brock. *Pasteur and Modern Science*. Madison, WI: Science Tech Publishers, 1988.

Ducourau, Vincent. *Léon Bonnat, 1833–1922: portraits d'apogée*. Bayonne: Musée Bonnat, 1998.

Dufour, Philippe. *Le Réalisme: de Balzac à Proust*. Paris: Presses universitaires de France, 1998.

Elkins, James. *On Pictures and the Words That Fail Them*. Cambridge: Cambridge University Press, 1998.

Elkins, James. *Pictures of the Body: Pain and Metamorphosis*. Stanford, CA: Stanford University Press, 1999.

Ellenbogen, Josh. *Reasoned and Unreasoned Images: the Photography of Bertillon, Galton, and Marey*. University Park, PA: Pennsylvania State University Press, 2012.

Ellis, Jack D. *The Physician-Legislators of France: Medicine and Politics in the Early Third Republic, 1870–1914*. Cambridge: Cambridge University Press, 1990.

Elsner, John and Roger Cardinal (eds). *The Cultures of Collecting*. London: Reaktion Books, 1993.

Emery, Elizabeth. *Photojournalism and the Origins of the French Writer House Museum (1881–1914)*. Aldershot: Ashgate, 2012.

English, Donald E. *Political Uses of Photography in the Third French Republic, 1871–1914*. Ann Arbor, MI: University of Michigan Press, 1984.

Evans, Martha Noel. *Fits and Starts: A Genealogy of Hysteria in Modern France*. Ithaca, NY: Cornell University Press, 1991.

Facos, Michelle. 'Richard Bergh: Natural Science and National Art in Sweden', *Interdisciplinary Science Reviews*, 35 (2010), 39–50.

Farley, John. *Bilharzia: A History of Imperial Tropical Medicine*. Cambridge: Cambridge University Press, 1990.

Fend, Mechthild. 'Bodily and Pictorial Surfaces: Skin in French Art and Medicine, 1790–1860', *Art History*, 28:3 (June 2005), 311–339.

Fend, Mechthild. 'Portraying Skin Disease: Robert Carswell's Dermatological Watercolours', in Kevin Siena and Jonathan Reinarz (eds), *A Medical History of Skin*. London: Pickering and Chatto, 2013, pp. 147–164.

Ford, Brian J. *Images of Science: A History of Scientific Illustration*. London: The British Library, 1992.

Forrest, Derek William. *Hypnotism: A History*. London: Penguin, 2000.

Christopher E. Forth and Bertrand Taithe (eds), *French Masculinities: History, Culture, and Politics*. New York: Palgrave Macmillan, 2007.

Foucault, Michel. *Naissance de la clinique*. Paris: Presses universitaires de France, 1963.

Foucault, Michel. *Madness and Civilization: A History of Insanity in the Age of Reason*. Translated by Richard Howard. London: Tavistock, 1965.

Foucault, Michel. *The History of Sexuality*. Translated by Robert Hurley. London: Penguin Books, 1990.

Fox, Robert, and George Weisz (eds). *The Organization of Science and Technology in France 1808–1914*. Cambridge: Cambridge University Press, 1980.

Freund, Gisèle. *Photography and Society*. Translated by David Godine. Boston, MA: D.R. Godine; London: Gordon Fraser Gallery, 1980.

Fried, Michael. *Realism, Writing, Disfiguration on Thomas Eakins and Stephen Crane*. Chicago: University of Chicago Press, 1987.

Fried, Michael. *Courbet's Realism*. Chicago: University of Chicago Press, 1990.

Fried, Michael. *Manet's Modernism, or, the Face of Painting in the 1860s*. Chicago: University of Chicago Press, 1996.

Fried, Michael. *Menzel's Realism: Art and Embodiment in Nineteenth-Century Berlin*. New Haven, CT: Yale University Press, 2002.

Gallagher, Catherine and Thomas Laqueur (eds). *The Making of the Modern Body: Sexuality and Society in the Nineteenth Century*. Berkeley, CA: University of California Press, 1987.

Gamwell, Lynn. *Exploring the Invisible: Art, Science and the Spiritual*. Princeton, NJ: Princeton University Press, 2000.

Garb, Tamar. *Bodies of Modernity: Figure and Flesh in Fin-de-Siècle France*. London: Thames and Hudson, 1998.

Garb, Tamar. *The Painted Face: Portraits of Women in France, 1814–1914*. New Haven, CT: Yale University Press, 2007.

Gebauer, Gunter and Christoph Wulf. *Mimesis: Culture, Art, Society*. Translated by Don Reneau. Berkeley, CA: University of California Press, 1992.

Geison, Gerald L. *The Private Science of Louis Pasteur*. Princeton, NJ: Princeton University Press, 1995.

Geison, Gerald. 'Organizations, Products, and Marketing in Pasteur's Scientific Enterprise'. *History and Philosophy of the Life Sciences*, 24:1 (2002), 37–51.

Geison, Gerald L. (ed.). *Professions and the French State, 1700–1900*. Philadelphia, PA: University of Pennsylvania Press, 1984.

Gilman, Sander L. *Seeing the Insane: A Cultural History of Madness and Art in the Western World*. New York: John Wiley & Sons, 1982.

Gilman, Sander L. *Disease and Representation: Images of Illness from Madness to Aids*. Ithaca, NY: Cornell University Press, 1987.

Gilman, Sander L. *The Case of Sigmund Freud: Medicine and Identity at the fin-de-siècle*. Baltimore, MD: Johns Hopkins University Press, 1993.

Gilman, Sander L. *Health and Illness: Images of Difference*. London: Reaktion Books, 1995.

Gilman, Sander L, Helen King, Roy Porter *et al. Hysteria Beyond Freud*. Berkeley, CA: University of California Press, 1993.

Goetz, Christopher G., Michel Bonduelle, and Toby Gelfand. *Charcot: Constructing Neurology*. Oxford: Oxford University Press, 1995.

Goldstein, Jan. *Console and Classify: The French Psychiatric Profession in the Nineteenth Century*. Cambridge: Cambridge University Press, 1987.

Goldstein, Jan. 'The Uses of Male Hysteria: Medical and Literary Discourse in Nineteenth-Century France', *Representations*, 34 (Spring 1991), 134–165.

Goodbody, Bridget L. '"The Present Opprobrium of Surgery": *The Agnew Clinic* and Nineteenth-Century Representations of Cancerous Female Breasts', *American Art* (Winter 1994), 33–51.

Goodman, Nelson. *Languages of Art: An Approach to a Theory of Symbols*. Indianapolis, IN: Bobbs-Merrill, 1968.

Green, Nicholas. *The Spectacle of Nature: Landscape and Bourgeois Culture in Nineteenth-Century France*. Manchester: Manchester University Press, 1990.

Grosz, E.A. *Volatile Bodies: Toward a Corporeal Feminism*. Bloomington, IN: Indiana University Press, 1994.

Haeger, Knut. *The Illustrated History of Surgery*. London: Harold Starke, 1989.

Hannaway, Caroline and Ann La Berge (eds). *Constructing Paris Medicine*. Amsterdam; Atlanta, GA: Rodopi, 1998.

Hansen, Bert. 'America's First Medical Breakthrough: How Popular Excitement about a French Rabies Cure in 1885 Raised New Expectations for Medical Progress', *The American Historical Review*, 103:2 (April 1998), 373–418.

Hansen, Bert. *Picturing Medical Progress from Pasteur to Polio: A History of Mass Media Images and Popular Attitudes in America*. New Brunswick, NJ: Rutgers University Press, 2009.

Hargrove, June Ellen and Neil McWilliam (eds). *Nationalism and French Visual Culture, 1870–1914*. New Haven, CT: Yale University Press, 2005.

Harrington, Anne. *Medicine, Mind, and the Double Brain: A Study in Nineteenth-Century Thought*. Princeton, NJ: Princeton University Press, 1987.

Harris, Ruth. *Murders and Madness: Medicine, Law, and Society in the Fin de Siècle*. Oxford: Clarendon, 1989.

Harsin, Jill. *Policing Prostitution: In Nineteenth-Century Paris*. Princeton, NJ: Princeton University Press, 1985.

Harsin, Jill. 'Syphilis, Wives, and Physicians: Medical Ethics and the Family in late Nineteenth-Century France', *French Historical Studies*, 16:1 (Spring 1989), 72–95.

Hawthorne, Melanie. *Rachilde and French Women's Authorship: From Decadence to Modernism*. Lincoln, NE: University of Nebraska Press, 2001.

Héran, Emmanuelle *et al. Le Dernier Portrait*. Paris: Réunion des musées nationaux, 2002.

Hildreth, Martha L. *Doctors, Bureaucrats, and Public Health in France, 1888–1902*. New York: Garland, 1987.

Hollier, Denis (ed.). *A New History of French Literature*. Cambridge, MA: Harvard University Press, 1989.

Holmes, Diana. *Rachilde: Decadence, Gender and the Woman Writer*. Oxford: Berg, 2001.

Hopwood, Nick. *Embryos in Wax: Models from the Ziegler Studio*. Cambridge: Whipple Museum of the History of Science, University of Cambridge, 2002.

Huet, Marie-Hélène. *Monstrous Imagination*. Cambridge, MA: Harvard University Press, 1993.

Hustvedt, Asti. *Medical Muses: Hysteria in Nineteenth-Century Paris*. New York: W.W. Norton & Co., 2011.

Iversen, Margaret. *Alois Riegl: Art History and Theory*. Cambridge, MA: MIT Press, 1993.

Jammes, André. 'A Glaring Act of Scientific Piracy?', in Andrea P. Belloli (ed.), *Photography: Discovery and Invention, Papers Delivered at a Symposium Celebrating the Invention of Photography*. Malibu, CA: J. Paul Gerry Museum, 1990, pp. 63–70.

Johns, Elizabeth. *Thomas Eakins: The Heroism of Modern Life*. Princeton, NJ: Princeton University Press, 1983.

Jonas, S. *Cent portraits de médecins illustres*. Paris: Masson et Cie, 1960.

Jones, Colin, and Roy Porter (eds). *Reassessing Foucault: Power, Medicine, and the Body*. London: Routledge, 1994.

Jordanova, Ludmilla. *Sexual Visions: Images of Gender in Science and Medicine between the Eighteenth and Twentieth Centuries*. Madison, WI: University of Wisconsin Press, 1989.

Jordanova, Ludmilla. *Nature Displayed: Gender, Science and Medicine 1760–1820*. London; New York: Longman, 1999.

Jordanova, Ludmilla. *Defining Features: Scientific and Medical Portraits, 1660–2000*. London: Reaktion Books, 2000.

Kahane, Claire. *Passions of the Voice: Hysteria, Narrative, and the Figure of the Speaking Woman, 1850–1915*. Baltimore, MD: Johns Hopkins University Press, 1995.

Keller, Evelyn Fox. *Reflections on Gender and Science*. New Haven, CT: Yale University Press, 1985.

Kemp, Martin and Marina Wallace. *Spectacular Bodies: The Art and Science of the Human Body from Leonardo to Now*. London: Hayward Gallery, 2000.

Kete, Kathleen. '*La Rage* and the Bourgeoisie: The Cultural Context of Rabies in the French Nineteenth Century', *Representations*, 22 (Spring 1988), 89–107.

Kirkup, John. *The Evolution of Surgical Instruments: An Illustrated History from Ancient Times to the Twentieth Century*. Novato, CA: Norman Publishers, 2003.

Knibiehler, Yvonne and Catherine Fouquet. *La Femme et les médecins: analyse historique*. Paris: Hachette, 1983.

Komesaroff, Paul A. (ed). *Troubled Bodies: Critical Perspectives on Postmodernism, Medical Ethics, and the Body*. Durham, NC: Duke University Press, 1995.

Krauss, Rosalind. 'Tracing Nadar', *October*, 5 (Summer 1978), 29–47.

Krell, Alan. 'Dirt and Desire: Troubled Waters in Realist Practice', in Richard Hobbs (ed.), *Impressions of French Modernity*. Manchester: Manchester University Press, 1998, pp. 135–147.

Kromm, Jane. '"Marianne" and the Madwoman', *Art Journal*, 46:4 (Winter 1987), 299–304.

La Berge, Ann F. *Mission and Method: The Early Nineteenth-Century French Public Health Movement*. Cambridge: Cambridge University Press, 1992.

La Berge, Ann F., and Mordechai Feingold (eds). *French Medical Culture in the Nineteenth Century*. Amsterdam and Atlanta, GA: Rodopi, 1994.

Laqueur, Thomas. *Making Sex: Body and Gender from the Greeks to Freud*. Cambridge, MA: Harvard University Press, 1990.

Larson, Barbara. 'Evolution and Degeneration in the Early World of Odilon Redon', *Nineteenth-Century Art Worldwide* 2 (Spring 2003), www.19thc-artworldwide.org, accessed 28 April 2015.

Larson, Barbara. *The Dark Side of Nature: Science, Society, and the Fantastic in the Work of Odilon Redon*. University Park, PA: Pennsylvania State University Press, 2005.

Lathers, Marie. *Bodies of Art: French Literary Realism and the Artist's Model*. Lincoln, NE: University of Nebraska Press, 2001.

Latour, Bruno. *The Pasteurization of France*. Cambridge, MA: Harvard University Press, 1988.

Latour, Bruno and Steve Woolgar. *Laboratory Life: The Construction of Scientific Facts*. Princeton, NJ: Princeton University Press, 1979.

Lehning, James R. *To Be a Citizen: The Political Culture of the Early French Third Republic*. Ithaca, NY: Cornell University Press, 2001.

Lellouch, Alain. *Jean Martin Charcot et les origines de la gériatrie*. Paris: Payot, 1992.

Lemagny, Jean-Claud and André Rouillé (eds). *A History of Photography: Social and Cultural Perspectives*. New York: Cambridge University Press, 1986.

Léonard, Jacques. *La France médicale: médecins et malades au XIXe siècle*. Paris: Gallimard/Julliard, 1978.

Levin, Miriam R. *Republican Art and Ideology in Late Nineteenth-Century France*. Ann Arbor, MI: UMI Research Press, 1986.

Levine, George (ed.). *Realism and Representation: Essays on the Problem of Realism in Relation to Science, Literature, and Culture, Science and Literature*. Madison, WI: University of Wisconsin Press, 1992.

Lorber, Judith. *Gender and the Social Construction of Illness*. Thousand Oaks, CA: Sage Publications, 1997.

Lunbeck, Elizabeth and Lorraine Daston (eds). *Histories of Scientific Observation*. Chicago: University of Chicago Press, 2010.

Lupton, Deborah. *Medicine as Culture: Illness, Disease and the Body in Western Societies*. London: Sage, 1994.

Luxenberg, Alisa. 'Léon Bonnat (1833–1922)'. PhD dissertation, New York University, 1990.
Mackaman, Douglas Peter. *Leisure Settings: Bourgeois Culture, Medicine, and the Spa in Modern France*. Chicago: University of Chicago Press, 1998.
Mainardi, Patricia. *Art and Politics of the Second Empire: The Universal Expositions of 1855 and 1867*. New Haven, CT: Yale University Press, 1987.
Mainardi, Patricia. *The End of the Salon: Art and the State in the Early Third Republic*. Cambridge: Cambridge University Press, 1993.
Majumdar, Margaret A. *Postcoloniality: The French Dimension*. New York: Berghahn Books, 2007.
Martin, Marc. *Trois siècles de publicité en France*. Preface by Jean-Noël Kapferer. Paris: Editions Odile Jacob, 1992.
Matlock, Jann. *Scenes of Seduction: Prostitution, Hysteria, and Reading Difference in Nineteenth-Century France*. New York: Columbia University Press, 1994.
Mayer, Andreas. *Sites of the Unconscious: Hypnosis and the Emergence of the Psychoanalytic Setting*. Translated by Christopher Barber. Chicago: University of Chicago Press, 2013.
Mayeur, Jean-Marie and Madeleine Rebérioux. *The Third Republic from Its Origins to the Great War, 1871–1914*. Translated by J.R. Foster. Cambridge: Cambridge University Press, 1984.
McGrath, Roberta. *Seeing Her Sex: Medical Archives and the Female Body*. Manchester: Manchester University Press, 2002.
McMillan, James F. 'Clericals, Anticlericals and the Women's Movement in France under the Third Republic', *The Historical Journal*, 24:2 (June 1981), 361–376.
McPherson, Heather. *The Modern Portrait in Nineteenth-Century France*. Cambridge: Cambridge University Press, 2001.
McQueen, Alison. *The Rise of the Cult of Rembrandt: Reinventing an Old Master in Nineteenth-Century France*. Amsterdam: Amsterdam University Press, 2003.
McQuillan, Melissa. *Impressionist Portraits*. London: Thames and Hudson, 1986.
Melberg, Arne. *Theories of Mimesis*. Cambridge: Cambridge University Press, 1995.
Micale, Mark S. 'The Salpêtrière in the Age of Charcot: An Institutional Perspective on Medical History in the Late Nineteenth Century', *Journal of Contemporary History*, 20:4 (October 1985), 703–731.
Micale, Mark S. 'Hysteria and its Historiography – A Review of Past and Present Writing', *History of Science*, 27 (1989), 223–261.
Micale, Mark S. 'Charcot and the Idea of Hysteria in the Male', *Medical History*, 34:4 (1990), 363–411.
Micale, Mark S. 'On the "Disappearance" of Hysteria: A Study in the Clinical Deconstruction of a Diagnosis', *Isis*, 84:3 (September 1993), 496–526.
Micale, Mark S. *Approaching Hysteria: Disease and Its Interpretations*. Princeton, NJ: Princeton University Press, 1995.
Micale, Mark S. (ed.). *The Mind of Modernism: Medicine, Psychology, and the Cultural Arts in Europe and America, 1880–1940*. Stanford, CA: Stanford University Press, 2004.

Micale, Mark S. and Roy Porter (eds). *Discovering the History of Psychiatry*. New York: Oxford University Press, 1994.

Monnais, Laurence. 'Preventing Medicine and "Mission Civilisatrice": Uses of the BCG Vaccine in French Colonial Vietnam between the Two World Wars', *International Journal of Asia Pacific Studies*, 2:1 (May 2006), 40–66.

Morgan, Jayne. 'Eadweard Muybridge and W.S. Playfair: an Aesthetics of Neurasthenia', *History of Photography*, 23:3 (Autumn 1999), 225–231.

Moulin, Anne Marie. 'Patriarchal Science: The Network of the Overseas Pasteur Institute', in Patrick Petitjean, Catherine Jami, and Anne Marie Moulin (eds), *Science and Empires: Historical Studies about Scientific Development and European Expansion*. Dordrecht: Kluwer Academic Publishers, 1992, pp. 307–322.

Mulvey, Laura. *Visual and Other Pleasures*. Bloomington, IN: Indiana University Press, 1988.

Murray, Gale. *Toulouse-Lautrec: The Formative Years 1878–1891*. Oxford: Clarendon Press, 1991.

Nardin, Anne, Françoise Salaün Ramalho and Hélène Couot. *'De l'audace, encore de l'audace, toujours de l'audace': La chirurgie hospitalière à Paris à la fin du XIXe siècle à travers une acquisition*. Paris: Assistance Publique – Hôpitaux de Paris, 2000.

Nead, Lynda. *The Female Nude: Art, Obscenity and Sexuality*. London: Routledge, 1992.

Nicole-Genty, Geneviève, M. Chapuis, J. Chapuis *et al. Les Premières Femmes médecins en France*. Paris: Académie national médecin, 1975.

Nochlin, Linda. *Realism*. Harmondsworth: Penguin Books, 1971.

Nochlin, Linda. 'Courbet's "L'origine du monde": the Origin without an Original', *October*, 37 (Summer 1986), 76–86.

Nochlin, Linda. *Women, Art, and Power: And Other Essays*. New York: Harper & Row, 1988.

Nord, Philip. 'The Welfare State in France, 1870–1914', *French Historical Studies*, 18:3 (Spring 1994), 821–838.

Nord, Philip. *The Republican Moment: Struggles for Democracy in Nineteenth-Century France*. Cambridge, MA: Harvard University Press, 1995.

Nye, Robert A. *Crime, Madness, and Politics in Modern France: The Medical Concept of National Decline*. Princeton, NJ: Princeton University Press, 1984.

Nye, Robert. 'Honor, Impotence, and Male Sexuality in Nineteenth-Century French Medicine', *French Historical Studies*, 16 (Spring 1989), 48–71.

Nye, Robert A. *Masculinity and Male Codes of Honor in Modern France*. New York: Oxford University Press, 1993.

Nye, Robert A. 'Medicine and Science as Masculine "Fields of Honor"', *Osiris*, 2:12 (1997), 60–79.

O'Connor, Erin. 'Camera Medica: Towards a Morbid History of Photography', *History of Photography*, 23:3 (Autumn 1999), 232–244.

Offen, Karen. 'Depopulation, Nationalism, and Feminism in Fin-de-Siècle France', *The American Historical Review*, 89:3 (June 1984), 648–676.

Olin, Margaret. *Forms of Representation in Alois Riegl's Theory of Art*. University Park, PA: Pennsylvania State University Press, 1992.

Oppenheimer, Margaret. 'The Charming Spectacle of the Cadaver: Anatomical and Life Study by Women Artists in Paris', *Nineteenth-Century Art Worldwide*, 6:1 (Spring 2007), www.19thc-artworldwide.org.

Orwicz, Michael R. (ed.) *Art Criticism and Its Institutions in Nineteenth-Century France*. Manchester: Manchester University Press, 1994.

Owen, A.R.G. *Hysteria, Hypnosis and Healing: The Work of J.-M Charcot*. London: Dobson, 1971.

Panzanelli, Roberta and Julius Ritter von Schlosser (eds). *Ephemeral Bodies: Wax Sculpture and the Human Figure*. Los Angeles, CA: Getty Research Institute, 2008.

Papet, Édouard (ed.) *À fleur de peau: Le moulage sur nature au XIXe siècle*. Paris: Réunion des musées nationaux, 2001.

Pecker, André (ed.) *La Médecine à Paris au XIIIe au XXe siècle*. Paris: Hervas, 1984.

Pedersen, Jean Elisabeth. 'Regulating Abortion and Birth Control: Gender, Medicine, and Republican Politics in France, 1870–1920', *French Historical Studies*, 19:3 (Spring 1996), 673–698.

Pernick, Martin S. *A Calculus of Suffering: Pain, Professionalism, and Anesthesia in Nineteenth-Century America*. New York: Columbia University Press, 1985.

Petherbridge, Deanna, and L.J. Jordanova. *The Quick and the Dead: Artists and Anatomy*. London: National Touring Exhibitions/Berkeley, CA: University of California Press, 1997.

Petrey, Sandy. *In the Court of the Pear King: French Culture and the Rise of Realism*. Ithaca, NY: Cornell University Press, 2005.

Pilbeam, Pamela M. *Madame Tussaud and the History of Waxworks*. London: Hambledon and London, 2002.

Pingeot, Anne (ed.). *Le Corps en morceaux*. Paris: Ministère de la culture, de la communication, des grands travaux et du bicentenaire; Réunion des musées nationaux, 1990.

Pointon, Marcia R. *Naked Authority: The Body in Western Painting, 1830–1908*. Cambridge: Cambridge University Press, 1990.

Pointon, Marcia. 'Casts, Imprints and the Deathliness of Things: Artefacts at the Edge', *Art Bulletin*, 96:2 (June 2014), 170–195.

Pointon, Marcia, and Kathleen Adler (eds). *The Body Imagined: The Human Form and Visual Culture Since the Renaissance*. Cambridge: Cambridge University Press, 1993.

Pollock, Griselda. *Differencing the Canon: Feminist Desire and the Writing of Art's Histories*. London: Routledge, 1999.

Prendergast, Christopher. *The Order of Mimesis: Balzac, Stendhal, Nerval, Flaubert*. Cambridge: Cambridge University Press, 1986.

Price, Roger. *A Social History of Nineteenth-Century France*. New York: Holmes & Meier, 1987.

Richardson, Ruth. *Death, Dissection and the Destitute*. London: Kegan Paul; Routledge, 1987.

Ritzenthaler, Cecil. *L'École des Beaux-Arts du XIXe siècle: Les Pompiers*. Paris: Editions Mayer, 1987.

Roquebert, Anne. *Le Paris de Toulouse-Lautrec*. Paris: Hachette: Réunion des musées nationaux, 1992.

Rosario, Vernon A. 'Pointy Penises, Fashion Crimes, and Hysterical Mollies: The Pederasts' Inversion', in Jeffrey Merrick and Bryant T. Ragan (eds), *Homosexuality in Modern France*. New York: Oxford University Press, 1996, pp. 146–176.

Rose, Jacqueline. *Sexuality in the Field of Vision*. London: Verso, 1986.

Rosenblum, Robert. 'Portraiture: Fact versus Fiction', in Sébasatian Allard and Robert Rosenblum, *Citizens and Kings: Portraits in the Age of Revolution 1760–1830*. London: Royal Academy of Arts, 2007, pp. 14–24.

Roth, Nancy L. and Katie Hogan (eds). *Gendered Epidemic: Representations of Women in the Age of Aids*. New York: Routledge, 1998.

Rothfield, Lawrence. *Vital Signs: Medical Realism in Nineteenth-Century Fiction*. Princeton, NJ: Princeton University Press, 1992.

Rouillé, André. *L'Empire de la photographie: Photographie et pouvoir bourgeois, 1839–1870*. Paris: Le Sycomore, 1982.

Rouillé, André and Bernard Marbot. *Le Corps et son image: Photographies du dix-neuvième siècle*. Paris: Contrejour, 1986.

Ruiz-Gómez, Natasha. 'The "Scientific Artworks" of Doctor Paul Richer', *Medical Humanities*, 39:1 (June 2013), 4–10.

Ruiz-Gómez, Natasha. 'A Hysterical Reading of Rodin's *Gates of Hell*', *Art History*, 36:5 (September 2013), 994–1017.

Sawday, Jonathan. *The Body Emblazoned: Dissection and the Human Body in Renaissance Culture*. London: Routledge, 1995.

Schalk, David L. 'Tying up the Loose Ends of an Epoch: Zola's Docteur Pascal', *French Historical Studies*, 16:1 (Spring 1989), 202–216.

Schehr, Lawrence R. *Rendering French Realism*. Stanford, CA: Stanford University Press, 1997.

Schickore, Jutta. *The Microscope and the Eye: A History of Reflections, 1740–1870*. Chicago: University of Chicago Press, 2007.

Schiebinger, Londa. *The Mind has no sex? Women and the Origins of Modern Science*. Cambridge, MA: Harvard University Press, 1989.

Schnalke, Thomas. *Diseases in Wax: The History of the Medical Moulage*. Translated by Kathy Spatschek. Chicago: Quintessence Publishers, 1995.

Schnalke, Thomas. 'Casting Skin: Meanings for Doctors, Artists, and Patients', in Soraya de Chadarevian and Nick Hopwood (eds), *Models: The Third Dimension in Science*. Stanford, CA: Stanford University Press, 2004, pp. 207–241.

Schor, Naomi. *Breaking the Chain: Women, Theory and French Realist Fiction, Gender and Culture*. New York: Columbia University Press, 1985.

Schor, Naomi. *Reading in Detail: Aesthetics and the Feminine*. New York: Methuen, 1987.

Schultheiss, Katrin. *Bodies and Souls: Politics and the Professionalization of Nursing in France, 1880–1922*. Cambridge, MA: Harvard University Press, 2001.

Schwartz, Vanessa R. *Spectacular Realities: Early Mass Culture in Fin-De-Siècle Paris*. Berkeley, CA: University of California Press, 1998.

Sedgwick, Eve Kosofsky. *Between Men: English Literature and Male Homosocial Desire.* New York: Columbia University Press, 1985.
Sekula, Alan. 'The Body and the Archive', in Richard Bolton (ed.), *The Contest of Meaning*. Cambridge, MA: MIT Press, 1989.
Shapiro, Ann-Louise. *Breaking the Codes: Female Criminality in Fin-De-Siècle Paris.* Stanford, CA: Stanford University Press, 1996.
Shaw, Jennifer L. 'The Figure of Venus: Rhetoric of the Ideal and the Salon of 1863', *Art History*, 14:4 (December 1991), 540–570.
Shaw, Jennifer L. *Dream States: Puvis De Chavannes, Modernism and the Fantasy of France*. New Haven, CT: Yale University Press, 2002.
Sheehan, Tanya. *Doctored: The Medicine of Photography in Nineteenth-Century America*. University Park, PA: Pennsylvania University Press, 2011.
Shiff, Richard. 'Art History and the Nineteenth Century: Realism and Resistance', *The Art Bulletin*, 70:1 (March 1988), 25–48.
Showalter, Elaine. *The Female Malady: Women, Madness, and Culture in England, 1830–1980*. New York: Pantheon Books, 1985.
Showalter, Elaine. *Sexual Anarchy: Gender and Culture at the Fin De Siècle*. London: Penguin Books, 1990.
Showalter, Elaine. *Hystories: Hysterical Epidemics and Modern Culture*. London: Picador, 1997.
Sigsworth, E.M. 'Science and the Brewing Industry, 1850–1900', *The Economic History Review*, 17:3 (1965), 536–50.
Silverman, Debora. *Art Nouveau in Fin-De-Siècle France: Politics, Psychology, and Style.* Berkeley, CA: University of California Press, 1989.
Simon-Dhouailly, Nadine. *La Leçon de Charcot – voyage dans une toile*. Cahours: Imprimerie Tardy Quercy, 1986.
Sinding, Christiane. 'Claude Bernard and Louis Pasteur: Constructing Images through Public Commemorations', *Osiris*, 2:14 (1999), 61–85.
Snow, Stephanie J. *Blessed Days of Anaesthesia: How Anaesthetics Changed the World.* Oxford: Oxford University Press, 2008.
Snyder, Joel. 'Visualization and Visibility', in Peter Galison and Caroline Jones (eds), *Picturing Science, Producing Art*. New York: Routledge, 1998, pp. 379–397.
Solomon-Godeau, Abigail. *Male Trouble: A Crisis in Representation*. London: Thames and Hudson, 1997.
Sontag, Susan. *On Photography*. New York: Farrar, Straus & Giroux, 1973.
Sournia, Jean-Charles. *Histoire de la médecine et des médecins*. Paris: Larousse, 1991.
Spongberg, Mary. *Feminizing Venereal Disease: The Body of the Prostitute in Nineteenth-Century Medical Discourse*. Basingstoke: Macmillan, 1997.
Stafford, Barbara Maria. *Body Criticism: Imaging the Unseen in Enlightenment Art and Medicine*. Cambridge, MA: MIT Press, 1991.
Sterling, Charles. *Expositions des collections artistiques de la faculté de médecine de Paris*. Preface by Paul Valéry. Paris: Faculté de médecine, 1935.
Stewart, Mary Lynn. *For Health and Beauty: Physical Culture for Frenchwomen, 1880s–1930s*. Baltimore, MD: Johns Hopkins University Press, 2000.

Suleiman, Susan R. (ed.). *The Female Body in Western Culture: Contemporary Perspectives*. Cambridge, MA: Harvard University Press, 1986.

Surkis, Judith. *Sexing the Citizen: Morality and Masculinity in France, 1870–1920*. Ithaca, NY: Cornell University Press, 2006.

Tagg, John. *The Burden of Representation: Essays on Photographies and Histories*. Basingstoke: Palgrave Macmillan, 1988.

Tagg, John. *Grounds of Dispute: Art History, Cultural Politics and the Discursive Field*. Minneapolis, MN: University of Minnesota Press, 1992.

Tagg, John. *The Disciplinary Frame: Photographic Truths and the Capture of Meaning*. Minneapolis, MN: University of Minnesota Press, 2009.

Taithe, Bertrand. *Defeated Flesh: Welfare, Warfare and the Making of Modern France*. Manchester: Manchester University Press, 1999.

Terry, Jennifer, and Jacqueline Urla (eds). *Deviant Bodies: Critical Perspectives on Difference in Science and Popular Culture*. Bloomington, IN: Indiana University Press, 1995.

Thomson, Richard, Claire Frèches-Thory, Anne Roquebert, and Danièle Devynck. *Toulouse-Lautrec*. London: Hayward Gallery, 1991.

Thomson, Richard. *The Troubled Republic: Visual Culture and Social Debate in France, 1889–1900*. New Haven, CT: Yale University Press, 2004.

Thomson, Richard. *Art of the Actual: Naturalism and Style in Early Third Republic France, 1880–1900*. New Haven, CT: Yale University Press, 2012.

Thuillier, Jean. *Monsieur Charcot de la Salpêtrière*. Paris: R. Laffont, 1993.

Tilles, Gérard. 'Histoire des bibliothèques médicales et des musées des hôpitaux de l'Assistance publique. L'exemple de l'hôpital Saint-Louis', PhD dissertation, Université de Paris XII, 1995.

Tilles, Gérard and Daniel Wallach. *Le Musée des moulages de l'hôpital Saint-Louis*. Paris: Doin-AP-HP, 1996.

Tilles, Gérard and Daniel Wallach. *Les Musées de médecine: histoire, patrimoine et grandes figures de la médecine en France*. Toulouse: Privat, 1999.

Tucker, Jennifer. *Nature Exposed: Photography as Eye Witness in Victorian Science*. Baltimore, MD: Johns Hopkins University Press, 2005.

Vaisse, Pierre. 'Between Convention and Innovation: the Portrait in France in the Nineteenth Century', in Félix Baumann, Maurianne Karabelnik and Jean Sutherland Boggs (eds), *Degas Portraits*. London: Merrell Holberton, 1994, pp. 118–127.

Vallery-Radot, Maurice. *Pasteur, dessins et pastels*. Paris: Editions Hervas, 1987.

Vallery-Radot, Maurice. *Pasteur savant et artiste*. Paris: Editions Hervas, 1995.

Vallery-Radot, Pierre. 'La Médecine et les Médecins dans l'œuvre de Toulouse-Lautrec', *La Presse Médicale*, 59:48 (14 July 1951), 1021–1022.

Vallery-Radot, René. *Pasteur dessinateur et pastelliste (1836–1842)*. Paris: Publications André Marty, É. Paul, 1912.

Vigarello, Georges. *Concepts of Cleanliness: Changing Attitudes in France since the Middle Ages*. Cambridge: Cambridge University Press, 1988.

Wangensteen, Owen H. and Sarah D. Wangensteen. *The Rise of Surgery: From Empiric Craft to Scientific Discipline*. Folkestone: Dawson, 1978.

Waller, John. *The Discovery of the Germ: Twenty Years That Transformed the Way We Think About Disease*. Cambridge: Icon Books, 2002.

Waller, Susan. 'Censors and Photographers in the Third Republic of France', *History of Photography*, 23:3 (Autumn 1999), 222–235.

Waller, Susan. *Invention of the Model: Artists and Models in Paris, 1830–1870*. Aldershot: Ashgate, 2005.

Warner, John Harley. 'The History of Science and the Sciences of Medicine', *Osiris*, 10:1 (1995), 164–193.

Warner, John Harley. *Against the Spirit of the System: The French Impulse in Nineteenth-Century American Medicine*. Princeton, NJ: Princeton University Press, 1998.

Warner, John Harley and James M. Edmonson. *Dissection: Photographs of a Rite of Passage in American Medicine, 1880–1930*. New York: Blast Books, 2009.

Weber, Eugen Joseph. *France: Fin de Siècle*. Cambridge, MA: Belknap Press, 1986.

Wechsler, Judith. *A Human Comedy: Physiognomy and Caricature in 19th-Century Paris*. Chicago: University of Chicago Press, 1982.

Weisberg, Gabriel. *The Realist Tradition: French Painting and Drawing 1830–1900*. Cleveland, OH: Cleveland Museum of Art, 1980.

Weisberg, Gabriel P (ed.) *The European Realist Tradition*. Bloomington, IN: Indiana University Press, 1982.

Weisberg, Gabriel P. *Against the Modern: Dagnan-Bouveret and the Transformation of the Academic Tradition*. New York: Dahesh Museum of Art, 2002.

Weisberg, Richard. 'The Representation of Doctors at Work in Salon Art of the Early Third Republic'. PhD dissertation, New York University, 1995.

Weisberg, Yvonne M.L. and Gabriel P. Weisberg. *The Realist Debate: A Bibliography of French Realist Painting, 1830–1885*. New York: Garland, 1984.

Weisz, George. *The Emergence of Modern Universities in France, 1863–1914*. Princeton, NJ: Princeton University Press, 1983.

Weisz, George. *The Medical Mandarins: The French Academy of Medicine in the Nineteenth and Early Twentieth Centuries*. New York: Oxford University Press, 1995.

Weisz, George. *Divide and Conquer: A Comparative History of Medical Specialization*. New York: Oxford University Press, 2004.

Werbel, Amy. *Thomas Eakins: Art, Medicine, and Sexuality in Nineteenth-Century Philadelphia*. New Haven, CT: Yale University Press, 2007.

White, Hayden. *Figural Realism: Studies in the Mimesis Effect*. Baltimore, MD: Johns Hopkins University Press, 1999.

Wilder, Kelly. *Photography and Science*. London: Reaktion Books, 2009.

William, Guy. *The Age of Miracles: Medicine and Surgery in the Nineteenth Century*. London: Constable, 1981.

Woodall, Joanna (ed.). *Portraiture: Facing the Subject*. Manchester: Manchester University Press, 1997.

Woodfield, Richard (ed.) *Framing Formalism: Riegl's Work*. Amsterdam: G+B Arts International, 2001.

Worboys, Michael. *Spreading Germs: Disease Theories and Medical Practice in Britain, 1865–1900*. New York: Cambridge University Press, 2000.

Worboys, Michael. 'Practice and the Science of Medicine in the Nineteenth Century', *Isis* 102:1 (March 2011), 109–115.
Wrotnowska, Denise. 'Pasteur et l'art', *Médecine de France,* 66 (August 1955), 9–16.
Young, Katherine. *Presence in the Flesh: The Body in Medicine.* Cambridge, MA: Harvard University Press, 1997.

Index